HOW MUCH IS THE COST OF CODING ERRORS?

A Study on Factors Influencing Quality of Clinical Coding in Implementation of MY-DRGs Casemix System in Hospital Services

**PROFESSOR EMERITUS DR SYED MOHAMED ALJUNID
AND
DR SITI ATHIRAH ZAFIRAH**

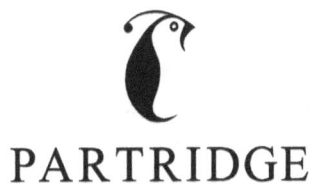

PARTRIDGE

Copyright © 2023 by Professor Emeritus Dr Syed Mohamed Aljunid & Dr Siti Athirah Zafirah

ISBN: Softcover   978-1-5437-7299-9
       eBook   978-1-5437-7300-2

All rights reserved. No part of this book may be used or reproduced by any means, graphic, electronic, or mechanical, including photocopying, recording, taping or by any information storage retrieval system without the written permission of the author except in the case of brief quotations embodied in critical articles and reviews.

Because of the dynamic nature of the Internet, any web addresses or links contained in this book may have changed since publication and may no longer be valid. The views expressed in this work are solely those of the author and do not necessarily reflect the views of the publisher, and the publisher hereby disclaims any responsibility for them.

Print information available on the last page.

To order additional copies of this book, contact
Toll Free +65 3165 7531 (Singapore)
Toll Free +60 3 3099 4412 (Malaysia)
orders.singapore@partridgepublishing.com

www.partridgepublishing.com/singapore

Contents

List of Abbreviations xxv
Acknowledgement xxvii

Chapter 1 Introduction 1

    1.1   Introduction 1
    1.2   Study Background 1
    1.3   DRGs and Coding Process 4
    1.4   Problem Statements 5
    1.5   Research Objectives 6
    1.5.1 General Objective 6
    1.5.2 Specific Objectives 7
    1.6   Hypothesis 7
    1.7   Study Justification 8
    1.8   Conceptual Framework 10

Chapter 2 Literature Review 14

    2.1   Introduction 14
    2.2   Healthcare Financing 15
    2.3   Casemix System 18
    2.4   Diagnosis Related Group (DRG) 20
    2.5   Clinical Coding 24
    2.5.1 Clinical Coding Process 26
    2.5.2 Steps in Assigning Codes 29
    2.5.3 The Coders 31
    2.6   Clinical Coding Errors 33
    2.6.1 Type of Clinical Coding Errors 36
    2.6.2 Factor Influencing the Clinical Coding Errors ... 38
    2.7   Improving the Quality of Coding 43

	2.8	Implications of Clinical Coding Errors 45

Chapter 3 Methodology 48

	3.1	Introduction 48
	3.2	Study Background 48
	3.3	Study Design 49
	3.4	Sample Unit 50
	3.5	Sampling Method 50
	3.5.1	PMR 50
	3.5.2	Coders 50
	3.5.3	Doctors 50
	3.6	Sample Size Calculation 51
	3.7	Inclusion And Exclusion Criteria 52
	3.7.1	Inclusion Criteria for PMR 52
	3.7.2	Exclusion Criteria for PMR 52
	3.8	Study Tools 53
	3.8.1	PMR 53
	3.8.2	Data Abstraction Sheet 53
	3.8.3	Checklist for 14 Casemix Variables 53
	3.8.4	Survey Form on Clinical Coder's Demographic Data 54
	3.8.5	Information Sheet on Doctor's Demographic Data 54
	3.8.6	MY-DRG® Grouper 55
	3.8.7	Procedure of Data Collection 55
	3.9	Methodology of the Re-Coding Process 57
	3.10	Definition of Coding Errors 58
	3.11	Definition of the Type of Coding Errors ... 59
	3.11.1	Type of Coding Errors in Primary Diagnosis Code 59
	3.11.2	Type of Coding Errors in Secondary Diagnosis Code 61
	3.11.3	Type of Coding Errors in Primary Procedure Code 63
	3.11.4	Type of Coding Errors in Secondary Procedure Code 65
	3.12	Data Analysis 67

	3.12.1	Data Analysis on the Incidence of Clinical Coding Errors in UKMMC 67
	3.12.2	Data Analysis on the Economic Impact of Coding Errors 70
	3.13	Variables 72
	3.13.1	Dependent Variables 72
	3.13.2	Independent Variables 72
	3.14	Variables Operational Definition 73
	3.14.1	Dependent Variables 73
	3.14.2	Independent Variables 74

Chapter 4 Results 79

4.1	Introduction 79
4.2	Profile of Patients 79
4.3	Coding Errors Rate in UKMMC 81
4.3.1	Coding Errors in Primary Diagnosis Code 83
4.3.2	Coding Errors of Secondary Diagnosis Code 95
4.3.3	Coding Errors of Primary Procedure Code 104
4.3.4	Coding Errors of Secondary Procedure Code ... 118
4.4	Coding Erros by Case-Type 127
4.4.1	Coding Errors of Medical Case-Type 129
4.4.2	Coding Errors of Surgical Case-Type 160
4.4.3	Coding Errors of O&G Case-Type 188
4.4.4	Coding Errors of Paediatric Case-Type 220
4.5	Coding Errors by Severity Level 253
4.6	Coding Errors by Type of CMG 254
4.7	Coding Errors by MY-DRG® Groups 257
4.8	Coding Errors by Completeness of Admission Form 260
4.9	Coding Errors by Completeness of Discharge Summary 260
4.10	Coding Erros by Coder's Characteristic 262
4.11	Coding Errors by Doctor's Characteristic 263
4.12	Multiple Logistic Regression on Factors Influencing Coding Errors 265
4.13	UKMMC's Potential Hospital Revenue 268
4.13.1	Total Potential Hospital Revenue by

Case-Type 269
4.13.2 Total Potential Hospital Revenue by Severity Level 273
4.13.3 Top 10 MY-DRG® with Highest Total Potential Hospital Revenue 277
4.13.4 Top 10 CMGs With Highest Total Potential Hospital Revenue 281
4.14 Bivariate Analyses on Factors Influencing Loss of Potential Hospital Revenue in Casemix System 283
4.14.1 Association between Coding Errors of Primary Diagnosis Code and Potential Loss of Hospital Revenue 284
4.14.2 Association between Coding Errors of Secondary Diagnosis Code Potential Loss of Hospital Revenue 285
4.14.3 Association between Coding Errors of Primary Procedure Code and Potential Loss of Hospital Revenue 286
4.14.4 Association between Coding Errors of Secondary Procedure Code and Potential Loss of Hospital Revenue 287
4.14.5 Association between Coding Error Cases with Errors of Severity Level and Potential Loss of Hospital Revenue 287
4.14.6 Association between Coding Error Cases with Errors of Case-Type and Potential Loss of Hospital Revenue 288
4.14.7 Association between Cases with Incomplete Admission Form Potential Loss of Hospital Revenue 289
4.14.8 Association between Cases with Discharge Summary and Potential Loss of Hospital Revenue 289
4.15 Multiple Logistic Regression on Factors Influencing Accuracy of Assignment of Potential Hospital Tariff 290

Chapter 5   Discussion 293

    5.1   Introduction 293
    5.2   Evaluation of Quality of Clinical Coding
           In UKMMC 293
    5.2.1 Quality of the Discharge Summary 295
    5.2.2 Coders' Knowledge on Coding Process 297
    5.2.3 Implications of Doctors' Demographic
           towards Clinical Coding 300
    5.2.4 Evaluation Method 304
    5.3   Issue of Under-Coding 306
    5.3.1 Poor Enforcement of Casemix System 308
    5.3.2 Unclear Rules and Guidelines 310
    5.3.3 Structural Limitations of Discharge Summary . 312
    5.3.4 Ambiguities in Interpretation 314
    5.4   Economic Implication 315
    5.4.1 Ungroupable Case 318
    5.4.2 Importance of Birthweight 319
    5.5   Study Limitations 320

Chapter 6   Conclusions and Recommendations 322

    6.1   Introduction 322
    6.2   Conclusions of Study's Findings 322
    6.3   Recommendations 324
    6.3.1 Hospital Managers 325
    6.3.2 Coders 326
    6.3.3 Doctors 327
    6.3.4 Primary Reference of Clinical Coding 328

References 331

List of Appendices

Appendix A   Study Tools 351

Appendix B   List of Top 50 Assigned Primary
             Diagnosis Code 355

Appendix C   List of Top 50 Assigned Secondary
             Diagnosis Code 359

Appendix D   List of Top 50 Assigned Primary
             Procedure Code 363

Appendix E   List of Top 50 Assigned Secondary
             Procedure Code 367

Appendix F   List of Top 50 Cases with Highest
             Potential Loss of Revenue 371

List of Figures

Figure 1.1 Flow of Casemix System 4

Figure 1.2 Conceptual Framework 13

Figure 2.1 Example of MY-DRG Code 21

Figure 3.1 Flow of the Study 56

Figure 4.1 Distributions of Coded Case by Case-Type 80

Figure 4.2 Distributions of Coded Cases by Age 80

Figure 4.3 Distributions of Coded Cases by Severity Level 81

List of Tables

Table 2.1 Definition of Components in Calculation of Hospital Tariff 23

Table 2.2 Percentage of Coding Errors in Previous Studies 34

Table 2.3 Type of Clinical Coding Errors 36

Table 2.4 Profit Loss due to Clinical Coding Errors 46

Table 3.1 UKMMC's Patient Data from 2002 to 2013 49

Table 4.1 Distribution of Coding Errors Rate 83

Table 4.2 Type of Coding Errors Among Primary Diagnosis Code 84

Table 4.3 Example of Error Cases Among Primary Diagnosis Code 86

Table 4.4 Top 10 Primary Diagnosis Codes Assigned Before and After the Re-Coding Process 90

Table 4.5 Changes in the Assignment of Top 10 Primary Diagnosis Code Before the Re-Coding Process due to Coding Errors 93

Table 4.6 Distributions of the Number of Secondary Diagnosis Codes Assigned Before and After the Re-Coding Process 95

Table 4.7 Number of Secondary Diagnosis Codes Assigned Per Patient Before and After the Re-Coding Process..98

Table 4.8 Distributions of Error Cases by Number of Secondary Diagnosis Code 99

Table 4.9 Type of Coding Errors of Secondary Diagnosis Code..99

Table 4.10 Examples of Coding Errors Cases of Secondary Diagnosis Code 101

Table 4.11 Distributions of Top 10 Secondary Diagnosis Codes Assigned Before and After the Re-Coding Process..... 105

Table 4.12 Distributions of the Type of Coding Errors within Primary Procedure Codes...106

Table 4.13 Examples of Error Cases in the Assignment of Primary Procedure Codes 107

Table 4.14 Top 10 Code Assigned as Primary Procedure Code Before and After the Re-Coding Process....................... 111

Table 4.15 Changes in Top 10 Code Assigned as Primary Procedure Code Due to Coding Error...................... 114

Table 4.16 Distributions of Total Number of Secondary Procedure Code Assigned to Patient Before and After the Re-Coding Process 118

Table 4.17 Distributions of Coding Error Cases by Number of Secondary Procedure Code................................... 119

Table 4.18 Comparisons of Number of Secondary Procedure Code Assigned per Patient Before and After the Re-Coding Process 121

Table 4.19 Distributions of Type of Coding Errors in
Secondary Procedure Code 122

Table 4.20 Example of Error Cases in the Assignment
of Secondary Procedure Code 123

Table 4.21 Top 10 Code Assigned as Secondary
Procedure Code Before and After the Re-Coding Process 126

Table 4.22 Distributions of Coding Errors by MY-
DRG® Case-Type 127

Table 4.23 Distributions of Cases by MY-DRG® Case-
Type After Audit 128

Table 4.24 Distributions of Coding Error Cases by
Coding Item in Medical Case-Type 130

Table 4.25 Distribution of Type of Coding Errors
Among Primary Diagnosis Code in Medical Case-Type 131

Table 4.26 Primary Diagnosis Code Assigned Before
and After Audit within Medical Case-Type 134

Table 4.27 Changes in the Assignment of Top 10
Primary Procedure Code within Medical Case-Type 135

Table 4.28 Distributions of the Number of Secondary
Diagnosis Codes Assigned Before and After the Re-
Coding Process within Medical Case-Type 136

Table 4.29 Comparisons of Number of Secondary
Diagnosis Code Assigned per Patient Before and After
the Re-Coding Process in Medical Case-Type 139

Table 4.30 Distributions of Coding Error Cases by
Number of Secondary Diagnosis Codes 140

Table 4.31 Distributions of Type of Coding Errors in
Secondary Diagnosis Code within Medical Case-Type 141

Table 4.32 Comparisons of Top 10 Secondary Diagnosis
Code Assigned within Medical Case-Type 143

Table 4.33 Distributions of the Type of Coding Errors
within Primary Procedure Codes in Medical Case-Type 145

Table 4.34 Comparisons of Top 10 Primary Procedure
Code Assigned Before and After the Audit within
Medical Case-Type 147

Table 4.35 Changes in the Assignment of Top 10
Highest Frequency Primary Procedure Code before the
Audit within Medical Case-Type 150

Table 4.36 Distributions of Total Number of Secondary
Procedure Code Assigned to Patient Before and After
the Re-Coding Process within Medical Case-Type 152

Table 4.37 Distributions of Coding Errors Cases by
Number of Secondary Procedure Code within Medical
Case-Type 153

Table 4.38 Comparison of Number of Secondary
Procedure Code Assigned per Patient Before and After
the Re-Coding Process within Medical Case-Type 155

Table 4.39 Distributions of Type of Coding Errors in
Secondary Procedure Code within Medical Case-Type 156

Table 4.40 Comparisons of Top Secondary Procedure
Code Assigned within Medical Case-Type 159

Table 4.41 Distributions of Coding Error Cases by
Coding Item in Surgical Case-Type 160

Table 4.42 Distribution of Type of Coding Errors Among Primary Diagnosis Code in Surgical Case-Type 161

Table 4.43 Top Primary Diagnosis Code Assigned Before and After Re-Coding Process within Surgical Case-Type 164

Table 4.44 Changes in the Top 10 Primary Diagnosis Code Assigned Before the Re-Coding Process in Surgical Case-Type 165

Table 4.45 Distributions of the Number of Secondary Diagnosis Codes Assigned Before and After the Re-Coding Process within Surgical Case-Type 166

Table 4.46 Comparisons of Number of Secondary Diagnosis Code Assigned per Patient Before and After the Re-Coding Process in Surgical Case-Type 168

Table 4.47 Distributions of Coding Errors Cases by Number of Secondary Diagnosis Codes in Surgical Case-Type 169

Table 4.48 Distributions of Type of Coding Errors in Secondary Procedure Code within Surgical Case-Type 170

Table 4.49 Comparisons of Top 10 Secondary Diagnosis Code within Surgical Case-Type 172

Table 4.50 Distributions of the Type of Coding Errors within Primary Procedure Codes in Surgical Case-Type 174

Table 4.51 Comparisons of Top 10 Highest Frequency Primary Procedure Code Before and After the Re-Coding Process within Surgical Case-Type 176

Table 4.52 Changes Among the Top 10 Primary
Procedure Code Assigned Among Surgical Case-Type
due to Coding Errors 177

Table 4.53 Distributions of Total Number of Secondary
Procedure Code Assigned to Patient Before and After
the Re-Coding Process within Surgical Case-Type 180

Table 4.54 Distributions of Coding Errors Cases by
Number of Secondary Procedure Code within Surgical
Case-Type 181

Table 4.55 Comparison of Number of Secondary
Procedure Code Assigned per Patient Before and After
the Re-Coding Process within Surgical Case-Type 183

Table 4.56 Distributions of Type of Coding Errors in
Secondary Procedure Code within Surgical Case-Type 185

Table 4.57 Comparisons of Top 10 Secondary Procedure
Code Assigned within Surgical Case-Type 187

Table 4.58 Distributions of Coding Error Cases by
Coding Item in O&G Case-Type 188

Table 4.59 Distribution of Type of Coding Errors of
Primary Diagnosis Code in O&G Case-Type 190

Table 4.60 Top 10 Primary Diagnosis Code Assigned
Before and After Re-Coding Process within O&G
Case-Type 192

Table 4.61 Changes in the Top 10 Primary Diagnosis
Code Assigned Before the Re-Coding Process in O&G
Case-Type due to Coding Errors 193

Table 4.62 Distributions of the Number of Secondary Diagnosis Codes Assigned Before and After the Re-Coding Process within O&G Case-Type 198

Table 4.63 Comparisons of Number of Secondary Diagnosis Code Assigned per Patient Before and After the Re-Coding Process in O&G Case-Type............................200

Table 4.64 Distributions of Coding Errors Cases by Number of Secondary Diagnosis Codes in O&G Case-Type.201

Table 4.65 Distributions of Type of Coding Errors in Secondary Diagnosis Code within O&G Case-Type 202

Table 4.66 Comparisons of Top 10 Secondary Diagnosis Code Assigned within O&G Case-Type 205

Table 4.67 Distributions of the Type of Coding Errors of Primary Procedure Codes in O&G Case-Type 207

Table 4.68 Comparisons of Top 10 Primary Procedure Code Assigned Before and After the Re-Coding Process within O&G Case-Type...209

Table 4.69 Changes Among the Top 10 Primary Procedure Code Among O&G Case-Type due to Coding Errors 210

Table 4.70 Distributions of Total Number of Secondary Procedure Code Assigned to Patient Before and After the Re-Coding Process within O&G Case-Type 212

Table 4.71 Distributions of Coding Error Cases by Number of Secondary Procedure Code within O&G Case-Type..213

Table 4.72 Comparison of Number of Secondary Procedure Code Assigned per Patient Before and After the Re-Coding Process Within O&G Case-Type 215

Table 4.73 Distributions of Type of Coding Errors of Secondary Procedure Code within O&G Case-Type 216

Table 4.74 Comparisons of Top Secondary Procedure Code Assigned within O&G Case-Type 219

Table 4.75 Distributions of Coding Errors Cases by Coding Item in Paediatric Case-Type 220

Table 4.76 Distribution of Type of Coding Errors of Primary Diagnosis Code in Paediatric Case-Type 221

Table 4.77 Top 10 Primary Diagnosis Code Assigned Before and After Re-Coding Process within Paediatric Case-Type 224

Table 4.78 Changes in the Top 10 Primary Diagnosis Code Assigned Before the Re-Coding Process in Paediatric Case-Type due to Coding Errors 226

Table 4.79 Distributions of the Number of Secondary Diagnosis Codes Assigned Before and After the Re-Coding Process within Paediatric Case-Type 229

Table 4.80 Comparisons of Number of Secondary Diagnosis Code Assigned per Patient Before and After the Re-Coding Process in Paediatric Case-Type 231

Table 4.81 Distributions of Coding Errors Cases by Number of Secondary Diagnosis Codes in Paediatric Case-Type 232

Table 4.82 Distributions of Type of Coding Errors in
Secondary Diagnosis Code within Paediatric Case-Type 233

Table 4.83 Comparisons of Top 10 Secondary Diagnosis
Code Assigned within Paediatric Case-Type 236

Table 4.84 Distributions of the Type of Coding Errors
of Primary Procedure Codes in Paediatric Case-Type 238

Table 4.85 Comparisons of Top 10 Primary Procedure
Code Assigned Before and After the Re-Coding
Process within Paediatric Case-Type 240

Table 4.86 Changes Among the Top 10 Primary
Procedure Code Assigned Among Paediatric Case-Type
due to Coding Errors 243

Table 4.87 Distributions of Total Number of Secondary
Procedure Code Assigned to Patient Before and After
the Re-Coding Process within Paediatric Case-Type 245

Table 4.88 Distributions of Coding Errors Cases by
Number of Secondary Procedure Code within Paediatric
Case-Type 246

Table 4.89 Comparison of Number of Secondary
Procedure Code Assigned per Patient Before and After
the Re-Coding Process within Paediatric Case-Type 248

Table 4.90 Distributions of Type of Coding Errors of
Secondary Procedure Code within Paediatric Case-Type 249

Table 4.91 Comparisons of Top 10 Secondary Procedure
Code Assigned within Paediatric Case-Type 252

Table 4.92 Distributions of Error Cases by Severity Level 253

Table 4.93 Distributions of Severity Level After the Re-coding Process 254

Table 4.94 Top 10 Highest Frequency CMG Before and After the Re-Coding Process..256

Table 4.95 Top 10 Highest MY-DRG® Code Before and After The Re-Coding Process 259

Table 4.96 Distributions of Error Cases by Completeness of Admission Form 260

Table 4.97 Distributions of Coding Error Cases by Completeness of Discharge Summary 261

Table 4.98 Distributions of Coding Errors by Coder's Characteristic 262

Table 4.99 Distributions of Coding Errors by Doctor's Characteristic 264

Table 4.100 Description of Variables used in Multiple Logistic Regression 266

Table 4.101 Multiple Logistic Regression of Factors Influencing Coding Errors...267

Table 4.102 Comparisons of Total Potential Hospital Revenue Before and After the Re-Coding Process..................269

Table 4.103 Comparisons of Total Potential Hospital Revenue Before and After the Re-Coding Process by Case-Type...270

Table 4.104 Comparisons of Total Potential Hospital Revenue Before and After the Re-Coding According to Severity Level..274

Table 4.105 Comparisons of the Top 10 MY-DRG® Group With Highest Potential Hospital Revenue Before and After the Re-Coding Process 279

Table 4.106 Top 10 Cases with Highest Potential Loss of Revenue 280

Table 4.107 Comparisons of the Top 10 CMGs With Highest Potential Hospital Revenue Before and After the Re-Coding Process 282

Table 4.108 Distributions of Factors Influencing Loss of Potential Hospital Revenue is Casemix System 283

Table 4.109 Description of Variables used in Multiple Logistic Regression 291

Table 4.110 Results of the Analysis Using Multiple Logistic Regressions on Factors Influencing the Hospital Tariff 292

List of Abbreviations

UKMMC	Universiti Kebangsaan Malaysia
DRG	Diagnosis Related Group
MY-DRG®	Malaysia Diagnosis Related Group
CBG	Case Based Group
CMG	Casemix Group
O&G	Obstetric & Gynecology
ICD	International Classification of Disease
ICD 9 CM	International Classification of Disease Ninth Revision Clinical Modification
ICD 10	International Classification of Disease 10th Revision
ISC	Independent Senior Coder
PMR	Patient Medical Record
HT	Hospital Tariff

Acknowledgement

First and foremost praise to the Almighty Allah swt for all his blessing for giving us the patience and good health to complete this book.

We acknowledge the contributions of Associate Professor Dr Amrizal Muhammad Nur and Professor Dr Sharifa Ezat Wan Puteh in the research project that resulted in this book. They have provided great insights and constructive comments when we embarked on the project to analyse huge collection of data from the casemix database in the hospital.

Dr Siti Athirah would like to mention roles played her lovely Mama, Junaidah Kamarruddin, her late father Abdul Rashid Shaharudin, and her dear "ibu", Maizura Zainal by providing continuous motivation and support throughout the three-year period to complete the research project. She also want to express her deepest gratitude to her supporting husband, Mohd Izhar Hafiz Abdul Latiff for all his patience and supports. Thank you for never cutting her wings whenever she wanted to fly and for taking care of their kids; Irfan Harith and Alya Zahra in allowing her to concentrate on her writings.

Last but not least, we would like to thank our fellow colleagues in International Centre for Casemix and Clinical Coding (ITCC-UKM) for the valuable tips and tricks. May whatever we gained throughout our journey, we could contribute it back to our society. May Allah bless all of us.

INTRODUCTION

1.1 Introduction

The first chapter of the book is divided into six sections. The first section gave a brief introduction to the background of the study. The second section discussed the problem statement followed by the objectives of the study. In the fourth section, the hypothesis of the study is presented. At the end of this chapter, the study justification and conceptual framework of the study is being discussed.

1.2 Study Background

Globally, the sharp escalation of healthcare costs due to the rising of lifestyle diseases and extended longevity has risen attention towards the importance of healthcare financing. In Malaysia, the economic burden of chronic non-communicable disease (CNCDs) is estimated to be as high as USD221.7 constituting 12.5% of the nation's Gross Domestic Product (GDP). However, despite the escalation of the cost in the healthcare sector, in 2013, the government spending in the healthcare sector is only 4.0% of the nation's GDP (Min 2013). With the current demographic shift such as the increment of the non-communicable diseases in Malaysia, it is essential to increase the budget allocation in the healthcare sector to ensure sufficient resources could be rendered to the citizen. As a necessity for population's health improvement and healthcare resources management, this nation required a health system reform. Subsequently, in 2017, the Ministry of Health Malaysia announced to launch Voluntary Health Insurance (VHI) Scheme in the year 2018 with the assurance to resolve all issues in the healthcare sector including cost, coverage and products (Bernama 2017).

Currently, the healthcare financing programme employed by public health facilities in Malaysia is mainly through general taxation whereas for private services is out-of-pocket payments and some private insurance. To reach a better health care resources management and to ensure the success of VHI scheme, a reformation of the healthcare financing system is needed. For example, casemix system could be implemented in this country. The employment of casemix system is believed could help in utilising the available resources for a better outcome including the efficiency of the care management, efficiency of hospital management and also the efficiency of the healthcare financing. Evidently, Malaysia neighbouring country ; Republic of Indonesia has successfully implemented Social Health Insurance through casemix system in 2004 with the purpose to meet the goal of universal health coverage and to ensure fairness in health care financing (Thabrany 2008).

Casemix system is a patient classification system, which was developed in 1967 by Bob Fetter and Jon Thompson from Yale University. This system works as a tool to classify patient treatment episode, designed to form groups that are relatively homogeneous in view of resources and contains patient with similar characteristic. Through casemix system, a powerful tool called Diagnosis Related

Group (DRG) were developed as a mean of relating the type of patients of a hospital treats to the cost incurred by the hospital (Goldfield 2010; Palmer & Reid 2001). In using casemix system as the provider payment tool, each episode of care would be assigned to a DRG code according to their clinical condition generated through the clinical coding process. Accordingly, each DRG code is assigned to a pre-determined hospital tariff. Figure 1.1 below shows the flow of the Casemix system.

Historically, casemix system was introduced in Malaysia in 1998. This system was officially introduced in University Kebangsaan Malaysia Medical Centre (UKMMC) in July 2002. UKMMC is the first hospital in Malaysia that took the initiative to implement casemix system. During the early implementation of this system, 2 full-time Clinical Coordinators and 5 full-time coders were employed by the Hospital to run the unit. Coordinators and coders were given intensive training of casemix system. In September 2002, the unit was officially launched and took over the coding process from the ward clerks and Assistant Medical Record Officers. Based on Casemix Progress Report in UKMMC, the implementation of this system led to the improvement of quality in care services and has increased financial resources. Parallel with that, the implementation of this system resulted in positive outcomes towards hospital activities as well as the treatment that is available from many disciplines and expertise (Saperi et al., 2005). Up to date, this system is used in this hospital for research purposes and is not being used for budgeting purposes.

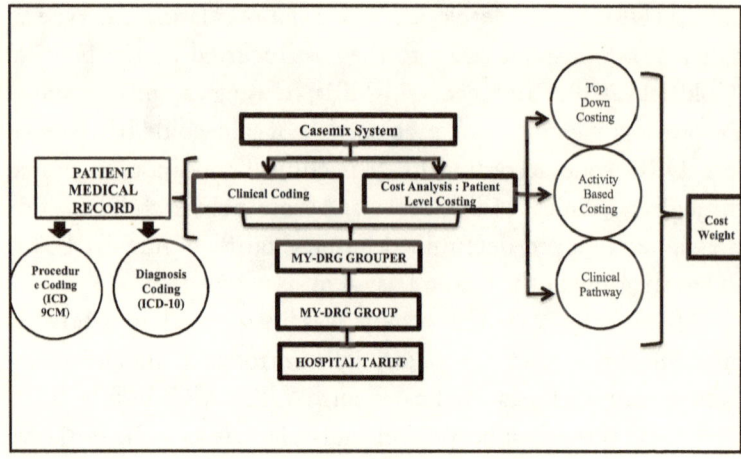

Figure 1.1 Flow of Casemix System

1.3 DRGs and Coding Process

Diagnosis Related Groups (DRGs) are one of the main components in Casemix (Goldfield 2010). DRGs help to classify groups of patients using systematic code and was developed as a means of relating the type of patients that a hospital treat to the cost incurred by hospitals. DRGs are derived from codes of diagnosis and procedure coding. Thus the accuracy of clinical coding of diagnosis and procedure are crucial in determining the DRGs codes.

In UKMMC, codes are assigned using the International Classification of Disease (ICD). The diagnosis code is assigned according to the International Classification of Disease 10th (ICD-10), meanwhile, the procedure code is assigned according to the International Classification of Disease 9th revision Clinical Modification (ICD-9-CM). In the year of 2013, the clinical coding process was conducted in Health Informatics Department (HID) by trained coders. After assigning the code, the clerk from HID will key in both clinical and demographic information of the patient in the Health Information System (HIS), finally all the information will be key in into a software called grouper. This grouper will then, produce the DRG codes. However, since 2017, the clinical coding process was conducted in International Centre for Casemix and Clinical Coding (ITCC).

In using casemix system as the provider payment tool, the DRGs groups play a vital role in determining patient's cost of treatment (Paul et al. 2008). Thus, in preparing UKMMC to officially implement Casemix system as the provider payment tool, the accuracy of clinical coding is crucial since it is the key in determining the accuracy of hospital revenue. Clinical coding errors would lead to the misclassification in DRG codes and this may cause the hospital to receive inappropriate amount of hospital revenue.

1.4 Problem Statements

Casemix system was launched in UKMMC in the year of 2002. This system was only use for research purposes and not officially used in the structure of the hospital's governance. However, in 2012, UKM has granted their title as the autonomy university by the Government of Malaysia (Sivaselvam 2012). This has led to the preparation of this university in fully governing their administrative and financial aspects. In using casemix system in the hospital governance, the quality of clinical coded data is a pivotal subject to ensure the effectiveness of this system in governing the hospital.

In casemix system, clinical coded data plays a critical role in determining the reimbursement group of the patient. The errors in the assignment of clinical codes could relates to adverse impact whereby a hospital may receive an inaccurate amount of hospital revenue. It is also important to note that the clinical coded data also could be beneficial for the hospital governance. The hospital managers could utilise the information generated from the clinical coding process to constitute monitoring programme in increasing the efficiency of the treatment provided to the patient.

It is also worth to mention that up to date in UKMMC, there no clear rules and guidelines on the clinical coding process constitute by the hospital managers. This has led to the question of the effectiveness of the clinical coding process conducted by the clinical coders in UKMMC. The unclear rules and guidelines on the clinical coding process could cause the coding process conducted by the clinical coders to become an error-prone process. However, without assessing the regular clinical coding process in UKMMC, it is difficult to identify problems that are occurring during the clinical coding process, and the constitution of proper rules and guidelines for the clinical coding process would become challenging.

From 2009 to 2013, more than 180,000 cases were coded by the clinical coding staff at UKMMC. However, before the commencement of this study, the evaluation of the accuracy of these coded data was never conducted. Therefore, the accuracy of these data is still unknown. In determining the actual cost of treatment through the casemix system, the accuracy of clinical coding data needs to be assessed. Without the accuracy of the clinically coded data, it could possibly lead to a loss of revenue for the hospital. This may be due to the inaccurate assignment of hospital tariffs, according to which the patient's might be assigned to a higher or lower hospital tariff.

1.5 Research Objectives

1.5.1 General Objective

The aim of this study is to analyse the economic impact of diagnosis and procedure coding errors in the implementation of MY-DRG® Casemix System in University Kebangsaan Malaysia Medical Centre (UKMMC).

1.5.2 Specific Objectives

1. To measure the coding errors rate in UKMMC.
2. To identify type of coding errors of diagnosis and procedure classification in the implementation of Casemix in UKMMC.
3. To determine the factors influencing coding errors rate. These include training level and experience of coders, complexity of cases, type of cases and doctor's experience.
4. To measure the economic impact of coding errors in the use of Casemix system for hospital reimbursement.
5. To determine factors influencing accuracy of the assignment of hospital tariff.
6. To recommend mechanism to improve coding errors rate in UKMMC.

1.6 Hypothesis

1. Coding errors rate among primary procedure code is more likely to be higher than primary diagnosis code.
2. Coding errors rate among cases with a higher number of secondary diagnoses codes is more likely to be higher than cases with a lower number of secondary diagnosis codes.
3. Coding errors rate among cases with incomplete admission form and discharge summary is more likely to be higher than cases with complete admission form and discharge summary.
4. Coding errors are more likely to be higher among coder with less experience, low of training and lower level of educational level.
5. Coding errors rate is more likely to be higher among doctor with less experience and lower level of educational level.
6. Coding errors leading to misclassification of case in MY-DRG® will cause to substantial loss of revenue in UKMMC.
7. The accurate assignment of hospital tariff is more likely to be influenced by the accuracy of the diagnosis code.

1.7 Study Justification

This study aims to investigate the economic impact of clinical coding errors in the implementation of casemix system (MY-DRG®) in UKMMC. The justifications of this study are as follow:

The clinical coding process plays a vital role in determining the cost incurred to a patient per hospital visit. Erroneous assignment of clinical codes would cause the wrong assignment of MY-DRG®, and it is believed it would negatively impact the calculation of hospital revenue. However, to date, there is no evaluation of the quality of the clinical coding process conducted in this hospital. In addition, research on the quality of clinical coding in the casemix system is also lacking in Malaysia. As a pioneer hospital that is using the casemix system, it is crucial for UKMMC to identify the current quality of clinical coding in this hospital. The outcome of this study would help UKMMC determine the necessary measures to improve the quality of coding and reach a high level of coding accuracy. By having a high degree of coding accuracy, UKMMC would become the benchmark for other public and private hospitals to measure their quality of coding. The high quality of clinical coding could also help UKMMC be a source of reference for other hospitals in improving their quality of clinical coding.

i) This study explores the interactions between clinical coding errors and coders. Coders are the most important personnel during the coding process. However, how the coders affect the quality of coding has rarely been reported in Malaysia. The output of this study will provide a valuable outcome to hospital managers in Malaysia in terms of evaluating and improving coders' performance.
ii) Besides coders, doctors also play a vital role in ensuring the high quality of clinical coding. As clinical coding accuracy is influenced by the quality of the documentation, it is critical to

assess doctors' awareness of the importance of clinical coding, specifically their awareness of clinical coding in the context of the casemix system. Therefore, this study also explores the interactions between doctors and the quality of the documents that were used in the clinical coding process. The output of this study is to identify doctors' level of awareness of their important role in the implementation of clinical coding in the Casemix system, which could be used by hospital managers in instituting a programme on the awareness of the importance of clinical coding among doctors.

iii) In this study, although in UKMMC the in-house coder is using the discharge summaries alone during the coding process, the quality of clinical coding is being accessed by examining the entire patient medical records for the selected episode of care because the quality of coding is at its best when referring to the whole medical record (Reid et al. 2017a). The methodology used in this study could help hospital administrators decide the best clinical coding practise to produce a better quality of clinical coding output

iv) In January 2012, UKMMC was granted autonomy warrant by the government of Malaysia (Sivaselvam 2012). Parallel to this, hospital revenue and expenditures need to be calculated precisely as the decision-making power will be transferred from federal agencies and the ministry to the university. This study is expected to help UKMMC achieve its status as a full autonomy research university in Malaysia by focusing on the economic impact of coding errors in both diagnosis and procedure coding. Furthermore, with rising healthcare costs, effective resource management in the healthcare sector is critical. In implementing the casemix system, the accurate cost of treatment could not be determined without accurate clinical coding codes. As this study investigates the economic impact of clinical coding errors, it is hoped that it will serve as a resource for other health care facilities as they implement the casemix system as a provider payment tool.

1.8 Conceptual Framework

In this study, it was hypothesised that there are four major factors influencing clinical coding errors. The factors are clinical coders, clinicians, medical records and the structure of hospital governance. Figure 1.2 below illustrates the conceptual framework of this study.

The first factor that could influence the quality of clinical coding is the clinical coders themselves. The quality of clinical coding output depends on the experience of the clinical coder. Clinical coders with a shorter length of service may produce more clinical coding errors due to their limited understanding of the clinical coding process. Therefore, a clinical coding process that is being conducted by experienced clinical coders could mitigate the probability of coding errors occurring. The lack of experience among junior clinical coders could contribute to the erroneous interpretation of the patient's clinical condition and procedure reported by the doctors. Furthermore, the clinical coder's participation in clinical coding training may have an impact on clinical coding errors. This study believes that coders with a higher number of clinical coding training could diminish clinical coding errors. Coders that are actively involved in clinical coding's training would be equipped with the current rules and guidelines of the clinical coding process. Thus, subsequently, it would help them produce accurate clinical coding output. Also, this study believes that the educational level of the coder could influence the clinical coding errors. Coders with a lower educational level are argued to produce clinical coding errors.

The second factor that this study believes could influence the clinical coding error is the clinicians. Commonly, clinicians are the leading actor in the healthcare environment. Clinicians are the most important people during the patient's episode of treatment. In the era of the Value-Based Health Care especially in using the Casemix system as the provider payment tools, clinicians is not only the key person in treating patient but also the key person in ensuring a good quality of clinically coded data. In the Casemix system, the veracity of the clinically coded data is imperative to get the correct amount of hospital revenue. Therefore, this study believes the clinician's duration of service provision is imperative as it could influence the accuracy of the diagnosis and procedure assigned by the clinicians. In addition, the type of clinician's educational level also could influence the clinical coding errors. The higher the educational level of the clinicians, the lower the potential of the case attend by the clinicians to be coded wrongly. This is linked to the clinicians' level of knowledge on the importance of medical documentation and level of knowledge on the importance of clinical coding. This study holds that higher educated clinicians would be aware of the importance of medical documentation and the importance of clinical coding. Therefore, the medical documentation attended by these clinicians is assumed to have more clarity and accuracy that could ease the clinical coding process among the clinical coders.

The third important factor that could relate to the clinical coding errors is the clinical documentation. Firstly, the clinical coding errors could be due to the type of case in the clinical documentation. For instance, a surgical case could have a higher tendency to be assigned with a wrong code compared to the medical case. Also, the severity level of the case could also influence the clinical coding errors, where the coding process for higher severity cases are more complicated than for lower severity cases. More importantly, the clinical coding errors could be influenced by the accuracy and the clarity of the information written in the clinical documentation. The quality of the clinical documentation that is being used as the primary documentation of the clinical coding process plays a crucial role in mitigating the clinical coding errors cases.

This study believes that the last important factor that could contribute to the clinical coding errors is the structure of the hospital's governance. The visibility of the importance of the clinical coding process among the hospital's managers is pivotal in determining the quality of clinical coding. The unavailability of the clinical coding process in the structure of the hospital's governance could prevent hospital managers from allocating an adequate budget for the clinical coding process. For example, without a sufficient budget, clinical coders would be unable to purchase updated reference material for the clinical coding process. Furthermore, when clinical coding is excluded from hospital governance, hospital managers will find it difficult to develop clear rules and guidelines for the clinical coding process. The absence of clinical coding's process in the structure of the hospital's governance could also cause difficulties among the hospital's managers in conducting regular monitoring of the clinical coding process.

In implementing the Casemix system as the provider payment tool, the incidence of clinical coding errors could lead to far-reaching consequences. Firstly, without accurate information from clinically coded data, the hospital's revenue might not reflect actual revenue. It is worth mentioning that the wrong assignment of clinical codes would relate to the wrong assignment of the patient's DRG group, which may relate to a higher or lower reimbursement. This may have financial ramifications for the hospital. In addition, the clinical coding errors could also relate to the poor quality of a treatment rendered to the patient. Data retrieved from the clinical coding could help the hospital determine the direction of the treatment provided to the patient. However, incorrect clinical coding information could mislead the hospital's manager's direction or planning in increasing the efficiency of patient treatment.

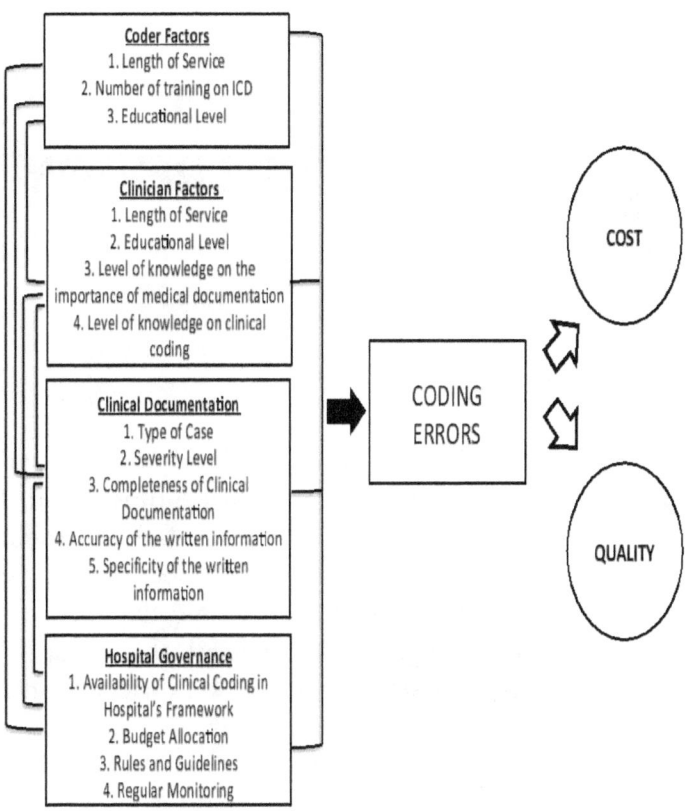

Figure 1.2 Conceptual Framework

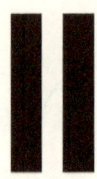 **LITERATURE REVIEW**

2.1 Introduction

In this literature review, instances which prove the casemix system's role as the provider payment tool, primarily on the purpose of identifying the hospital tariff through clinical coding, is investigated. Healthcare financing is the focus of the first section in this, along with studies regarding the approaches implemented for provider payment, particularly the utilisation of DRG through casemix system as the tool for provider payment. Following that, the clinical coding role in casemix system is emphasised here. In the third section, the errors occurring in the clinical coding, including its description and types, are elaborated in depth in the third section. Last but not least, reviews on the impacts of errors in clinical coding are presented in the last section.

2.2 Healthcare Financing

The increase of diseases attributed to lifestyle, which increases the cost needed for healthcare, has made the restructuring of healthcare delivery important. Due to the increase in healthcare cost, access to healthcare which is especially required by many developing countries is hindered (Robyn et al. 2013). To illustrate this, in 2015, from the Malaysia's Gross Domestic Product (GDP) amounted to RM 1, 156.9 billion, the percentage of the amount used by the healthcare sector was only 4.55% (Mathauer & Wittenbecher 2013). It was reported that a number of developed countries such as France, Japan and the United Kingdom spent significantly for health, where their expenditure percentage were 11.7%, 10.3% and 9.1%, respectively (Jaafar et al. 2013). In acquiring the efficiency and fairness healthcare resources administration among the population, the implementation of an appropriate reimbursement system is highly important.

Past study has highlight that the possible definition of reimbursement system in healthcare is the method used by those who pay for healthcare to allocate money to the care providers (Jegers et al. 2002). Furthermore, prospective and retrospective payment system are the most well-known reimbursement systems which become a topic of debate among researchers in the healthcare industry in the recent years (Jegers et al. 2002; Lehtonen 2007; McClellan & Rivlin 2014). These two systems of payment are distinguished according to the association between method of reimbursement and the activities carried out at the hospital.

Depending on the diagnosis of patient's discharge and how the medical procedures and treatment are conducted during their stay, the utilisation of the retrospective payment system for the cost to be paid by the patient is determined after treatment are provided by the hospital. However, with this payment system, hospitals would be incapable of facing the risk of profit loss. It also discourages the participation of hospitals into any cost reduction programme, as the funder fully covers the cost of the services (Jegers et al.

2002; Lehtonen 2007). Although the adoption of retrospective payment will demotivate the hospital from "cost effectiveness" programme, the quality of care for this type of payment system is rarely debated. Moreover, with this payment system, hospitals will provide treatment without being affected by profit loss. This situation will avoid discrimination towards patients who pay significantly for treatment (Chok et al. 2018).

Fee for service payment is one of the retrospective payment system types which is often increased by the researcher (Busse et al. 2011; Jewish Healthcare & Pittsburgh Regional 2007; Lehtonen 2007; Robinson 2001). This is an approach of payment where the service provider will receive reimbursement after the treatment given to the patient. With this payment method, the reimbursed value often increases, which results to doctors getting overworked. This is due to the association between the income and the quantity of services which the patients receive (Jegers et al. 2002; Robyn et al. 2013). Consequently, this is possibly related to the exceeding duration of stay for patients in the hospital. This unnecessary admission results in maximum monetary gain for the hospital, along with the significant administrative cost which the hospital needs to sustain as the doctors and other clinical staff work for unnecessary long durations.

On the other hand, as for the prospective payment system, there is flat rate between the cost charged on the patients and the actual cost. However, the cost is pre-determined before the provision of treatment. Furthermore, past study by Jeggers et al. (2002) highlighted that, in this system, estimation of the actual treatment cost charged on patients could be performed by computing the average amount of cost charged on patients of different groups but with same clinical characteristic. However, in the aspect of the resources used for treatment, homogeneity in the patient's classification scheme is necessary (Jegers et al. 2002). With this system, provided that the hospital takes over the funder's responsibility over the cost, cost effectiveness is a highly important matter. For this reason, at hospitals where prospective payment system is implemented in their reimbursement programme, cost reduction programme holds high significance (Ma 1994; Robyn et al. 2013).

The quality and cost of health treatment is important. Furthermore, it is a complicated subject within healthcare where prospective payment system is implemented. This is due to the argument regarding the tendency of this type of reimbursement programme to be aimed towards patients who are provided with low-cost treatment for a significant amount of reimbursement (Jegers et al. 2002; Ma 1994; Preston et al. 1997). The challenge to get the balance between cost and quality in each series of treatment has made the employment of casemix system became favourable among hospital that is adopting prospective payment system in their reimbursement programme (Goldfield 2010; Paul et al. 2008). Moreover, Diagnosis Related Group (DRG) is an instrument present in the casemix system which aids the hospital in balancing treatment quality and cost (Averill et al. 1998; Goldfield 2010; Pongpirul & Robinson 2013).

Economic burden is a prevalent issue within society, particularly in the healthcare sector. Based on the perspective of healthcare provider, retrospective payment system often leads to high cost and cost uncertainty in spite of the maximum profit gaining which is guaranteed to the hospital. Besides, not only significant financial risk to the provider comes along with it, it could also lead to exceeding working hours for hospital staff, as well as patients' exceeding duration of stay at hospitals. On the contrary, despite the risky financial situation faced by hospitals through prospective payment system, the estimation of how much each treatment is charged could be done in advance, which helps hospitals to perform necessary actions in the prevention of monetary loss as well as unnecessary labours' service. Through the implementation of the casemix system in hospital reimbursement programme, balancing the quality and cost of each healthcare is possible by employing the casemix system. This discussion is followed by the next section which presents the details regarding the implementation of casemix system as a tool for provider payment.

2.3 Casemix System

The generic description of casemix is a system which classifies patients into particular groups according to a series of treatment provided in a healthcare setting. With this system, patients who have similar clinical characteristics are classified under one homogenous costing group known as Diagnosis Related Group (DRG). According to Hopfe et al. (2016), Professor Robert Bob Fetter and Jon Thompson originally developed Casemix system, in the 1970s at Yale University with the aims to manage patients in acute hospital. Therefore, in accordance to the application of the prospective payment system under Medicare in the United States of America, the implementation of this system was with the purpose of offering a transparent, efficient, and quality medical treatment provision (Hopfe et al. 2016; Lehtonen 2007).

Based on previous studies, it is indicated that Casemix system consists of two primary components which are cost analysis and patient classification system (Goldfield 2010; Pongpirul, Walker, Winch, et al. 2011; Preyra 2004; Turner-Stokes et al. 2012). As for the classification system of patients in the casemix system, it consists of procedure coding and diagnosis coding (Goldfield 2010; Pongpirul, Walker, Winch, et al. 2011). In patient classification system, which is the casemix system's first component, the codification of each disease into alpha and alphanumeric code is performed based on the International Classification of Disease (ICD). As for the second element of casemix system which is the analysis of cost, the calculation of the cost charged for patient's stay at hospital is performed before the provision of healthcare, which is based on the information developed from the process of clinical coding. Step-Down Costing and Activity Based Costing (ABC) are the approaches of costing which are frequently implemented under casemix system (Roszita et al. 2017).

Casemix system is a multi-purpose system where it functions as an instrument of provider payment as well as a tool used for numerous objectives within the health care industry, particularly for the contribution towards hospitals' quality improvement (Gong et al. 2004). As shown in previous studies, it is possible to use the information obtained from this system for the assessment and monitoring of performance, guarantee of quality, aids provided for hospitals' internal management programme, and healthcare quality benchmark (Goldfield 2010; Moshiri et al. 2010; Roger France 2003).

Information extracted from casemix system could be utilised in evaluating performance monitoring and quality assurance as well as facilitate the hospital for internal management programme and benchmarking the quality of care (Goldfield 2010; Moshiri et al. 2010; Roger France 2003). Furthermore, it has a remarkable ability of attracting countries, especially middle and low-income countries for the redevelopment of their health care industry's programmes. Moreover, it has been reported that the countries which apply the casemix system for their reimbursement purposes consist of around 70% of all Organisation for Economic Cooperation and Development (OECD) and more than 25 middle and low-income countries (Hopfe et al. 2016).

With the requirement of casemix for the redevelopment of every component of hospitals including the improvement of clinical documentation within their health care, previous literatures have come up with a number of obstacles in implementing the casemix system. The application of the concept of casemix among the staff of hospitals, especially doctors, is one of the issues which have become frequent topic of argument (Dowling et al. 1995). In this system, the cooperation of doctors and other clinical staff including laboratory staff is needed to gather casemix's minimum data set such as patient's primary and secondary diagnosis phrases, patient's activities during their hospital stay and patient's demographic information for full application of this system (Busse et al. 2011). Additionally, the primary obstacles in the implementation of casemix system as the tool for provider payment are the completion of these minimum data set information, which is essentially regarding patients' procedural and diagnostic phrases

(Chin et al. 2013). The implementation of this system could be interrupted when information from the minimum data set is lost. This is due to the dependability of the construction of Diagnosis Related Groups (DRG) on this recorded information.

2.4 Diagnosis Related Group (DRG)

The Diagnosis Related Groups (DRG) code is the basis in the casemix system for the assignment of the hospital tariff for an episode of care. Therefore, DRG is essential for the application of the casemix system as the instrument for provider payment. Initially, DRG was the first grouping system created under casemix system which functioned as a way of association between the types of receiver of medical treatment to the cost charged by the hospital (Averill et al. 1998; Goldfield 2010; Palmer & Reid 2001). Recently, there has been a wide scale of this system implementation by many countries worldwide, each having their own version of DRGs. Examples of such countries are Malaysia (Malaysia Diagnosis Related Group; MY-DRG®), Australia (Australia Refined Diagnosis Related Group; AR-DRG), the United Kingdom (Healthcare Resources Groups; HRG), and Germany (G-DRG) (Busse et al. 2011; Gong et al. 2004; Saperi et al. 2005).

Malaysia Diagnosis Related Group (MY-DRG®) is used in UKMMC. This system is a casemix classification type where MY-DRG® casemix grouper is involved. The development of MY-DRG® casemix grouper is conducted by a number of researchers from United Nations University-International Institute for Global Health (UNU-IIGH) and International Training Centre for Casemix and Clinical Coding (ITCC) (Moshiri et al. 2010; Zafirah et al. 2017). In accordance to Figure 2.1, the DRG code created by the grouper is a composition of 5 alphanumeric codes, where four numbers and one letter are present in this system (Zafirah et al. 2018). The body systems, which are labelled as Casemix Main Group (CMG), are indicated by the first digit.

Meanwhile, the second digit represents the type of case for the patient (1 = surgical case, 4 = medical case, 8 = O&G case, 9 = paediatric case). On the contrary, the third and fourth digit of the code are known as Case-Based Group (CBG), followed by the last digit of the code which indicates how severe the illness of the patient is (I = mild, II = moderate, III = severe).

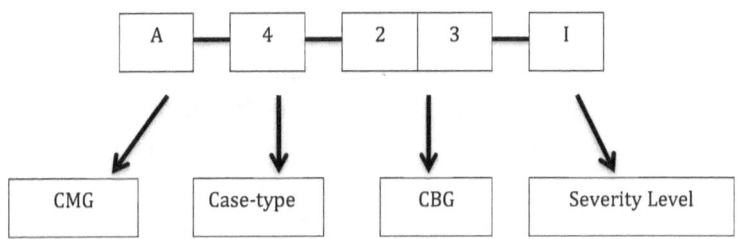

Figure 2.1 Example of MY-DRG Code

Based on the recent literature reviews regarding the usage of DRG in the health financing they provide, positive results can be seen from most of the studies in countries where this system is implemented in their reimbursement programme (Jameson & Reed 2007; Mathauer & Wittenbecher 2013; Or. 2014; Rosenberg & Browne 2001). Past study highlight that among the countries where DRG is applied in their reimbursement programme, there has been a relative increase in the General Government Health Expenditure (GGHE) after DRG was implemented as the tool for provider payment. Examples of those countries are Estonia, where the involvement has risen from 66.8% to 78.7%, Thailand where it has increased from 63.5% to 75.0%, and Kyrgyzstan where the increase is from 41.1% to 56.2% (Mathauer & Wittenbecher 2013). Based on previous studies, it can be seen that due to the application of DRG, the money spent by the government for the healthcare sector had increased. It was possible that the calculated amount of expenditure was lower than the actual amount before DRG was implemented. Overall, this proves that, with the retrospective payment through DRG, access to health care to the entire nation has been facilitated, which diminishes the possible occurrence of inequality in healthcare provision.

The DRG is a multipurpose tool which can be used by the healthcare industry. It is also a tool which, aside from healthcare financing, can be used for measurement and assessment of the performance of hospital and investigation into health services (Hensen et al. 2005; Lowe 2001). Based on a study past study, DRG is defined as an approach of enhancing the productivity of hospitals while maintaining the same service quality (Radu et al. 2010). Meanwhile, DRG is defined by previous studies as an instrument to identify the products used by hospitals, and an approach for the hospital to acquire the understanding regarding control resource and utilize it (Chok et al. 2018; Lehtonen 2007). Based on a similar research by Lehtonen (2007), it has been emphasized that, with focus placed on the outcome of the quality of care and financial outcome of hospitals, the effective utilisation of intermediate services is possible with the DRG control framework comprising of the DRG-based casemix accounting systems and prospective payment (Lehtonen 2007). Evidently, after the implementation of DRG in Swiss health care, the gradual decrease of the average duration of stay for ICU patients was reported (Chok et al. 2018). This showed that the reduction of the duration of the patient's stay through identification of the effective treatment essential to the patient is possible according to the DRG.

As for the use of DRG as the instrument for provider payment tools through the implementation of casemix system, while each patient will be placed under a DRG group, the amount of hospital tariff imposed on the patient is represented by this group. With this system, the specification of the DRG group for each patient is based on the patient's clinical characteristic (Mathauer & Wittenbecher 2013; Wallis et al. 2009). Therefore, the allocation of each DRG code was conducted to a constant amount of hospital tariff. The calculation of this amount was conducted in costing analysis where the calculation of the adjustment factor, base rate, and cost weight was performed. In accordance to previous studies, what is displayed in Table 2.1 provides the description of adjustment factor, base rate, and cost weight (Goldfield 2010; Mathauer & Wittenbecher 2013). Through the implementation of DRG in the casemix system, it is of high importance to obtain accuracy in the assignment of DRG code in order to ensure the accuracy of the cost of treatment charged on patients. Accordingly, the accuracy of the information regarding the clinical condition of patients and accurate costing analysis calculation are the determiners of the accuracy of DRG code allocation (Chin et al. 2013; Schreyögg et al. 2006). Therefore, clinical costing and coding analysis has a crucial role in the implementation of DRG as the tool for payment provider through the casemix system.

Table 2.1 Definition of Components in Calculation of Hospital Tariff

No	Item	Definition
1.	Cost Weight	Relative measurement which indicates the resources' relative use which are associated to a particular DRG in comparison to other DRG
2.	Base Rate	Monetary value. The value is the same for all DRGs
3.	Adjustment Factor	Instrument for the adjustment of the payment rate of DRG bases

Despite the employment of DRG as the instrument for provider payment being preferable by countries where prospective payment system is implemented, a number of significant challenges are still present and need to be overcome. It has been highlighted from previous studies that comprehensive clinical documentation, particularly information regarding procedure and diagnosis phrases, is crucial for an optimum DRG allocation. However, the inaccuracy of its clinical information is frequently found in the clinical documents (Burns et al. 2012; Chin et al. 2013; Hennessy et al. 2010; B. Reid & Sutch 2008). The importance of clinical coding was rarely highlighted among the medical staff relating to the lack of reporting of this crucial information namely diagnostic and procedural phrases (Farhan et al. 2005). With this, the hospital revenue would be impacted, which would lead to possible adverse outcomes, such as the insufficiency of reimbursement rate. For this reason, it is highly important to put emphasis on the significance of clinical coding in the implementation of DRG. With this, the accuracy of the allocation of DRG code, which is a significant factor of hospital's revenue, will be guaranteed. This is followed by the next section of this chapter, where details on clinical coding from the perspective of casemix system will be described.

2.5 Clinical Coding

Clinical coding is a process of translating written medical terms into numeric and alphanumeric codes. Clinical coding is a standard language used by health care practitioners to describe treatment and services that they provide to a patient (Bajaj et al. 2007; O'Malley et al. 2005; Sherri et al. 2003). To illustrate this, International Classification of Disease 10th Revision (ICD 10) states that code I10 represents hypertension. Meanwhile, International Classification Disease 9th Revision – Clinical Modification (ICD-9-CM) agrees that code 87.44 represents the procedure of chest x-ray for patients. Clinical coded data usually presents the essential clinical condition of the patient during their episode of care and each clinical condition is labelled with a standardised labels (Cresswell et al. 2012; Heywood et al. 2016; Tai et al. 2007). With the process of clinical coding, easy access to written information in medical records is easily obtainable, which subsequently makes optimal utilisation of clinical information possible. Moreover, utilisation of clinical coded data by people of various backgrounds, even those without high medical knowledge, is possible with simplification of the medical terms into the standardised term.

In healthcare sector, clinically coded data is a multipurpose data where its usage is possible in many aspects of hospital's governance. This data functions in enhancing hospital's productivity by conducting continuous supervision on the daily activities conducted there. With the yearly expenditure of healthcare being carried out at a fast rate, hospital's productivity is important for equal distribution of high quality healthcare services. In addition, it is an informative tool where benchmarking process of daily activities conducted at hospitals can be utilized (Nouraei et al. 2009). Meanwhile, past study highlighted that when daily activities at hospitals are continuously supervised from coded data, it will be a dependable information source for better health treatment and improved productivity of hospitals (Rudman 2000). To illustrate this, with the data acquired from the coding process, identification and elimination of procedures with lack of efficiency can be performed by hospitals. The same case goes to the elimination of operations which could risk the misuse of human or financial resources. Besides, hospital managers will be able to receive assistance for the creation of hospital's governance framework based on operation and procedure which could bring hospital's productivity to the optimum level.

Aside from monitoring purposes, the data obtained from the coding process is also useful for research development. Furthermore, it is believed that researchers will be assisted in extracting information for the development of research when clinical coding information is present. Besides, with the availability of this information, dependency on complex medical records is unnecessary (Preda et al. 2012). With the increasing number of research, it is possible for hospital's management to establish a clinical programme which would aid the improvement in the treatment provided by hospitals in terms of efficiency. Moreover, hospital managers are able to acquire statistical data regarding mortality rate at hospitals through output from clinical coding (Lowe 2001). With the availability of data regarding mortality rate, observation on the adherence of a medical operation for areas with higher mortality rate is possible for hospitals. The same case goes to surveillance on saturated occurrence of disease in areas with higher mortality rate.

Information extracted from the clinical coding process is also beneficial for hospital's health financing. As an example, the main function of data from clinical coding in the United States of America and Canada is for billing (Cresswell et al. 2012). Furthermore, when DRG is used through casemix system as the instrument for provider payment, clinical coding has a crucial role. This is due to the identification of the patient costing group being based on the information regarding the clinical characteristic of patients, which are acquired through the clinical coding process (Lowe 2001). When DRG is used as the tool for provider payment, the tariff allocated to the patient is calculated based on how the patients are clinically faring based on the report by the coded data. However, loss of the coded data would resulted in inaccurate hospital tariff allocation to patients which, as a result, may be associated with hospital's potential revenue loss.

To summarise, the clinical coding process is a primary component which should be focused by the governance of hospitals. With this data, the productivity and hospital's health financing will be enhanced. Nevertheless, the challenge in utilising this data is to maintain its quality due to its lengthy procedure. This will be followed by the next section which discusses on the reference of clinical coding which are involved during the coding process, along with the procedures taken during the allocation of codes to the procedural and diagnose phrases.

2.5.1 Clinical Coding Process

This process consists of two primary components namely diagnosis coding and procedure coding (Goldfield 2010; O'Malley et al. 2005). The process for the former takes place through the allocation of patient's primary and secondary diagnosis, while the process for the latter takes place through the allocation of code for procedures which are conducted on the patients during their stay at hospital (Goldfield 2010; Pongpirul, Walker, Winch, et al. 2011; Razik et al. 2013; Sherri et al. 2003; Zafirah et al. 2017). The coding process is normally performed in accordance to the International Classification of Disease (ICD).

William Farr, an English doctor, established a disease classification in 1825 for the codification of mortality data for death certificates (Preda et al. 2012). Preda et al. (2012) emphasize that International Congress of Statistics in Brussels acknowledged the importance of standardization in disease specification in 1853. This was followed by approval by the World Health Organization on a complete list of regulations for deciding on the causes of morbidity and death in 1949. This list was compiled in a document named "Manual of Classification of Diseases, Accidents and Causes of Death", where the generic name for it is ICD (International Classification of Diseases) (Preda et al. 2012). Based on a report of different study by Adeleke et al. (2014), the study of ICD commenced in the 16th century in order to provide authorisation of comparison of mortality and morbidity data, systematic interpretation, analysis, and recording, which were gathered in different areas or countries and separate times (Adeleke et al. 2014).

The adaptation of ICD has been done since 1949, as well as its periodical update. Following that, the establishment of ICD 9 was done by WHO in 1978. In order increase the functionality of it at the hospitals in America, modification of ICD 9 into ICD 9 Clinical Modification (ICD-9-CM) was done by the U.S Public Health Service (O'Malley et al. 2005). Aside from ICD, it has been indicated by a number of literatures that Health Care Common Procedural Coding System (HCPCS), CPT 4th Edition, Health Care Financing Administration (HCFA), and American Medical Association's Current Procedure Terminology are part of the nosologies which are prevalent in the sector of healthcare (Busse et al. 2011; Hywel Dda University 2014; O'Malley et al. 2005).

In casemix system, the allocation of the codes for diagnosis phrases is conducted according to International Classification of

Disease 10th Revision (ICD 10). The introduction of ICD 10 as an alternative to ICD 9 was made in 1993. Supposedly, the introduction of ICD 10 should be made in 1985. Nevertheless, due to the case of alphanumerical code and development of digital version, the introduction was delayed (Aljunid et al. 2012). Besides consisting of the regulations needed for the coding and recording, the diseases classified under it amount to 24 chapters (WHO 2008; Aljunid et al. 2012). There are three volumes under ICD, which are Volume 1 (main classification), Volume 2 (regulations required for ICD user), and Volume 3 (alphabetical index to the classification) (WHO 2008). In accordance to WHO (2008), the purpose of ICD 10 is for;

a) Primary Diagnosis:

1. The condition diagnosed at the end of episode healthcare primarily responsible for patient need for treatment or investigation;
2. The condition responsible for the greatest utilization of resources during patient's stay;
3. The conditions that best justify the length of stay.

b) Secondary Diagnosis:

1. Co-morbidities (condition which exist prior to admission);
2. Complications (conditions which occur in hospital).

The allocation of the code for the procedures undergone by patient during the hospital stay is according to International Classification Disease 9th Revision – Clinical Modification (ICD-9-CM). Even so, the allocation of procedure code is according to the Office of Population Censuses and Surveys (OPCS) in the United Kingdom (Haliasos et al. 2010). The specification of disease for a statistical purpose is enabled through ICD-9-CM, when it is used so that the claim examiner and medical biller are able to transform conditions such as illnesses into a numeric code. Furthermore, Alexander (2004) agrees that ICD-9-CM consists of three volumes, which are Volume I (a tabular listing of illnesses), Volume II (an alphabetical listing of illnesses, with details in English), and Volume III (an alphabetical and numerical listing of surgical and non-surgical operations which doctors may conduct) (Julie Levin Alexander 2004). In accordance to ICD-9-CM, surgical operations are categorized in rubrics 01-86, while non-surgical operations are categorized in rubrics 87-99.

In the coding process, a number of steps and tremendous cooperation provided by hospital staff from every level are necessary. The important steps of the allocation of clinical codes according to ICD-9-CM and ICD 10 are presented in the next sub-topic.

2.5.2 Steps in Assigning Codes

A number of steps of code allocation consist of commitment given by many hospital staff of many levels in the coding process. Based on a previous study, it has been shown that coding process is a multi-step procedure which needs overlapping roles in the disciplines of health professionals (Pongpirul et al. 2011). Moreover, it has been claimed by past studies that the commencement of coding process takes place when patients are admitted to hospitals. This process ends after the recording of the diagnosis admitted to the allocated ICD codes after the release of patients (Johnson et al. 2014; O'Malley et al. 2005). For this reason, previous literatures have emphasised the importance of determining high accuracy of clinical coding, aside from information regarding patient's clinical condition upon the phase of treatment, the information provided when patients are admitted to hospitals is also essential.

With accurate documentation of information during every stage of patients' admission, the accuracy of data, which are coded after patients are released, would be guaranteed. Therefore, the coding process commences after the discharge of patients from hospitals. In this stage, the doctor in charge will gather the diagnosis and all clinical activities into a discharge summary. This is followed by the allocation of certified coders allocated to the fitting ICD-10 and ICD-9-CM codes according to the information obtained from discharge summary and demographic information on patient's clinical condition from Health Information System (HIS). This code will be input into a software known as grouper. Through this software, a DRGs code suitable for the patient will be created (Farhan et al. 2005; Pongpirul et al. 2011; Pongpirul et al. 2011).

Based on the Casemix Online Course organised by United Nation University, the allocation of procedure coding and diagnosis consists of seven steps (UNU IIGH 2008). Below are the procedures for the coding of diagnosis according to ICD-10:

1. Identify the type of statement to be coded and refer to the appropriate section of the alphabetical index (disease/nature of injury, external causes, drugs and chemical, procedures);
2. Locate the lead term. Read and be guided by any note that appears under the lead term;
3. Read any terms enclosed in parentheses after the lead term, as well as any essential modifiers – ensure all parts of the diagnosis are considered;
4. Follow carefully any cross - references found in the index (volume 3);
5. Refer to the tabular list (volume 1);
6. Be guided by any inclusion or exclusion terms under the selected code, chapter, block or category heading;
7. Finally assign the code.

Below are the steps of procedure coding:

1. Identify the procedure phrase to be coded;
2. Decide the lead term;
3. Look up the lead term in the alphabetical index;
4. Locate any modifiers;
5. Check the code given in the index with tabular list;

6. Check for inclusion and exclusion terms;
7. Assign the code.

Based on previous literatures, the issue regarding the documents which are the most effective as primary references during the clinical coding process has been argued upon. It is important to consider that detailed regulations on the selection of documents as the primary reference for clinical coding procedure are absent. Subsequently, the selection of the primary reference for clinical coding procedures would be vague, in spite of the possibility for discharge summary to be utilised by some hospitals as the primary reference. Meanwhile, complete medical records may be used by a number of hospitals as the primary reference of clinical coding process (Ghaffari et al. 2010). Even though compared to the discharge summary, the medical records contained specific and accurate patient's clinical information, the voluminous medical record could also lead to difficulties among coders to conduct the clinical coding process in an accurate manner (Farhan et al. 2005; Ghaffari et al. 2010; Peng et al. 2016). Nevertheless, medical records as the primary reference of clinical coding are still suggested by past study due to the reliability of the information present in medical records in comparison to the information in the discharge summary (B. A. Reid et al. 2017a). It is also worth to note that in UKMMC, the coding process is conducted by using the discharge summary as the primary reference of clinical coding process (Zafirah et al. 2017). From the past studies it is shown that the absent of the clear rules on the selection of primary reference of clinical coding process has caused discordance of the documents referred during the clinical coding process.

2.5.3 The Coders

Coding process is usually conducted by personnel who expertise in coding fields such as clinical coders. The important function of the coder is specifying the accurate code representing every clinical information of patients shown in the medical record (Hassan. A et al. 2002; Lorence & Ibrahim 2003).

It has been shown from previous literatures that people from various levels would be enrolled as the clinical coder by different countries. As an example, the doctor will be in charge of the coding process in France (Paul et al. 2008). As for Thailand, coding task is conducted by medical statisticians who are enrolled by several hospitals. Besides, a number of hospitals in Thailand also allocate the coding process to doctor and nurses (Pongpirul et al. 2011). Based on a study by Ghaffari et al. (2010), as doctors will be in charge of procedure coding, clinical coders will be responsible for diagnosis coding. In UKMMC, Malaysia, all the clinical coding task will be done by a trained clinical coders (Saperi et al. 2005). On the other hand, it was reported by Razik et al. (2013) that in a Orthopaedic Day Sugery Department in United Kingdom, the coding task is performed by the professional coders without the involvement of clinical staff.

Past studies have raised issues on the qualification of coders and the reliability of the clinical coding conducted by these coders. Bramley and Reid have raised that commonly coders have not received an adequate education on coding and most of the coders only received on-the-job training on clinical coding (Bramley & Reid 2005). In the same study by Bramley and Reid, it was reported that Diploma Programmes constitute Clinical Coding as the core subject is only available in Australia, United States of America and Canada. The lack of awareness regarding the significance of clinical coding, particularly in the developing countries, is evident from the absence of proper coding programmes there. This idea received support from past studies which emphasised that clinical coding has been perceived as insignificant as a task associated with the negligence of the significance of clinical coding among hospital managers (Heywood et al. 2016; Preda et al. 2012). This has resulted in the clinical coders getting employed without having medical background and not receiving appropriate training in clinical coding. This consequently leads to the issue concerning the quality of clinical coding.

2.6 Clinical Coding Errors

Clinical coding is a complex process where not only it requires precise assignment of ICD codes, it is also important for medical records to be complete in order to determine its accuracy. For the ICD codes to be allocated, patients' clinical information written in the medical records is required (Rosenstein et al. 2009). For this reason, in specifying the precision of ICD code allocation, precise and complete information regarding patient's illness by the doctor is essential for the clinical coding process. Besides, accurate discernment by the clinical coder is also important for the allocation of relevant ICD codes for the procedural and diagnostic phrases present in the medical record by the doctor. Moreover, incorrect presumption regarding the allocation of the ICD codes presented by clinical coders would possibly lead to errors in clinical coding. Subsequently, negative consequences will take place in hospital revenue and administration.

Generally, the clinical coding errors could be defined as diagnosis or procedure code assigned by in-house coder for one episode of care differs from those assigned by independent reviewer (Campbell et al. 2001b; O'Malley et al. 2005). In spite of this fact, depending on countries, clinical coding error is described differently (Bajaj et al. 2007; Campbell et al. 2001b; Haliasos et al. 2010; Hywel Dda University 2014; Zafirah et al. 2017). To illustrate this, as for the United Kingdom, the amount of errors committed in the assignment of the code's first and second digit level is lower due to higher consciousness regarding clinical coding. For this reason, the measurement of the coding error here is based on the concordance of the code allocated by the independent coder and in-house coder who range from the third digit to the fifth digit level of the code (Bajaj et al. 2007; Hywel Dda University 2014). On the other hand, there was study reported definition of coding errors as code assigned by the in-house coder differs from those assigned by independent reviewer up to the third digit level of the code relating acceptance of coding error at the assignment of the fourth digit level and fifth digit level of the code (Campbell et al. 2001b; Tucker et al. 2016). Aljunid and Zafirah (2016) highlighted that the coding errors among novice countries adopting Casemix system needs to be measured at every level of the code.

Based on previous studies, the range of variations on the rate of clinical coding errors was wide. As presented in Table 2.2, the range of the rate of coding errors was from 16.0% to 84.5%, with 39.2% average (Bajaj et al. 2007; Campbell et al. 2001a; Curtis et al. 2002; Farhan et al. 2005; Mehrdad et al. 2010; Nouraei et al. 2015, 2009; Ping et al. 2009). Based on a report by Ping et al. (2009), the United States of America had the highest rate of coding error. However, Campbell et al. (2001) reported that this country had the lowest coding error rate in 2001. Despite the extensive literature regarding coding errors in developed countries, there were relatively insufficient amount of evidences found from developing countries.

Table 2.2 Percentage of Coding Errors in Previous Studies

Year	Coding Errors (%)	Country	Source
2001	16.0	United Kingdom	Campbell et al. 2001
2002	28.0	Australia	Curtis et al. 2002
2004	34.3	United States of America	Mehrdad et al. 2010
2005	30.0	Saudi Arabia	Farhan et al. 2005
2005	84.5	United States of America	Ping et al. 2009
2007	46.0	United Kingdom	Bajaj et al. 2007
2009	24.1	United Kingdom	Nouraei et al. 2009
2014	51.0	United Kingdom	Nouraei et al. 2015

In the literature review, comparison between the rate of coding errors and each coding items which are the codes of primary procedure, secondary procedure, primary diagnosis, and secondary diagnosis code is challenging. There has been reports from majority of the preceding studies regarding the overall rate of coding errors, with the exclusion of the rate of coding errors for each coding items in a particular manner (Curtis et al. 2002; Mehrdad et al. 2010; Nouraei et al. 2015, 2009; Ping et al. 2009). However, the possible conclusion drawn from these studies was that there is a high chance for the coding errors to occur during the secondary diagnosis code allocation, in comparison to other coding elements. This conclusion was supported by past studies which highlighted that allocation of case is most likely to imprecise secondary diagnosis code compared to other coding elements (Heywood et al. 2016; Pongpirul, Walker, Winch, et al. 2011). Accordingly, Farhan et al. (2005) has reported a higher coding errors rate among secondary diagnosis code compared to primary diagnosis code and procedure code (43.2% vs 28.5% and 28.3%, respectively) (Farhan et al. 2005). Also, study by Heywood et al. also has highlighted a higher coding errors rate in the assignment of secondary diagnosis code (38.4%) compared to the other coding items (Primary Diagnosis Code; 30.8%, Primary Procedure Code ; 21.9% and Secondary Procedure Code ; 22.1%) (Heywood et al. 2016).

Additionally, based on previous studies, primary diagnosis code exhibit higher quality in comparison to the quality shown by the primary procedure code. As a proof, it was reported in Bajaj et al.'s study in 2007 that the rate of coding error among primary procedure codes, which amounted to 86.0%, were higher than the rate of primary diagnosis code, which were 84.0%. The possible factor to this was high consciousness that primary diagnosis code has more significance than primary procedure code. Besides, a notable finding from previous studies was the frequent highlight on the significance of diagnosis coding, particularly on primary diagnosis compared to procedure coding (Kirkman et al. 2009; Pine et al. 2009; Preyra 2004). The lack of study reporting on the importance of primary procedure code have resulted in the insufficient awareness on the quality of other coding items, particularly the procedure code. Therefore, the rate of coding errors in the allocation of primary procedure code is usually higher than the ones in primary diagnosis code due to less consciousness on the significance of primary procedure code (Beckley et al. 2009).

2.6.1 Type of Clinical Coding Errors

Based on observation from previous studies, types of errors in clinical coding can be specified into two major categories. Coder error is the former, while the latter represents the non-coder error. The literatures focusing on these two primary categories of errors in clinical coding will be discussed below.

The coder error is an error caused by the coder's erroneous judgement of the input provided by the doctor in the primary reference of clinical coding process as well as discordance of coding's guidelines among coders during the clinical coding process (Hywel Dda University 2014). Table 2.2 below summarised the type of coding errors due to coder error that usually used in the preceding studies (Bajaj et al. 2007; Hywel Dda University 2014; Silverman & Skinner 2004; Zafirah et al. 2017). From the table, it is notable that the coder error is involving the assignment of any digit of the clinical coding code. In this type of error, the input given by doctor is considered as the gold-standard and the coder has misinterpreted those input leading to the error in the assignment of the code. The coder error is also caused by the discordance of the coding's guideline set by the hospital's governance (Hywel Dda University 2014). For example, there is a clear mandate by the hospital's governance of using patient's case note as the primary reference of clinical coding process but instead, the coder is using discharge summary as the primary reference of clinical coding process.

Table 2.3 Type of Clinical Coding Errors

No.	Type of Coding Errors	Definition
1.	Error at first digit level	Discordance at the first digit level of the code.
2.	Error at second digit level	Discordance at the second digit level of the code.
3.	Error at third digit level	Discordance at the third digit level of the code.
4.	Error at fourth digit level	Discordance at the fourth digit level of the code.

5.	Error at fifth digit level	Discordance at the fifth digit level of the code.
6.	Primary diagnosis (PDX) or Primary procedure (PP) code incorrectly sequenced	The accurate PDX code and PP code was listed as secondary diagnosis or secondary procedure by the in-house coder.
7.	Up-coding	The in-house coder has assigned irrelevant code that may lead to a higher level of severity or higher reimbursement.
8.	Under-coding	The in-house coder has assigned irrelevant code that may lead to a lower level of severity or lower reimbursement.

On the other hand, a non-coder error is an error caused by the factor external to the clinical coder such as accuracy of the input written by the doctors or hospital policy which requires coders to assign codes discordance to the national standards. For example, a doctor might document a wrong primary diagnosis phrase in the primary reference of clinical coding process that caused a wrong selection of code by the coders (Mckenzie et al. 2005; Shin et al. 2003; Tang et al. 2017). The less specific information written by a doctor on patient's clinical condition also could relate to coding errors (Heywood et al. 2016; Hywel Dda University 2014). The non-coder error could also be influenced by the structure of hospital governance which are motivated by the profit gain where this situation is called as DRG Creep (Or. 2014). The DRG Creep is a situation where the hospital managers instructed the coder to assign irrelevant codes for an episode of care to gain a higher reimbursement rate (Pongpirul, Walker, Winch, et al. 2011).

From the past studies, it could be concluded that various factors could influence the quality of clinical coding. Firstly, coder's knowledge and experience plays a vital role in determining the accuracy of code according to the input given by the doctors. Nevertheless, the fact that the input provided by doctors influences the output provided by coders is a worthy point to be considered. Besides, the policy set by hospital's governance is also a factor of the quality of the coding created by the coders. For this reason, for a clinical coding of excellent quality, it is important for hospital staff from every level to work together. Following this, the challenges in acquiring clinical coding of excellent quality will be presented in the next section.

2.6.2 Factor Influencing the Clinical Coding Errors

The quality of clinical coding could be influenced by various factors. Based on the past study, the roots of errors are placed between the diagnosis by the clinician and the clinical condition of the patient. It is also placed between the code and diagnosis allocated by medical coders (O'Malley et al. 2005). From the review of past literatures, it could be concluded that there are four major barriers in attaining a good quality of clinical coding (Mehrdad et al. 2010; Ping et al. 2009; Pongpirul, Walker, Rahman, et al. 2011; Razik et al. 2013; Santos et al. 2008). The challenges start with the knowledge and skills of the coder in order to perform clinical coding. This is followed by accuracy in reporting the clinical condition of patients at the level of doctors. Then, the quality of the document utilised as the clinical coding process' main reference is the third factor. Lastly is the structure of hospital's governance framework. In this section, literatures which focus on these four challenges will be presented.

a. Clinical Coders

In order to create clinical coding with excellent quality, it is important for the coder to possess knowledge and skill in order to conduct coding process. The knowledge necessary for the coders not only concerns on clinical coding process, but the knowledge on clinical practice is equally important. Furthermore, based on previous studies, inadequate knowledge of the guidelines of clinical coding, medical terminologies, and clinical practice will significantly obstruct coders from obtaining clinical coding with good quality (Ping et al. 2009; Razik et al. 2013). It is proven in a study by Razik et al. (2013) that clinical coding errors, especially the complicated cases associated with it, are mostly due to the coder's inadequate knowledge of clinical practice (Razik et al. 2013). It has also been proven in a study by Beckley et al. (2009) in a Urology Department that the coder's insufficient knowledge of urology procedures in depth have resulted in considerable amount of errors in the coding of procedure code, which ultimately lead to significant money loss. For this reason, the acquirement of clinical coding with good quality would be challenging without adequate knowledge in performing the coding process.

The duration of service provision is also the factor of the quality of clinical coding. To illustrate this, there will be a higher chance for the coding quality to improve when coders are gaining more experiences upon their service provision. Based on a report from a study by Mehrdad et al. (2010), the occurrence of clinical coding errors is highly possible when coders do not have at least five years of service duration. This is due to the high dependency on ICD 10 among junior coder especially in assigning codes for complicated cases. Besides, due to more familiarity with the clinical terms documented by the doctor in the clinical coding process' primary reference, experienced coders are more capable of reducing the rate of coding errors (Santos et al. 2008). Nevertheless, the fact that the issue regarding the employment of clinical coders is still new for most hospitals in developing countries should be taken into account (Pongpirul, Walker, Rahman, et al. 2011; Zafirah et al. 2017). With this reason, acquiring a clinical coding with excellent quality through experienced and knowledgeable clinical coders is challenging due to the scarce number of this type of clinical coders, especially in developing countries.

b. Doctors

The second influencing factor of clinical coding's quality is how accurate the report on the clinical condition of patients is.

Furthermore, it is a common knowledge that the primary task of a doctor is treating patients' illnesses. Due to the increase of global disease, being a doctor has become one of the busiest careers. Lenny (2014) has stated in his article submitted to the Washington Post magazine in 2014 that, in average, there are 11 to 30 patients who receive visits by doctors daily. Subsequently, doctor's busy work nature has led to the rising of issues on the accuracy of the diagnosis assigned by the doctor to the patient. Past study by Lorence and Ibrahim (2003b) has highlighted that, busy doctors frequently lack the time in attending patients tends to select incorrect diagnosis and this, without doubt, will lead to the error in clinical coding. In a report by West et al. in 2008, it is stated that a study by Woolf et al. (2008) revealed that over three-quarters of errors were reported for mistakes in treatment and diagnosis.

Additionally, the lack of consciousness of the significance of clinical coding is the result of doctor's busy nature of work. Besides, due to absence of consciousness of the significance of clinical coding, a number of issues associated with the reliability clinical documents regarding patients have surfaced. There have been frequent arguments on the lack of accuracy in the information on patient's condition reported in the clinical documentation by doctors (Callen et al. 2010; Chin et al. 2013; Ellen et al. 2006; Farhan et al. 2005; Tang et al. 2017). Although clinical information are crucial in assigning accurate clinical codes, doctors have a tendency to provide incomplete report on clinical information of patients (Farhan et al. 2005). The lack of consciousness among doctors of the significance of clinical coding has led to the process of documentation, which is crucial in the process of clinical coding, to lose its criticality among doctors. This is associated with the occurrence of errors in clinical coding.

c. **Quality of Clinical Documentation**

Quality of the clinical coding's main reference is the third influencing factor of errors in clinical coding. Furthermore, the significance of documentation with excellent quality as clinical coding's main reference has been emphasised by previous studies (Heywood et al. 2016; Jameson & Reed 2007). Clear documentation is paramount to ensure the accuracy of clinical coding. However, even though the importance of the good quality of primary reference of clinical coding process is unquestionable, the questions on the reliability of the documentation used as the primary reference of clinical coding continue to raise (Ghaffari et al. 2010; Hennessy et al. 2010). It has been reported in the study by Lorence and Ibrahim that when the list of diagnoses and procedures is not supported by the documentation in the medical record, conducting accurate clinical coding process would be challenging for coders (Lorence & Ibrahim 2003). Moreover, the influencing factor of documentation refers how high the consciousness of doctors is when reports are made on the patient's clinical condition. This is because documentation would be done poorly when the amount of attention given by doctors in documenting is insufficient (Hennessy et al. 2010). Therefore, clinical coding errors will most likely occur due to poor quality of documentation used as the main reference for the process of clinical coding.

Besides the issues on the quality of documentation, it is also worth to note that the question on the best selection of the primary reference of clinical coding is still unresolved. Past studies have highlighted that up to date there is no uniform structure on the primary reference used during the clinical coding process (Byrne et al. 2011; Johnson et al. 2014). Data are coded from a variety of sources such as discharge letters, patients' notes or other sources, for instance, computer based patient record systems (Wallis et al. 2009). Some hospitals may practice the coding process by referring to the discharge summary to reduce the time consumed by the coders during the clinical coding process. On the other hand, some hospital may practice the coding process by referring to patient's case note to increase the specificity of the code. Therefore without having clear standardised guidelines on the selection of primary reference used during the clinical coding process, it is difficult to choose on which documentation need to be prepared at the highest quality to ensure the good quality of clinical coding.

d. Structure of Hospital Governance

The last factor that could contribute to the clinical coding errors is due to the structure of the hospital governance's framework. The clinical coding plays a vital role in the health financing of the hospital that is employing casemix system as their provider payment tools (Cresswell et al. 2012). Accordingly, without the needs to utilise clinical coding to receive adequate hospital's revenue, the importance of clinical coding is rarely highlighted in the structure of the hospital governance's framework. Evidently, past study by Goldman et al. (2011) has reported that the quality of clinical coding is higher among profit hospital than teaching hospital as the governance of teaching hospital is not motivated by the profit gaining. The absent of the clinical coding in the structure of the hospital governance's framework has caused funding allocation for clinical coding's programmes becomes limited (Santos et al. 2008). This has subsequently retaliated the increment of knowledge among coders as they are lack of funding support by the hospital managers in the clinical coding's related programme.

The failure to see clinical coding as an important element of the hospital governance has related to the employment of the clinical coder as an unimportant subject among the hospital managers. In attaining a good quality of coding, it is essential for the hospital managers in providing clinical coding training among the clinical coders (Bramley & Reid 2005; Santos et al. 2008). The lack of training provided by the hospital managers could relate to a higher rate of clinical coding errors as the coders are not being updated with the current coding's rules and guidelines. Shepheard (2010) has highlighted in his study that it is important for the coders to receive continuous training in maintaining the good quality of clinical coding in the hospital. The continuous training not only will help to increase coder's knowledge but also works as a tool to increase coder's level of confidence in conducting clinical coding process.

It can be summarised that the quality of clinical coding process by the clinical coders are not only the main factor when errors occur in clinical coding, but doctors, hospital's governance, and the accuracy of patient's clinical information are also the influencing factors. For a better quality of clinical coding, it is highly important for every element in hospitals to be reconstructed. Following this is previous literatures where initiatives of improving the clinical coding quality is focused on, which will be presented in the next section of this chapter.

2.7 Improving the Quality of Coding

For guaranteed effectiveness of healthcare provided by hospitals to patients, clinical coding with excellent quality is highly important. Based on previous studies, it can be gathered that doctors, managers, and coders need to work together for a better quality of clinical coding. Previous studies which emphasised on the initiatives needed for a better quality of clinical coding, where hospital doctors, managers, and coders are the three important personnel for it, will be elaborated in this sub topic.

It has been suggested in previous studies that decisive intervention by hospital managers is important in order to obtain clinical coding of high quality (B. A. Reid et al. 2017a; Santos et al. 2008; Shin et al. 2003). This may include the effort of conducting a regular coding's audit to ensure the clinical coding process is conducted in an accurate manner. Past studies have stressed the importance of conducting a routine coding audit by hospital managers to improve the quality of clinical coding (Heywood et al. 2016; B. A. Reid et al. 2017a). For instance, in United Kingdom due to the implementation of Payment by Result (PbR) system, an Audit Commission was constituted to ensure a high quality of clinical coded data as the rewards given by National Health Service (NHS) to hospital is depending on the volumes of work reflected from the coded data (Beckley et al. 2009; Chiu GA & Woodwards 2011; Marini & Street 2007). Evidently, the regular clinical coding audit has proved to help in increasing the quality of coded data in a hospital (Adams et al. 2002; Heywood et al. 2016). Conducting a regular audit could help hospital managers in resolving the issue related to clinical coding process especially the problem on the quality of primary reference of clinical coding that subsequently will increase the quality of clinical coding in the hospital.

As the primary reference of clinical coding, documentation written by the doctor plays a vital role in improving the quality of clinical coding. Ghaffari et al. (2010), has highlighted that accuracy and completeness in documentation is highly essential to avoid any error during the assignment of codes. Therefore doctor's cooperation in submitting accurate and specific information of patient's clinical condition is pivotal to increase the quality of clinical coding. Reid et al. (2017a) have highlighted in their study on the importance of embedding the awareness of the importance of clinical coding among doctor to ensure the excellent quality of documentation. It is also essential for doctors to reduce the abbreviation used in documenting patient's clinical condition and also improve the clarity of their hand's writing to enhance the quality of the documentation (Adeleke et al. 2014; Mayo & Duncan 2004; O'Malley et al. 2005; Tang et al. 2017). This would subsequently improve the quality of clinical coding

Past studies also have highlighted that among the crucial efforts in improving the quality of clinical coding is by increasing the level of coder's knowledge in clinical coding process (Ghaffari et al. 2010; O'Malley et al. 2005; Ping et al. 2009; Shepheard 2010). It is widely known that the medical knowledge and diagnostic tools are an evolving nature. Parallel to that, codes and coding rules are also expanding and changing gradually. Thus coder delay in learning new skills will affect the accuracy of coding (O'Malley et al. 2005). Therefore, continuous training of the coders is highly important to prevent an error to occur during the coding process (Ghaffari et al. 2010). Coders with a limited understanding of medical terminology and techniques would reflect the quality of clinical coding in the hospital (Ping et al. 2009).

To sum it up, the efforts to improve the quality of clinical coding requires high cooperation between hospital managers, doctors and coders. The poor quality of clinical coding could relate to far-reaching consequences in both administrative and financial side of the hospitals. Therefore the importance of clinical coding needs to be embedded in these three significant personnel. A level of awareness of the importance of clinical coding needs to be increased to achieve a good quality of clinical coding. Next section will present past literature discussing the implications of clinical coding errors.

2.8 Implications of Clinical Coding Errors

The clinical coding errors could give an adverse impact towards the hospital's governance. Not only it would lead to the financial ramification, but the clinical coding errors also could affect the quality of management of the hospital. According to Haliasos et al. (2010), coding errors can cause failure in allocating the accurate budget to the hospital which would subsequently affect the management of the hospital (Haliasos et al. 2010). This sub-topic will present past studies that reported on the implications of the clinical coding errors.

The accuracy of clinical coding is a pivotal subject especially when the hospital is using casemix system as their provider payment tools. The incorrect assignment of clinical coding would relate to the wrong assignment of the DRG group (Curtis et al. 2002; Lorence & Richards 2002; Paul et al. 2008). Accordingly, the clinical coding errors would relate to danger on the sustainability of the budget allocated by the government to a hospital as coding errors could cause a hospital to receive a higher or lower reimbursement rate than the actual one (Wallis et al. 2009; Wockenfuss et al. 2009). Even though as reported by Marini and Street (2007) as well as Soonman (2003) that clinical coding errors such as up-coding could be beneficial to the health financing of the hospital, the adverse effect of the clinical coding is usually raised by the preceding studies.

Past studies have reported that the clinical coding errors have caused changes in the assignment of DRG which subsequently resulted in profit loss to the hospital (Chiu GA & Woodwards 2011; Kirkman et al. 2009; Ping et al. 2009; Zafirah et al. 2017). Table 2.4 below shows the summary of the studies that reported on profit loss due to the clinical coding errors (Bhasker & Coatesworth 2016; Murphy 2012; O'Malley et al. 2005; Razik et al. 2013; Tucker et al. 2016; Zafirah et al. 2017). From the table, it is notable that, the profit loss per month due to clinical coding errors is between RM 24, 515 to RM 30, 105 whereas the profit loss per case due to clinical coding errors is ranging between RM 1, 313 to RM 6, 563. The coding errors occurred among surgical discipline relates to the highest average profit loss amounting to RM 7, 950 per case (Tucker et al. 2016). It was reported in the same study by Tucker et al. (2016) that the wrong assignment of procedure code has caused changes in the assignment of hospital tariff in their study. It is also interesting to note that is an absence of research detailing the profit gain of clinical coding errors in a detailed manner. Subsequently, it relates to the assumptions that clinical coding errors is most likely would cause a loss of profit to the hospital.

Table 2.4 Profit Loss due to Clinical Coding Errors

Source (Year)	Department	Average Profit Loss*
O'Malley (2005)	Urinary Tract Infection	USD 2000 (RM 6,563) /case
Murphy et al. (2012)	Interventional Pulmonology	£ 5, 416 (RM 24, 515) / month
Razik et al. (2013)	Surgical	£ 290 (RM 1, 313) / case

Zafirah et al. (2016)	Medical, Surgical, O&G, Paediatric	RM 2,832/ case
Tucker et al. (2016)	Surgical	£ 1,756.41 (RM7,950) / case
Bhasker & Coatesworth (2016)	ENT	£ 6,651 (RM30,105) / month

*Exchange rate is according to rate of Central Bank of Malaysia on 31st December 2013 (http://www.bnm.gov.my/index.php?ch=statistic&task=converter)

Besides the healthcare financing, the clinical coding errors could also relates to the negative output of the hospital management. Coded data works not only for financial purposes but also represents the demographic details and diagnoses treated by the hospital (Cresswell et al. 2012; Stanfill et al. 2010). As reported by past study that, a poor quality of clinical coded data would leads to poor quality of information (Lorence & Richards 2002). Subsequently, this would become a barrier to the hospital managers in improving the quality of care in the hospital (Fisher et al. 1991; Heywood et al. 2016). The poor quality of information, would prevent the hospital management to evaluate the outcomes of hospital care as the information provided by the clinical coded data is less accurate.

An appropriate and completeness of coding is very important in governing the hospital. The good quality of clinical programmes is depending on the information from the clinical coded data. Ping et al. (2009) highlighted in their study that, coding will become the based in planning funding for public health programs, thus coding error will resulted inaccurate funding for public health programs. In addition, planning a good healthcare delivery is relies on good documentation in the medical record, through coding practice. Moje et al. (2006) point out in their study of the accuracy of injury coding in Victorian hospitals that, hospital need to maintain a good quality of coding as this will become the benchmark for quality and safety purposes in the hospital. Therefore without a good quality of clinical coding, the management could not fully utilised the resources presents in the hospital as the input provided by the clinical coded data is less accurate.

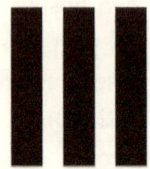 **METHODOLOGY**

3.1 Introduction

This chapter presents the methodology of this study covering study background, study design, sampling method and sample size calculation. The inclusion and exclusion criteria's of the selected samples are also presented in this chapter. This methodology chapter also discussed the study tools used by this study, procedure of the data collection and methodology employed for the re-coding process. At the end of this chapter, the definition of coding errors and its type, data analysis, also variables and its definitions are presented.

3.2 Study Background

This study was carried out in University Kebangsaan Malaysia Medical Centre (UKMMC). UKMMC formerly known as Hospital University Kebangsaan Malaysia (HUKM) started its operation since 1st July 1997. UKMMC which is located at

Bandar Tun Razak Cheras is among the oldest teaching hospital in Malaysia. In 1997, UKMCC has started their operational with 168 beds and has received 2517 patients' admissions with 2356 discharged patients. In the year of 2013, the number of beds has reached 845 and UKMMC has received total of 35 363 number of admission with 35 115 discharged patients. In the year of 2013, the coding process is conducted in Casemix Unit under the management of Health Informatics Department (HID). Based on data from 2009 up to July 2013, 173 536 cases were coded under this unit (Table 3.1).

Table 3.1 UKMMC's Patient Data from 2002 to 2013

Year	Total Admission	Number of Discharged Patient	Number of Bed	Bed Occupancy Rate	Average Length of Stay
2002	35 348	34 962	822	65.6	5.6
2003	35 596	35 429	834	66.6	5.7
2004	36 536	36 543	831	65.3	5.4
2005	35 857	36 008	852	63.9	5.4
2006	36 188	36 200	877	61.0	5.4
2007	35 801	35 946	875	62.2	5.5
2008	36 181	35 480	872	63.9	5.7
2009	37 056	36 972	888	61.7	5.4
2010	36 616	36 698	879	62.1	5.5
2011	35 171	35 303	827*	64.2	5.5
2012	34 473	34 207	837*	62.0	5.5
2013	35 263	35 115	845	64.4	5.6

* Special Ward was excluded during the survey

3.3 Study Design

A cross sectional descriptive study was conducted to analyse the incidence of clinical coding errors in UKMMC and its economic implication. The research was conducted mainly in Clinical Coding Unit, Health Informatic Department, UKMMC.

3.4 Sample Unit

There are three sample units of this study. The first sample unit was the coded Patient Medical Record (PMR) in the year of 2013. These selected records were among cases from four MY-DRG® Case-Type namely Medical, Surgical, O&G and Paediatric. The second sample unit was the coders who were responsible to codify the selected PMR. The third sample unit was the doctors who were responsible to complete the discharge summary of the selected PMR.

3.5 Sampling Method

3.5.1 PMR

A stratified random sampling method was applied for the selection of PMR. All the coded cases in the year of 2013 was stratified according to the MY-DRG® Case-Type namely Medical, Surgical, Obstetric & Gynaecologist (O&G) and Paediatric. Then, the cases were randomly selected from each of the case-type according to sample size requirement. The stratified sampling method according to the four MY-DRG® Case-Type have allowed the study to compare in detailed the clinical coding errors rate between each case-type.

3.5.2 Coders

A universal sampling method was applied for the selection of the coders. Therefore, all coders that involved in the coding process of the selected PMR.

3.5.3 Doctors

A universal sampling method was applied for the selection of the coders. Therefore, all doctors that responsible in completing the discharge summary of the selected PMR.

3.6 Sample Size Calculation

Sample size calculation for PMR to be included in the study is based on Lwanga and Lameshow (1991) scale. This formula is a standard formula used to identify the prevalence for particular incidence in health study (Agampodi et al. 2007, Lasserre et al. 2009, Livingston et al. 1998). The formula is as follows;

$$n = Z^2_{1-\alpha/2} P(1-P)/d^2$$

Whereby:

n = sample size
Z = value 1.96 for the level of confidence 95%, which is conventional
P = expected prevalence or proportion of 38.0% coding error rate or 0.38
d = precision (in proportion of one which is 5% or 0.05)

Therefore:

$$n = 1.96^2(0.38)(1-0.38)/(0.05)^2$$
$$= (3.84)(0.24)/(0.0025)$$
$$= 369$$

In this study:

a) Z statistic (z) : z value is 1.96, for the level of confidence 95% which is conventional.
b) Expected Proportion (P) : p value is 38.0% based on the average coding errors rate identified in four countries namely United Kingdom, Australia, United State of America and Saudi Arabia (Bajaj et al. 2007; Campbell et al. 2001b; Curtis et al. 2002; Farhan et al. 2005; Haliasos et al. 2010; Mehrdad et al. 2010; Ping et al. 2009). These

countries were selected due to the availability of literatures reported on the coding errors rate in these countries.
c) d : d is the absolute precision taken at 5 % or 0.05

Based on the formula, 369 samples was required for this study. Researchers have agreed to add another 15 per cent of sample to give a more reliable result. So finally 424 PMR was needed. Since there were four case-type in the study, 106 PMR was required per case-type. However, during the data collection, another 10 cases were added for each case-type to increase the accuracy of the data analysis. Finally there were 464 PMR was re-coded with 116 PMR per case-type.

3.7 Inclusion And Exclusion Criteria

3.7.1 Inclusion Criteria for PMR

1. All cases admitted starting from 1st January to 31st December 2013;
2. Cases from four case-type namely Medical, Surgical, O&G and Pediatric;
3. Cases with diagnoses and procedures have been coded by coders in UKMMC.

3.7.2 Exclusion Criteria for PMR

1. Cases admitted from UKMMC in 2013 but not coded by coders in UKMMC;
2. Cases discharges from UKMMC before year 2013 and after 2013;
3. Outpatient cases.

3.8 Study Tools

There were 6 types of study tools used by this study namely;

1. PMR
2. Data Abstraction Sheet
3. Checklist for 14 Casemix Variables
4. MY-DRG® Grouper
5. Survey Form on Clinical Coder's Demographic Data
6. Information Sheet on Doctor's Demographic Data

3.8.1 PMR

PMR was used to retrieve all the relevant information of the diagnosis and procedure phrases of the patient. These PMR will be collected retrospectively from January 2013 to December 2013. All the codes assigned to patient must be accordance to the information written in the PMR.

3.8.2 Data Abstraction Sheet

After identifying the PMR, the data in the records were re-abstracted and the new code was recorded in the data abstraction sheet. This sheet was based on the Clinical Documentation Improvement Toolkit recommended by past study (Maria et al. 2010).

3.8.3 Checklist for 14 Casemix Variables

This checklist was used to determine the level of completeness of the documentation used during the coding process. This checklist comprised all the 14 variables required for Casemix System: Patient's Identifier, Age, Gender, Birth Weight (for babies), Admission Date, Discharge Date, Length of Stay, Discharge Category, Patient Type, Principal Diagnosis, Secondary Diagnosis, Principal Procedure and Other Procedure.

In UKMMC, the coding process was conducted according to the information written in the discharge summary. Thus this study attempt to evaluate the completeness of the written information in the discharge summary in comparison to the information written in the PMR.

3.8.4 Survey Form on Clinical Coder's Demographic Data

This survey form was used to determine the association between clinical coder's demographic data and clinical coding errors. In the survey form, the coder was required to filled in below information;

a. Full Name
b. Identification Number
c. Length of Service
d. Job's position in the year of 2013
e. Job's grade in the year of 2013
f. Educational Level
g. Total number of clinical coding's training attended inside UKMMC
h. Total number of clinical coding's training attended outside UKMMC

3.8.5 Information Sheet on Doctor's Demographic Data

This information sheet was used to determine the association between doctor's demographic data and clinical coding errors. The information on doctor's demographic data was received from the Human Resource Department. The collected information were as below;

a. Full Name
b. Identification Number
c. Job's position in the year of 2013
d. Job's grade in the year of 2013
e. Educational Level

3.8.6 MY-DRG® Grouper

MY-DRG® grouper was used in this study to identify the new MY-DRG® group of the error cases identified in this study.

3.8.7 Procedure of Data Collection

This study was divided into two major parts. The first part was identifying the coding errors whereas the second part was to measure the economic implications of the coding errors.

At the first part, the data collection was done by using the PMR located in Clinical Coding Unit, UKMMC. An Independent Senior Coder who is unrelated to UKMMC was appointed to review and re-code the selected PMR. During the audit, a data abstraction sheet was used to record all the relevant diagnosis and procedure code according to the written information in the PMR. During the audit the Independent Senior Coder also simultaneously conducted a completeness checking of the PMR and discharge summary. The completeness checking was conducted according to the checklist of 14 Casemix Variables. After the audit by the Independent Senior Coder, all the new codes were sent to the casemix expert in International Centre for Casemix and Clinical Coding (ITCC) before it was used. If there was any ambiguity in the assignment of the new codes by the Independent Senior Coder, the casemix expert would re-examine the PMR.

In the second part of the study, to measure the economic implication of the coding errors, MY-DRG® grouper was used. After the casemix expert approved the new code, was re-grouped using the MY-DRG® grouper to identify if there is any change in the assignment of MY-DRG® group. When there was change in the assignment of MY-DRG® group, the new hospital tariff was assigned to the case in accordance to the new MY-DRG® group. The hospital tariff used by this study was calculated by the casemix expert located in ITCC. Figure 3.1 below summarised the study flow of this study.

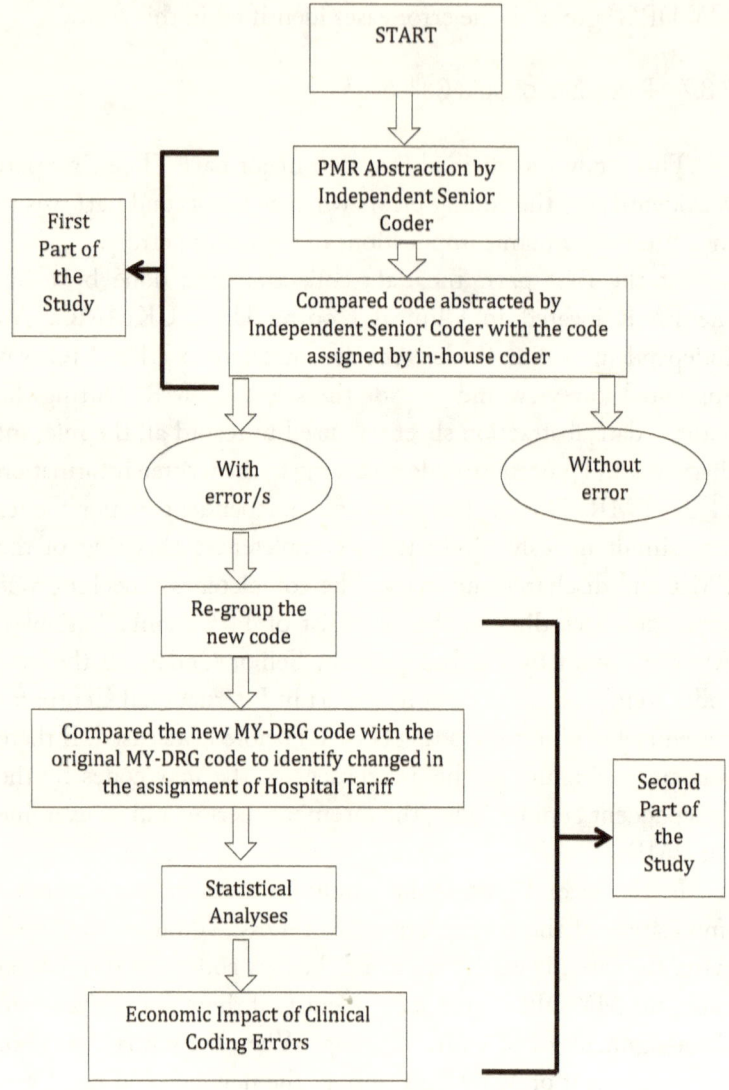

Figure 3.1 Flow of the Study

3.9 Methodology of the Re-Coding Process

There were enormous studies conducted by past studies on the clinical coding errors. However, the methodology applied during the re-coding process was varied according to studies. One of the methodology that were reported by past studies was by comparing two coded output and determine the level of agreement between two code (Donoghue 1992; Tucker et al. 2016). Another popular methodology was by re-analysing medical records and choose the right code (Bajaj et al. 2007; Curtis et al. 2002; Farhan et al. 2005; Haliasos et al. 2010). From the observation of past studies, the reported coding errors rate is more likely to be lower among studies that are employing internal doctors or coder to conduct the audit (Farhan et al. 2005; Haliasos et al. 2010; Nouraei et al. 2009). Donoghue also reported in his study in 1992 that the reported coding errors rate are lower among studies which the second coder had access to the original codes (Donoghue 1992).

To avoid above-mentioned issues on the methodology, a blinded re-coding process by an Independent Senior Coder was conducted by this study to evaluate the coding errors rate in UKMMC. A blind re-coding process is believed could avoid any bias judgement during the evaluation by the Independent Senior Coder. Also, the study also has appointed an Independent Senior Coder who is unrelated to UKMMC has more than ten years of experience in clinical coding. By employing an independent reviewer who is unrelated to the hospital, it also could eliminate the possibility of bias judgment during the audit. In addition to this, the selected Independent Senior Coder has undergone clinical coding's training at national and international level. The training received by the Independent Senior Coder is believed could increase the level of accuracy of the codes assigned during the audit.

However, even though the Independent Senior Coder is considered the expert in assigning the clinical coding code, there is also the tendency for the Independent Senior Coder to assign a wrong code to the patient. Thus, to avoid a wrong assignment of the code by the Independent Senior Coder, all the newly assigned codes were vetted by the casemix experts before it was used and accepted. If there is any ambiguity in the assignment of the codes, the experts will re-examine the PMR. These experts are the developer of the MY-DRG® grouper and were among the founders of the casemix system employed by UKMMC.

Another worth noting point in the methodology of the coding process is that the audit was conducted according to the information written in the PMR. Despite the culture in UKMMC of conducting the coding job according to the discharge summary alone, this study decided to conduct the audit based on the PMR. There were two main reasons relating to this decision. Firstly, as mentioned by the Pongpirul et al. in their study conducted in Thailand in 2011, the medical record is considered complete essential information of patient's demography as well as patient's health state (Pongpirul et al. 2011). Thus to evaluate the accurate coding errors rate in UKMMC, this study believed it is important to analyse the PMR. Secondly, by conducting the audit according to the PMR, this study could simultaneously examine the completeness of the written information in the discharge summary in comparison to the written information in the PMR. This could help to measure the effectiveness of the clinical coding process of using the discharge summary alone.

3.10 Definition of Coding Errors

In this study, the coding error was defined as diagnosis or procedure code that was assigned by the in-house coder that differ with those assigned by the Independent Senior Coder at any digit level of the code (Campbell et al. 2001b). If the code differed, the code assigned by the Independent Senior Coder that was vetted by the casemix expert was considered as the accurate code.

3.11 Definition of the Type of Coding Errors

During the audit, the codes were examined at the every digit level of the codes. The types of coding errors are defined according to the research on the clinical coding errors conducted by Zafirah et al. in 2017 (Zafirah et al. 2017).

3.11.1 Type of Coding Errors in Primary Diagnosis Code

There were six types of coding errors in the assignment of primary diagnosis code namely;

a. Wrong Selection of Primary Diagnosis Code

The primary diagnosis code selected by the Independent Senior Coder differs from those selected by the in-house coder. This indicates a wrong assignment at the first digit level of the code, which implies a wrong assignment of the ICD Chapter of the code. For example, a case was originally assigned by the in-house coder to code K12.1 (Other forms of stomatitis) but, the accurate code assigned by the Independent Senior Coder was G91.9 (Obstructive hydrocephalus).

b. Error at the Second Digit Level of the Code

The primary diagnosis has been assigned wrongly at the second digit level of the code. This indicates a wrong assignment of the category of the code. For example, a case was originally assigned by the in-house coder to code N18.1 (Chronic kidney disease, stage 1) but, the accurate code assigned by the Independent Senior Coder was N93.8 (Other specified abnormal uterine and vaginal bleeding).

c. Error at the Third Digit Level of the Code

The primary diagnosis has been assigned wrongly at the third digit level of the code. This indicates a wrong assignment of the category of the code. For example, a case was originally assigned by the in-house coder to code J12.9 (Viral pneumonia, unspecified) but, the accurate code assigned by the Independent Senior Coder was J18.9 (Pneumonia, unspecified organism).

d. Error at the Fourth Digit Level of the Code

The primary diagnosis has been assigned wrongly at the fourth digit level of the code. This indicates a wrong assignment of the sub-category of the code. For example, a case was originally assigned by the in-house coder to code P59.8 (Neonatal jaundice from other specified caused) but, the accurate code assigned by the independent senior codes was P59.9 (Neonatal jaundice, unspecified)

e. Error at the Fifth Digit Level of the Code

The primary diagnosis has been assigned wrongly at the fifth digit level of the code. This indicates a wrong assignment of the supplementary subdivisions of the code. For example, a case was originally assigned by the in-house coder to code M84.19 (Nonunion of fracture [pseudarthrosis], site unspecified) but, the accurate code assigned by the Independent Senior Coder was M84.16 (Nonunion of fracture [pseudarthrosis], lower leg).

f. Primary Diagnosis Code was Incorrectly Sequenced

The accurate primary diagnosis code has been wrongly sequenced by the in-house coder. Instead, it was listed as the secondary diagnosis code. For example, a case was originally assigned by the in-house coder to code O24.4 (Gestational diabetes mellitus) but, the accurate primary diagnosis code assigned by the Independent Senior Coder was O70.0 (First-degree perineal laceration during delivery). The accurate primary diagnosis code assigned by the Independent Senior Coder was listed at the secondary diagnosis code by the in-house coder.

3.11.2 Type of Coding Errors in Secondary Diagnosis Code

There were seven types of errors in the assignment of secondary diagnosis code namely;

a. Wrong Selection of Secondary Diagnosis Code

The secondary diagnosis code selected by the Independent Senior Coder differs from those selected by the in-house coder. This indicates a wrong assignment at the first digit level of the code, which implies a wrong assignment of the ICD Chapter of the code. For example, a case was originally assigned by the in-house coder to code L90.5 (Scar conditions and fibrosis of skin) but, the accurate code assigned by the Independent Senior Coder was Y86 (Sequelae of other accidents).

b. Error at the Second Digit Level of the Code

The secondary diagnosis has been assigned wrongly at the second digit level of the code. This indicates a wrong assignment of the category of the code. For example, a case was originally assigned by the in-house coder to code P70.1 (Syndrome of infant of a diabetic mother) but, the accurate code assigned by the Independent Senior Coder was P92.3 (Underfeeding of newborn).

c. Error at the Third Digit Level of the Code

The secondary diagnosis has been assigned wrongly at the third digit level of the code. This indicates a wrong assignment of the category of the code. For example, a case was originally assigned by the in-house coder to code Z37.0 (Single live birth) but, the accurate code assigned by the Independent Senior Coder was Z38.0 (Singleton, born in hospital).

d. Error at the Fourth Digit Level of the Code

The secondary diagnosis has been assigned wrongly at the fourth digit level of the code. This indicates a wrong assignment of the sub-category of the code. For example, a case was originally assigned by the in-house coder to code I95.9 (Hypotension, unspecified) but, the accurate code assigned by the independent senior codes was I95.2 (Hypotension due to drugs).

e. Error at the Fifth Digit Level of the Code

The secondary diagnosis has been assigned wrongly at the fifth digit level of the code. This indicates a wrong assignment of the supplementary subdivisions of the code. For example, a case was originally assigned by the in-house coder to code M81.97 (Osteoporosis, unspecified, ankle and foot) but, the accurate code assigned by the Independent Senior Coder was M81.99 (Osteoporosis, unspecified, site unspecified).

f. Up-coding

The in-house coder has assigned irrelevant code for the selected case that may lead to higher level of severity or higher reimbursement rate in casemix classification. For example, a case was originally assigned by the in-house coder to code Z51.1 (Chemotherapy session for neoplasm) but, the according to the Independent Senior Coder, the assignment secondary diagnosis code was unnecessary for this case.

g. Under-coding

The Independent Senior Coder identified additional codes that was missed by in-house coder that may lead to lever level of severity being assigned or the hospital may get lower level of reimbursement. For example, a case was originally unassigned to any secondary diagnosis code but, according to the Independent

Senior Coder, J45.9 (Asthma, unspecified) was a relevant secondary diagnosis code for this case.

3.11.3 Type of Coding Errors in Primary Procedure Code

There were seven types of coding errors in the assignment of primary procedure code namely;

a. Wrong Selection of Primary Procedure Code

The primary procedure code selected by the Independent Senior Coder differs from those selected by the in-house coder. This indicates a wrong assignment at the first digit level of the code, which implies a wrong assignment of the primary axis of the code. The primary axis of procedure code indicates the anatomical site of the procedure. For example, a case was originally assigned by the in-house coder to code 53.10 (Bilateral repair of inguinal hernia, not otherwise specified) but, the accurate code assigned by the Independent Senior Coder for this case was 17.24 (Laparoscopic bilateral repair of inguinal hernia with graft or prosthesis, not otherwise specified)

b. Error at the Second Digit Level of the Code

The primary procedure code was assigned wrongly at the second digit level of the code. This indicates a wrong assignment of the secondary axis of the code which is referring to the type of procedure undergone by patient. For example, a case was originally assigned by the in-house coder to code 73.6 (Episiotomy) but, the accurate code assigned by the Independent Senior Coder for this case was 75.69 (Repair of other current obstetric laceration).

c. Error at the Third Digit Level of the Code

The primary procedure code was assigned wrongly at the third digit level of the code. This indicates a wrong assignment of the tertiary axis of the code which is referring to the site or techniques of the procedure undergone by patient. For example, a case was originally assigned by the in-house coder to code 99.25 (Injection or infusion of cancer chemotherapeutic substance) but, the accurate code assigned by the Independent Senior Coder for this case was 99.04 (Transfusion of packed cells).

d. Error at the Fourth Digit Level of the Code

The primary procedure code was assigned wrongly at the fourth digit level of the code. This indicates a wrong assignment of the tertiary axis of the code which is referring to the site or techniques of the procedure undergone by patient. For example, a case was originally assigned by the in-house coder to code 53.02 (Other and open repair of indirect inguinal hernia) but, the accurate code assigned by the Independent Senior Coder for this case was 53.05 (Repair of inguinal hernia with graft or prosthesis, not otherwise specified).

e. Primary procedure code was Incorrectly Sequenced

The accurate primary procedure code has been wrongly sequenced by the in-house coder. Instead, it was listed as the secondary procedure code. For example, a case was originally assigned by the in-house coder to code 93.9 (Respiratory Therapy) but, the accurate primary procedure code assigned by the Independent Senior Coder was 87.44 (Routine chest x-ray, so described). The accurate primary procedure code assigned by the Independent Senior Coder was listed at the secondary procedure code by the in-house coder.

f. Up-coding

The in-house coder has assigned irrelevant primary procedure code for the selected case that may lead to higher level of severity or higher reimbursement rate in casemix classification. For example, a case was originally assigned by the in-house coder to code 45.26 (Open biopsy of large intestine) but, the according to the independent senior coder, the accurate primary procedure code for this case was 45.25 (Closed biopsy of large intestine).

g. Under-coding

The Independent Senior Coder identified additional codes that was missed by in-house coder that may lead to lever level of severity being assigned or the hospital may get lower level of reimbursement. For example, a case was originally unassigned to any primary procedure code but, according to the Independent Senior Coder, 88.78 (Diagnostic ultrasound of gravid uterus) was a relevant primary procedure code for this case.

3.11.4 Type of Coding Errors in Secondary Procedure Code

There were seven types of coding errors in the assignment of primary procedure code namely;

a. Wrong Selection of Secondary Procedure Code

The primary procedure code selected by the Independent Senior Coder differs from those selected by the in-house coder. This indicates a wrong assignment at the first digit level of the code, which implies a wrong assignment of the primary axis of the code. The primary axis of procedure code indicates the anatomical site of the procedure. For example, a case was originally assigned by the in-house coder to code 89.52 (Electrocardiogram) but, the accurate code assigned by the Independent Senior Coder for this case was 97.64 (Removal of other urinary drainage device).

b. Error at the Second Digit Level of the Code

The secondary procedure code was assigned wrongly at the second digit level of the code. This indicates a wrong assignment of the secondary axis of the code which is referring to the type of procedure undergone by patient. For example, a case was originally assigned by the in-house coder to code 87.71 (Diagnostic ultrasound of head and neck) but, the accurate code assigned by the Independent Senior Coder for this case was 88.75 (Diagnostic ultrasound of urinary system).

c. Error at the Third digit level of the code

The secondary procedure code was assigned wrongly at the third digit level of the code. This indicates a wrong assignment of the tertiary axis of the code which is referring to the site or techniques of the procedure undergone by patient. For example, a case was originally assigned by the in-house coder to code 88.78 (Diagnostic ultrasound of gravid uterus) but, the accurate code assigned by the Independent Senior Coder for this case was 88.38 (Other computerized axial tomography).

d. Error at the Fourth digit level of the code

The secondary procedure code was assigned wrongly at the fourth digit level of the code. This indicates a wrong assignment of the tertiary axis of the code which is referring to the site or techniques of the procedure undergone by patient. For example, a case was originally assigned by the in-house coder to code 88.74 (Diagnostic ultrasound of digestive system) but, the accurate code assigned by the Independent Senior Coder for this case was 88.75 (Diagnostic ultrasound of urinary system).

e. Up-coding

The in-house coder has assigned irrelevant secondary procedure code for the selected case that may lead to higher level of severity or higher reimbursement rate in casemix classification. For example, a case was originally assigned by the in-house coder to code 66.39 (Other bilateral destruction or occlusion of fallopian tubes) but, the according to the Independent Senior Coder, the assignment secondary procedure code was unnecessary for this case.

f. Under-coding

The Independent Senior Coder identified additional codes that was missed by in-house coder that may lead to lever level of severity being assigned or the hospital may get lower level of reimbursement. For example, a case was originally unassigned to any secondary procedure code but, according to the Independent Senior Coder, 57.94 (Insertion of indwelling urinary catheter), 97.64 (Removal of other urinary drainage device) was the relevant secondary procedure code for this case.

3.12 Data Analysis

There were two major parts of the data analysis in this study namely to explore the incidence of clinical coding errors rate in UKMMC and to measure the economic impact of coding errors towards UKMMC. In both analyses, the dependent variable and the independent variables differed.

3.12.1 Data Analysis on the Incidence of Clinical Coding Errors in UKMMC

In the first part of the data analysis, this study explores the incidence of clinical coding errors in UKMMC. This part includes the measurement of the coding errors rate, bivariate analysis on the level of agreement between the Independent Senior Coder and the in-house coder in the assignment of the codes, bivariate analysis on factor influencing coding errors and multivariate analysis on factor influencing coding errors.

a. Descriptive Analysis on Coding Errors Rate in UKMMC

This study imputed two level of coding errors rate calculation. In the first level of calculation, the coding error rate was based on the number of cases with error codes. The numerator was the total number of cases with errors, and the denominator was the total number of reviewed cases by the independent reviewer.

In the second level of calculation, the coding errors rate was calculated according to the total number of reviewed codes. The total number of error codes was the numerator, and the total number of codes reviewed by the independent reviewer was the denominator. The total number of error codes was inclusive all error codes at the first digit level, second digit level, third digit level, fourth digit level, fifth digit level as well as under-coded code and up-coded code. Each up-coded and the under-coded codes were counted as one error for each code. All the calculation was done using the Microsoft Excel 2010.

b. Bivariate Analysis on the Incidence of Coding Errors

At the first part of the data analysis, this study employed two types of bivariate analysis. Firstly the study has used A Cohen Kappa Test to identify the level of agreement between the Independent Senior Coder and the in-house coder. For primary diagnosis and primary procedure, the level of agreement was measured according to the code assigned to the selected PMR. On the other hand, for secondary diagnosis code and secondary procedure code, the level of agreement was evaluated according to the number of code assigned per coding item. Kappa value was interpreted as below (Burns et al. 2012; Zafirah et al. 2017) ;

i. 0.10 to 0.20 = poor agreement
ii. 0.21 to 0.40 = fair agreement
iii. 0.41 to 0.60 = moderate agreement
iv. 0.61 to 0.80 = substantial agreement
v. 0.81 to 1.0 = perfect agreement

Secondly, a Chi-Square test was conducted to identify the factors influencing coding errors. All analyses were conducted using IBM SPSS version 20.0 and p-value of <0.05 was considered as statistically significant.

c. **Identifying the Type of Coding Errors**

During the data analysis, SPSS syntax function using DO IF command was used to identify the type of coding errors. Examples of the syntax are as follow;

i) To identify if the accuracy of the code assigned by the in-house coder, below syntax was used;

DO IF (PDX_Original_Full_code = PDX_New_Full_code).
RECODE Dummy_variable (1=1) INTO Sameness_of_full_ code_PD1.
END IF.
EXECUTE.

RECODE Sameness_of_partial_code_PD1 (SYSMIS=0).
EXECUTE

The output of 1 indicated a coding error was identified in the assignment of the code.

ii) To identify in which level the error was found, below syntax was used;

DO IF (PDX_First_Digit_Level=PDX_First_Digit_Level).
RECODE Dummy_variable (1=1) INTO Sameness_of_first_digit_PD1.
END IF.
EXECUTE.

RECODE Sameness_of_first_digit_PD1 (SYSMIS=0).
EXECUTE.

If the output was 0, this syntax was applied to the next level of the code. The output of 1 indicated the error level of the code.

d. Multivariate Analysis

Lastly, in the first part of the data analysis, a multiple logistic regression was applied to examine the determinant factors influencing coding errors rate (Baram et al. 2008; Rangachari 2007). All analyses were conducted using IBM SPSS version 20.0 and p-value of <0.05 was considered as statistically significant.

3.12.2 Data Analysis on the Economic Impact of Coding Errors

In the second part of the analysis, this study explored the impact of coding errors towards hospital potential revenue. The analyses covering the total potential hospital revenue before and after the audit, bivariate analysis on the difference of the income before and after the audit, bivariate analysis on the factor influencing changes in the assignment of potential hospital tariff and lastly multivariate analysis on the factors influencing changes in the assignment of potential hospital tariff.

a. Calculation of the Total Potential Hospital Revenue Before and After

The calculation of total potential hospital revenue before and after the audit was accordance to the calculated hospital tariff per MY-DRG® group. This hospital tariff was calculated beforehand by the casemix expert and available in ITCC. Total potential hospital revenue before the audit was imputed according to the MY-DRG® group generated by MY-DRG® grouper according to the original code assigned by the in-house coder. On the other hand, the total potential hospital revenue after the audit was imputed according to the MY-DRG® group generated by MY-DRG® grouper according to the new code assigned by the Independent Senior Coder.

Univariate analysis was performed in SPSS to identify the total potential hospital revenue, mean potential revenue per patient, maximum potential hospital tariff per patient and minimum potential hospital tariff per patient before and after the audit.

b. Bivariate Analysis

In the second part of the data analysis, two types of bivariate analysis were performed namely paired sample t-test and Chi-square test. Paired sample t-test was employed to identify the significant difference of the total potential hospital revenue before and after the audit. On the other hand, Chi-squared test was performed to identify factors influencing changes in the assignment of potential hospital tariff. All analyses were conducted using IBM SPSS version 20.0 and p-value of <0.05 was considered as statistically significant.

c. Multivariate Analysis

Lastly, in the second part of the data analysis, a multiple logistic regression was applied to examine the determinant factors influencing the accuracy of the assignment of potential hospital tariff. All analyses were conducted using IBM SPSS version 20.0 and p-value of <0.05 was considered as statistically significant.

3.13 Variables

There were two dependent variables and several independent variables in this research. The variables are listed below.

3.13.1 Dependent Variables

The dependent variable for the first part of the data analysis was Cases with Coding Error. On the other hand, the dependent variable for the second part of the data analysis was Cases with Changes in the Assignment of Hospital Tariff due to Coding Errors.

3.13.2 Independent Variables

The independent variables for the first part of the data analysis were;

1. MY-DRG® Case-type
2. Severity Level
3. Casemix Groups (CMGs)
4. MY-DRG® Groups
5. Admission Form
6. Discharge Summary
7. Coder's Demographic
8. Doctor's Demographic

The independent variables for the second part of the data analysis were;

1. Coding Error Case in the Assignment of Primary Diagnosis Code
2. Coding Error Case in the Assignment of Secondary Diagnosis Code
3. Coding Error Case in the Assignment of Primary Procedure Code

4. Coding Error Case in the Assignment of Secondary Procedure Code
5. Coding Error Case in the Assignment of Severity Level
6. Coding Error Case in the Assignment of MY-DRG® Case-type
7. Cases with Incomplete Admission Form
8. Cases with Incomplete Discharge Summary

3.14 Variables Operational Definition

3.14.1 Dependent Variables

a. Cases with Coding Errors

A case with the coding error was measured based on the comparison the original code by the in-house coder and the new code by the Independent Senior Coder. The data were analysed as a categorical variable. Case without disparity in the assignment of the code was categorised as no error (0), and case with a difference in the assignment of the code was categorised as coding errors cases (1).

b. Case with Errors in the Assignment of the Hospital Tariff due to Coding Errors

A case with errors in the assignment of the hospital tariff due to coding errors was measured by comparing the originally assigned hospital tariff before the audit and newly assigned hospital tariff after the audit. The data were analysed as a categorical variable. Case without changes in the assignment of hospital tariff was categorised as no error cases (0) and case with changes in the assignment of hospital tariff was categorised as error cases (1).

3.14.2 Independent Variables

a. Independent Variables for the First Part of the Data Analysis

i. Case-Type

There was four case-type involved in the data analysis. The data were analysed as categorical data. Medical case was categorised as (4), the Surgical case was categorised as (1), the O&G case was categorised as (6), and the Paediatric case was categorised as (8).

ii. Severity Level

There was three severity involved in the data analysis. The data were analysed as categorical data. Severity Level I (mild) was categorised as (1), Severity Level 2 (moderate) was categorised as (2), and Severity Level III (severe) was categorised as (3).

iii. CMG Group

There were 21 types of CMG group involved in the data analysis. The data were analysed as categorical data. The list of the category could be found in the appendix.

iv. MY-DRG® Group

There were 164 types of MY-DRG® groups involved in the data analysis. The data were analysed as categorical data. The list of the category could be found in the appendix.

v. Completeness of Admission Form

The completeness of admission form was measured by identifying availability of these following information of the patient in the form; Identifier (Name and Medical Record Number), Age (age in days for infant below 1 year old), Gender, Birth Weight (for neonatal less than 28 days only), and Admission Date. The data were analysed as categorical variable whereby cases with the complete information above was categorised as (0) whereas cases without at least one completion of the information above were categorised as (1).

vi. Completeness of Discharge Summary

The completeness of discharge summary was measured by identifying availability of these following information of the patient in the form; Identifier (Name and Medical Record Number), Age (age in days for infant below 1 year old), Gender, Birth Weight (for neonatal less than 28 days only), Admission Date, Discharge Date, Length of Stay, Discharge Status (Home/ Transfer to Acute Facility/Against Medical Advice/ Died/Other or Unknown), Patient Type (Inpatient / Outpatient), Principal Diagnosis, All Secondary Diagnosis, Principal Procedure and Secondary Procedure. The data were analysed as categorical variable whereby cases with the complete information above was categorised as (0) whereas cases with at least one incomplete of the information above were categorised as (1).

vii. Coder's Characteristic

Coder's characteristic was analysed by looking at three main criteria namely, coder's length of service, coder's educational level and number of inside and outside training attended by coder's. All data was analysed as categorical variable. For coder's length of service there was two category namely More and Equal than 10 years (0) and Less than 10 years (1). On the other hand, for coder's educational level, the category was Non-degree Holder (0) and Degree Holder (1). Lastly, for the number of inside and outside training attended by coders, the category was More and Equal than 5 set of trainings (0) and less than 5 set of trainings. These categories were determined according to the distributions of the coder's demographic information.

viii. Doctor's Characteristic

Doctor's characteristic was analysed by looking at two main criteria namely, doctor's length of service and doctor's educational level. All data were analysed as a categorical variable. For doctor's length of service there was five category namely Less than 1 year (0), 1 year (1), 2 years (2), More and equal to 3 years (3), Data not found (4). On the other hand, for doctor's educational level, the category was Degree Holder (1), Master Holder (2) and Data not found (3). These categories were determined according to the distributions of the doctor's demographic information.

b. Independent Variables for the Second Part of the Data Analysis

i. Coding Error Case in the Assignment of Primary Diagnosis Code

Case without error in the assignment of primary diagnosis code was categorised as (0), and case with an error in the assignment of primary diagnosis code was categorised as (1). The data were analysed as a categorical variable.

ii. Coding Error Case in the Assignment of Secondary Diagnosis Code

Case without error in the assignment of secondary diagnosis code was categorised as (0), and case with an error in the assignment of secondary diagnosis code was categorised as (1). The data were analysed as a categorical variable.

iii. Coding Error Case in the Assignment of Primary Procedure Code

Case without error in the assignment of primary procedure code was categorised as (0), and case with an error in the assignment of primary procedure code was categorised as (1). The data were analysed as a categorical variable.

iv. Coding Error Case in the Assignment of Secondary Procedure Code

Case without error in the assignment of secondary procedure code was categorised as (0), and case with an error in the assignment of secondary procedure code was categorised as (1). The data were analysed as a categorical variable.

v. Coding Error Case with Changes in the Assignment of Severity Level

Coding error case without error in the assignment of the severity level was categorised as (0) and coding error case with the error in the assignment of severity level was categorised as (1). The data were analysed as a categorical variable.

vi. Coding Error Case with Changes in the Assignment of Discipline

Coding error case without error in the assignment of the discipline was categorised as (0) and coding error case with the error in the assignment of severity level was categorised as (1). The data were analysed as a categorical variable.

vii. Coding Error Case with Incomplete Admission Form

Coding error case with complete admission form was categorised as (0) and coding error case with incomplete admission form was categorised as (1). The data was analysed as categorical variable.

viii. Coding Error Case with Incomplete Discharge Summary

Coding error case with complete discharge summary was categorised as (0) and coding error case incomplete admission was categorised as (1). The data was analysed as categorical variable.

IV RESULTS

4.1 Introduction

This chapter presents the results of this study, which is divided into two major parts namely, the incidence of clinical coding in UKMMC and the economic impact of coding errors towards UKMMC potential hospital revenue.

4.2 Profile of Patients

In 2013, the total admission of patients in UKMMC was 35,263 of which 35,089 (99.5%) were inpatient cases that were coded by in-house coders. Out of these coded inpatient cases, 19,859 (56.6%) of the cases were categorised medical case-type, 7,338 (20.9%) cases were from surgical case-type, 2,982 (8.5%) cases were from O&G case-type, and the remaining 263 (0.7%) cases were cases from paediatric case-type. In addition to this, in the year 2013, there were 4,647 (13.2%) ungroupable cases. Figure 4.1 represent the distributions of the coded cases by each case-type.

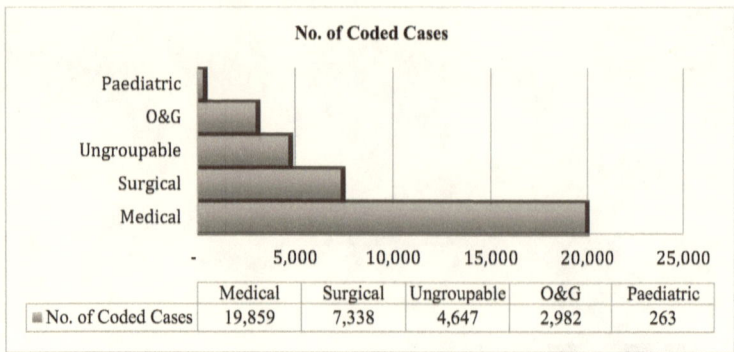

Figure 4.1 Distributions of Coded Case by Case-Type

From the 464 selected samples, 180 (38.8%) of the PMRs belong to male patients, and the remaining 284 (61.2%) of the PMRs belong to female patients. The mean age of the patient is 29 years old (SD: 24.1) with the minimum age being one day and maximum age being 89 years old. Figure 4.2 shows the distribution of the age for the samples.

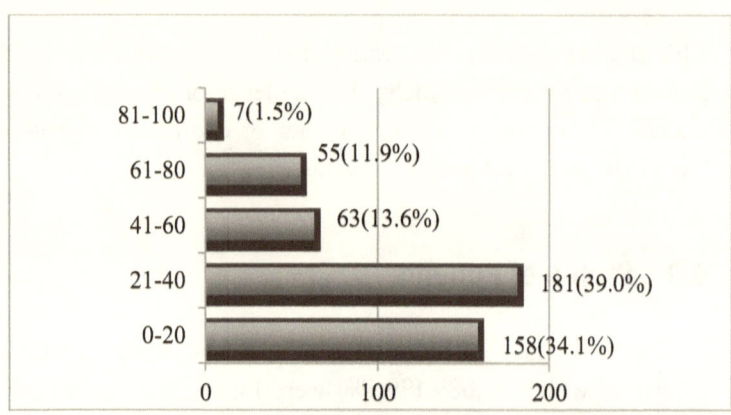

Figure 4.2 Distributions of Coded Cases by Age

The longest length of stay after the data trimming was 41 days. Meanwhile, the shortest length of stay was one day with the average mean of 4.3 days (SD: 3.7 days). From the selected sample, 297 (64.0%) of the cases were recorded as severity I cases, 124 (26.7%) of the cases were severity II cases, and 43 (9.3%) of the cases were severity III's cases.

The Figure 4.3 below shows the distribution of severity level for this selected data.

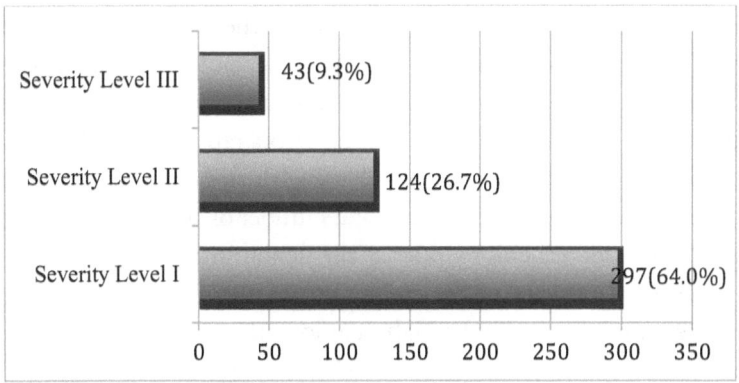

Figure 4.3 Distributions of Coded Cases by Severity Level

4.3 Coding Errors Rate in UKMMC

In this study, the 464 selected PMRs were reviewed and re-coded by the Independent Senior Coder. Before the re-coding process, all cases were assigned to the primary diagnosis code. From the 464 selected case, 349 (75.2%) of the cases were assigned to at least one secondary diagnosis code, 369 (79.5%) of the cases were assigned to primary procedure code and 235 (50.6%) of the cases were assigned to at least one secondary procedure code. After the re-coding process, the number of cases assigned to at least one secondary diagnosis code has increased to 421 (90.7%). Similarly, the number of cases assigned to primary procedure code has also increased to 451 (97.2%), and the number of cases assigned to at least one secondary procedure code has also shown a slight increment to 239 (51.5%) cases. In overall, data analysis from the present study revealed that 89.4% (415/464) of the selected PMR contained at least one error in the assignment of their diagnosis or their procedure code.

In this study, two level of coding errors calculation was imputed. At the first level of the coding errors calculation, the coding errors rate was based on the number coding error cases, which using the total number of the coding error cases as the numerator and the total number of case reviewed by the Independent Senior Coder as the denominator. On the other hand, at the second level of the coding errors calculation, the coding errors rate was based on the total number of error codes, which using the total number of error codes as the numerator and the total number of codes reviewed by the Independent Senior Coder as the denominator.

In the first level of the coding errors calculation, the coding errors were found to be the highest among the secondary diagnosis codes, which comprised 377 (81.3%) of error cases. The second highest number of coding error cases were recorded by secondary procedure codes covering 270 (58.2%) of the error cases. The third highest coding error cases were involved the primary procedure codes covering 236 (50.9%) of error cases. Among the coding items, primary diagnosis codes showed fewer error cases, covering 231 (49.8%) of error cases, respectively (Table 4.1).

As presented in Table 4.1, the level of agreement between the Independent Senior Coder and the in-house coder was higher in the assignment of the primary diagnosis code compared to the assignment of the primary procedure code (k= 0.495 vs k= 0.159). On the other hand, the level of agreement between the Independent Senior Coder and the in-house coder for the total number of codes assigned per patient is higher among secondary procedure code compared to secondary diagnosis code (k = 0.210 vs k = 0.108). Accordingly, from the four coding items, the only moderate agreement between the Independent Senior Coder and the in-house coder was for the assignment of the primary diagnosis code whereas the level of agreement for the other coding items was found to be fair or poor.

The data analysis from this study reveals that in the second level of coding errors calculation, the coding errors were the highest among secondary procedure codes where from 652 secondary procedure codes assigned in this study, 566 (86.8%) of the codes comprised of error codes. Coding errors among the secondary diagnosis codes were found to be the second highest in which out of 1,782 secondary procedure codes assigned in this study, 1,187 (66.6%) of the codes comprised of error codes. The third highest coding errors were found within the primary procedure codes whereby out of 451 primary procedure codes assigned in this study, 236 (52.3%) of the codes comprised of error codes. Lastly, assignment of the primary diagnosis codes showed fewer errors whereby out of 464 primary diagnosis code assigned in this study, only 231 (49.8%) of the codes comprised of error codes, respectively (Table 4.1). The different percentage of the errors in both levels of calculation were in respect to the different number of the denominator used in the first and second level of the calculation.

Table 4.1 Distribution of Coding Errors Rate

Coding Error Calculation	No. of Cases/ Codes Reviewed	No. of Errors (%)	Kappa Value	p Value
First Level of Calculation				
Primary Diagnosis	464	231 (49.8)	0.495	<0.001
Secondary Diagnosis	464	377 (81.3)	0.108	<0.001
Primary Procedure	464	236 (50.9)	0.159	<0.001
Secondary Procedure	464	270 (58.2)	0.210	<0.001
Second Level of Calculation				
Primary Diagnosis	464	231 (49.8)	N/A	N/A
Secondary Diagnosis	1,782	1,187 (66.6)	N/A	N/A
Primary Procedure	451	236 (52.3)	N/A	N/A
Secondary Procedure	652	566 (86.8)	N/A	N/A

4.3.1 Coding Errors in Primary Diagnosis Code

In the first level of coding errors calculation within the primary diagnosis codes, coding errors occurred in 231 (49.8%) of the selected cases. The second level of coding error calculation within the primary diagnosis codes also showed the same percentage of errors; 49.8% with respect to the similar total number of the denominator used in both level of calculations; n=464.

a. Type of Coding Errors among Primary Diagnosis Code

In the assignment of the primary diagnosis code, most of the codes were coded wrongly at the fourth digit level of the code, which comprised of 72 (15.5%) of the error cases. The second highest type of errors recorded are the errors that occur at the second digit level of the code, in which 47 (10.1%) of the cases contained this type of coding errors. The third highest type of coding errors are the errors at the third digit level of the code, covering 44 (9.5%) of the error cases. It is also apparent in Table 4.2 that the Independent Senior Coder has identified 40 (8.6%) of cases with a wrong selection of the primary diagnosis code. There were 26 (5.6%) cases with errors of primary diagnosis code which were incorrectly sequenced by the in-house coder, where they have assigned the appropriate primary diagnosis code as the secondary diagnosis code for the episode of care. In the assignment of the primary diagnosis code, the number of cases with an error at the fifth digit level of the code was the lowest; 2 (0.4%) error cases (Table 4.2).

Table 4.2 Type of Coding Errors Among Primary Diagnosis Code

Type of Errors	No. of Error Cases	%
Error at Fourth Digit Level	72	15.5
Error at Second Digit Level	47	10.1
Error at Third Digit Level	44	9.5
Wrong Selection of Primary Diagnosis Code	40	8.6
Primary Diagnosis Code Incorrectly Sequenced	26	5.6
Error at Fifth Digit Level	2	0.4

b. Examples of Errors Cases in the Assignment of Primary Diagnosis Codes

Table 4.3 shows two examples of cases with an error in the assignment of the primary diagnosis code. Case 1 was selected among the error cases without any changes in the assignment of the hospital tariff. In contrast, Case 2 was selected among error cases to demonstrate changes in the assignment of hospital tariff.

For Case 1, before the re-coding process by the Independent Senior Coder, this case was assigned to code K40.3 (Unilateral or unspecified inguinal hernia, with obstruction, without gangrene), but after the re-coding process, this case was re-assigned to code K43.0 (Ventral hernia with obstruction, without gangrene). The code assigned by the Independent Senior Coder and in-house coder showed discrepancies at the third digit level of the code. Besides that, error in the assignment of the primary diagnosis code also resulted in unnecessarily assigning of the code 88.19 (Other x-ray of abdomen) as its primary procedure code. However, despite the errors, the output of the re-grouping process using MY-DRG® grouper showed no changes in the assignment of MY-DRG® code for this case.

On the other hand, Case 2 is an example of a case with an error in the assignment of the primary diagnosis code, and this error has affected the assignment of the MY-DRG® code of this case. Before the re-coding process, code C73 (Malignant neoplasm of thyroid gland) was assigned as the primary diagnosis code for this case but, interestingly this code was listed as the secondary diagnosis code after the re-coding process by the Independent Senior Coder. The accurate primary diagnosis code was revealed as J39.8 (Other specified disease of upper respiratory tract). As seen in Table 4.3 beside the wrong sequence of the primary diagnosis code, this case also contained errors in the assignment of all the other coding items. For example, from the 4 secondary diagnosis codes assigned by the Independent Senior Coder, the in-house coder only assigned code Z51.1 (Radiotherapy session) as the secondary diagnosis code for this case. Also, the code 92.29 (Other radiotherapeutic procedure), which was listed by the Independent Senior Coder as the secondary procedure code for this case, was selected as the primary procedure code by the in-house coder. Subsequently, the combination of the errors identified in this case has affected the assignment of the MY-DRG® code. Before the audit, this case was assigned to MY-DRG® code E-4-13-I (Other disease of endocrine system - Mild) with the hospital tariff amounting to RM1, 758.78. After the audit, the case was re-assigned to MY-DRG® code U-4-13-II (Epiglottitis, upper respiratory tract infection laryngotracheitis & otitis media – Moderate) with the hospital tariff amounting to RM5,557.71. From the coding errors identified in this case, UKMMC could face a potential loss of revenue of RM3,798.93.

Table 4.3 Example of Error Cases Among Primary Diagnosis Code

	Before	After
Case 1		
MRN	M775165	M775165
Admission Date	08/09/13	08/08/09
Discharge Date	09/09/13	09/09/13
Primary Diagnosis Code	K40.3 (Unilateral or unspecified inguinal hernia, with obstruction, without gangrene)	K43.0 (Ventral hernia with obstruction, without gangrene)
Secondary Diagnosis Code	110 ([Essential] Hypertension), Z85.0 (Personal history of malignant neoplasm of digestive organs) 88.19 (Other x-ray of abdomen)	110 ([Essential] Hypertension), Z85.0 (Personal history of malignant neoplasm of digestive organs)
Primary Procedure Code	NIL	NIL
Secondary Procedure Code		NIL
MY-DRG Group	K-4-18-I (Other digestive system disorders –Mild)	K-4-18-I (Other digestive system disorders –Mild)

Hospital Tariff	RM1,380.38	RM1,380.38
Type of Error in Primary Diagnosis Code	Error at Third Digit Level	
Case 2		
MRN	N523935	N523935
Admission Date	14/11/13	15/11/13
Discharge Date	19/11/13	19/04/13
Primary Diagnosis Code	C73 (Malignant neoplasm of thyroid gland)	J39.8 (Other specified disease of upper respiratory tract)
Secondary Diagnosis Code	Z51.0 (Radiotherapy session),	R13 (Dysphagia), E89.2 (Postprocedural hypoparathyroidism), (Malignant neoplasm of thyroid gland), J38.0 (Paralysis of vocal cords and larynx), Z51.0 (Radiotherapy session)
Primary Procedure Code	92.29 (Other radiotherapeutic procedure)	22.5 (Other nasal sinusotomy)
Secondary Procedure Code	87.44 (Routine chest x-ray, so described)	43.23, (Other radiotherapeutic procedure), 93.75 (Other speech training and therapy), 92.29 (Other radiotherapeutic procedure)
MY-DRG Group	E-4-13-I (Other disease of endocrine system - Mild)	U-4-13-II (Epiglottitis, upper respiratory tract infection laryngotracheitis & otitis media – Moderate)
Hospital Tariff	RM1,758.	RM5,557.71
Type of Error	Primary Diagnosis Incorrectly Sequenced	

c. Top 10 Primary Diagnosis Codes Assigned Before and After the Re- Coding Process

Table 4.4 illustrates the top 10 primary diagnosis codes assigned in this study, both before and after the re-coding process by the Independent Senior Coder. As apparent in Table 4.4, due to the stratified sampling method employed in this study, the majority of the top 10 codes assigned before and after the re-coding process were among the Chapter 15 (Pregnancy, childbirth and the puerperium) and Chapter 16 (Certain conditions originating in the perinatal period) codes. As shown in Table 4.4, there was only one code, which was unrelated to Chapter 15 and 16 listed as one of the top 10 highly used primary diagnosis codes namely code H25.9 (Senile cataract, unspecified). The code H25.9 was the eight highest frequency a primary diagnosis codes before the audit. However after the re-coding process this code was unlisted as one of the highly assigned primary diagnosis code.

From Table 4.4, out of the 132 cases assigned to the top 10 primary diagnosis codes assigned before the re-coding process, 70 (53.0%) of the cases were assigned to a wrong primary diagnosis code. Subsequently, in comparison of the number of cases assigned to the primary diagnosis code before the re-coding process, the highest error rates were among cases assigned to code O68.9 (Labour and delivery complicated by fetal stress, unspecified) and H25.9 (Senile cataract, unspecified). All the cases that were assigned to code O68.8 (8 cases) and H25.9 (7 cases) before the re-coding process was assigned to a wrong primary diagnosis code resulting 100.0% of coding errors rate among these two codes. In contrast, the coding errors rate among twelve cases were assigned to code P22.1 (Transient tachypnoea of newborn) before the re-coding process was 0.0% as the primary diagnosis code for all the cases were assigned accurately by the in-house coder.

Another crucial outcome form Table 4.4 is the variation of the highest frequency of primary diagnosis code assigned before and after the re-coding process. The most assigned primary diagnosis code before the re-coding process was the code P59.9 (Neonatal jaundice, unspecified). On the other hand, the most assigned primary diagnosis code after the re-coding process was the code P59.8 (Neonatal jaundice from other specified causes). Both codes reflect that the highest volume of cases treated in paediatric cases was neonatal jaundice cases. However, the highest frequency code assigned after the audit was carried out by the Independent Senior Coder showed a more specific code whereby the cause of jaundice written in the medical record was identified by the Independent Senior Coder. Interestingly, although code P59.8 was the primary diagnosis code with the highest frequency of assignment after the re-coding, this code was not listed as the top 10 primary diagnosis codes with the highest frequency of assignment prior to the re-coding process by the Independent Senior Coder.

Table 4.4 Top 10 Primary Diagnosis Codes Assigned Before and After the Re-Coding Process

		Before Re-Coding Process				After Re-Coding Process		
		n = 464	n = *			n = 464	n = **	
No.	Primary Diagnosis Code	Description	n*(%)	No. of Cases with Coding Error (%)	Primary Diagnosis Code	Description	n**(%)	No. of Cases with Similar Primary Diagnosis Code as Before Re-Coding Process (%)
1.	P59.9	Neonatal jaundice unspecified	47 (10.1)	31 (66.0)	P59.8	Neonatal jaundice from other specific causes	28 (6.0)	0 (0.0)
2.	O70.0	First-degree perineal laceration during delivery	16 (3.4)	4 (25.0)	O70.0	First-degree perineal laceration during delivery	17 (3.7)	12 (70.6)
3.	O34.2	Maternal care due to uterine scar from previous surgery	12 (2.6)	6 (50.0)	P59.9	Neonatal jaundice unspecified	17 (3.7)	16 (94.1)
4.	P22.1	Transient tachypnoea of newborn	12 (2.6)	0 (0.0)	P22.1	Transient tachypnoea of newborn	14 (3.0)	12 (85.7)
5.	O68.9	Labour and delivery complicated by fetal stress, unspecified	8 (1.7)	8 (100.0)	O34.2	Maternal care due to uterine scar from previous surgery	11 (2.4)	6 (54.5)
6.	P23.9	Congenital pneumonia, unspecified	8 (1.7)	1 (12.5)	O36.3	Maternal care for signs of fetal hypoxia	10 (2.2)	0 (0.0)
7.	P36.9	Bacterial sepsis of newborn, unspecified	8 (1.7)	4 (50.0)	O80.0	Spontaneous vertex delivery	9 (1.9)	4 (44.4)
8.	H25.9	Senile cataract, unspecified	7 (1.5)	7 (100.0)	O32.1	Maternal care for breech presentation	7 (1.5)	6 (85.7)
9.	O80.0	Spontaneous vertex delivery	7 (1.5)	3 (42.9)	O75.7	Vaginal delivery following previous caesarean section	7 (1.5)	1 (14.3)
10.	O83.8	Other specified assisted single delivery	7 (1.5)	6 (85.7)	P23.9	Congenital pneumonia, unspecified	7 (1.5)	7 (100.0)

Kappa value = 0.495, p < 0.001

d. Changes in the Assignment of the Top 10 Primary Diagnosis Codes Due to Coding Errors

Data analysis from the descriptive study revealed that the 132 cases assigned to the top 10 diagnosis codes before the re-coding process consisted of 70 (53.0%) error cases. After the audit done by the Independent Senior Coder, these 70 error cases were re-assigned to other primary diagnosis codes. Table 4.5 shows the changes which occurred in the assignment of primary diagnosis codes of these 70 error cases.

The output from the data analysis revealed that all the cases that were assigned to the top 10 primary diagnosis codes before the re-coding process were assigned to an accurate first digit level of the code. This shows that the in-house coders are aware of the importance of the assignment of primary diagnosis code specifically on the assignment of the chapter of the code. However, from Table 4.5, it is visible that there was one case that was assigned to a wrong primary diagnosis code at the first digit level of the code indicating a wrong selection of the primary diagnosis code. The case was initially assigned by the in-house coder to code H25.9 (Senile cataract, unspecified) before the re-coding process and has re-assigned to code N20.0 (Calculus of kidney) after the re-coding process.

From Table 4.5, it is notable that the commonest type of errors identified among cases were assigned to the top 10 primary diagnosis codes prior to the re-coding process were the errors which occurred at the fourth digit level of the code. In total, there were 30 (42.9%) error cases which constituted errors at the fourth digit level of the code. Most of the error cases were involving the assignment of the code P59.9 (Neonatal jaundice unspecified). From the 47 (10.1%) cases assigned to code P59.9 as its primary diagnosis code before the re-coding process, 24 (51.1%) of the cases were assigned wrongly at the fourth digit level of the code. Specifically, 23 (48.9%) of the cases that were assigned to code P59.9 before the re-coding process were re-assigned to code P59.8

(Neonatal jaundice from other specified cause) after the re-coding process.

Data analysis also showed that the errors at the second digit level of the code were also prevalent among the cases that were assigned to the top 10 primary diagnosis codes before the re-coding process. In total there were 21 (30.0%) error cases which were identified with this type of errors, with the majority of the error cases involved the assignment of code O68.9 (Labour and delivery complicated by fetal stress, unspecified) as the primary diagnosis code. From Table 4.5, among the 8 cases that were assigned to code O68.9 before the re-coding process, 6 (75.0%) of the cases were re-assigned to code O36.3 (Maternal care for signs of fetal hypoxia) after the re-coding process.

To sum it up, cases that were assigned to the top 10 primary diagnosis codes assigned before the re-coding process were assigned to the accurate first digit level of the code. This implies a sufficient of coding skill in the assignment of primary diagnosis code among the in-house coders. However even though the in-house coder's performance in the assignment of the first digit level of the code is high, the attention towards the detail of the primary diagnosis is still lacking. This is proven with the common type of errors identified in Table 4.5 namely the fourth digit level of the code. The errors at the fourth digit level of the code indicating an erroneous interpretation of the specific condition of the patient such as the wrong selection of the cause of neonatal jaundice. Although commonly the error at the third and higher digit level of the primary diagnosis code does not affect the accuracy of the MY-DRG® code, it still affects the statistics of the morbidity in the hospital.

Table 4.5 Changes in the Assignment of Top 10 Primary Diagnosis Code Before the Re-Coding Process due to Coding Errors

No.	Before Re-Coding (n = 464)		After Re-Coding			
	Original Primary Diagnosis Code	No. of Cases (%)	No. of Cases with Unchanged Primary Diagnosis Code (%)	Cases With New Primary Diagnosis Code due to Coding Error		
				New Primary Diagnosis Code	Description	No. Cases(%)
1.	P59.9 (Neonatal jaundice, unspecified)	47 (10.1)	16 (34.0)	P59.8	Neonatal jaundice from other specified causes	23 (48.9)
				P55.1	ABO isoimmunization of fetus and newborn	2 (4.3)
				P58.4	Neonatal jaundice due to drugs or toxins transmitted from mother or given to newborn	2 (4.3)
				P58.8	Neonatal jaundice due to other specified excessive haemolysis	1 (2.1)
				P58.2	Neonatal jaundice due to infection	1 (2.1)
				P59.3	Neonatal jaundice from breast milk inhibitor	1 (2.1)
				P92.0	Vomiting in newborn	1 (2.1)
2.	O70.0 (First-degree perineal laceration during delivery)	16 (3.4)	12 (75.0)	O34.2	Maternal care due to uterine scar from previous surgery	1 (6.3)
				O42.0	Premature rupture of membranes, onset of labour within 24 hours	1 (6.3)
				O70.1	Second degree perineal laceration during delivery	1 (6.3)
				O70.9	Perineal laceration during delivery, unspecified	1 (6.3)
3.	O34.2 (Maternal care due to uterine scar from previous surgery)	12 (2.6)	6 (50.0)	O75.7	Vaginal delivery following previous caesarean section	2 (16.7)
				O14.1	Severe pre-eclampsia	1 (8.3)
				O32.1	Maternal care for breech presentation	1 (8.3)

#	Diagnosis	n (%)	Code	Sub-diagnosis	n (%)
4.	P22.1 (Transient tachypnoea of newborn)	12 (2.6)	0 (0.0)	O36.3	Maternal care for signs of fetal hypoxia	1 (8.3)
				O99.8	Other specified diseases and conditions complicating pregnancy, childbirth and the puerperium	1 (8.3)
5.	O68.9 (Labour and delivery complicated by fetal stress, unspecified)	8 (1.7)	0 (0.0)	NIL	NIL	NIL
				O36.3	Maternal care for signs of fetal hypoxia	6 (75.0)
				O68.1	Labour and delivery complicated by meconium in amniotic fluid	1 (12.5)
				O68.8	Labour and delivery complicated by other evidence of fetal stress	1 (12.5)
6.	P23.9 (Congenital pneumonia, unspecified)	8 (1.7)	7 (87.5)	P23.3	Congenital pneumonia due to streptococcus, group B	1 (12.5)
7.	P36.9 (Bacterial sepsis of newborn, unspecified)	8 (1.7)	4 (50.0)	P12.2	Epicranial subaponeurotic haemorrhage due to birth injury	1 (12.5)
				P22.1	Transient tachypnoea of newborn	1 (12.5)
				P70.4	Other neonatal hypoglycaemia	1 (12.5)
				P81.8	Other specified disturbances of temperature regulation of newborn	1 (12.5)
8.	H25.9 (Senile cataract, unspecified)	7 (1.5)	0 (0)	H26.9	Cataract, unspecified	4 (57.1)
				H28.0	Diabetic cataract	2 (28.6)
				N20.0	Calculus of kidney	1 (14.3)
9.	O80.0 (Spontaneous vertex delivery)	7 (1.5)	4 (57.1)	O75.7	Vaginal delivery following previous caesarean section	2 (28.6)
				O70.0	First degree perineal laceration during delivery	1 (14.3)
10.	O83.8 (Other specified assisted delivery)	7 (1.5)	1 (14.3)	O80.0	Single spontaneous delivery	4 (57.1)
				O24.1	Diabetes mellitus in pregnancy: Pre-existing diabetes mellitus, non-insulin-dependent	1 (14.3)
				O42.1	Premature rupture of membranes, onset of labour after 24 hours	1 (14.3)

4.3.2 Coding Errors of Secondary Diagnosis Code

In the first level of coding error calculation within the secondary diagnosis codes, coding errors occurred in 377 (81.3%) of the selected cases. In total, there were 1,782 codes reviewed by the Independent Senior Coder during the re-coding process. From these 1,782 codes, 1,187 (66.6%) of the codes were the error codes.

Before the re-coding process, the total numbers of codes assigned as secondary diagnosis code were 1,049 codes and had grossly increased to 1,740 codes after the re-coding process. This shows that the in-house coders missed around 691 secondary diagnosis or 65.8% of the secondary diagnosis. The cases were grossly under-coded by the in-house coder. Before the audit, the maximum number of code assigned per patient was 10 with the mean of 2.27 (SD: 2.07). The maximum number of code assigned per patient has also increased dramatically to 18 with the mean of 3.75 (SD: 2.97). The level of agreement between the Independent Senior Coder and in-house coder on the number of secondary diagnosis code assigned per patient was tested using Cohen's Kappa test, and the result showed a poor agreement with the kappa value of 0.108 (Table 4.6).

Table 4.6 Distributions of the Number of Secondary Diagnosis Codes Assigned Before and After the Re-Coding Process

No. of Secondary Diagnosis Code	Before	After	Kappa value	p value
			0.108	<0.001
Total No. of Code	1,049	1,740		
Max. Codes	10	18		
Mean (SD)	2.27 (2.07)	3.75 (2.97)		

a. **Comparison of Number of Secondary Diagnosis Code Before and After the Re-Coding Process**

Before the re-coding process by the Independent Senior Coder, there were 115 (24.8%) cases unassigned to any secondary diagnosis codes. Interestingly, after the audit, from these 115 cases, 76 (66.1%) of the cases were assigned to at least one secondary diagnosis code, and the remaining 39 (33.9%) of the cases remained without any secondary diagnosis code after the audit. However, as apparent in Table 4.7, after the re-coding process, besides these 39 cases, there were additional 4 cases that were unassigned to secondary diagnosis code. Apparently, before the re-coding process, these 4 cases were being up-coded by the in-house coder with irrelevant secondary diagnosis codes.

The original database before the re-coding process showed the highest number of secondary diagnosis code was 10 codes per patient. As shown in Table 4.8, there were 2 (0.4%) cases that were assigned to 10 secondary diagnosis codes before the audit. Subsequently, data analysis after the re-coding process revealed that from these 2 cases, only 1 (50.0%) case remained assigned to the similar number of secondary diagnosis code. On the other hand, the remaining 1 (50.0%) case was re-assigned to a higher number of secondary diagnosis codes after the re-coding process by the Independent Senior Coder. In addition, from Table 4.8, it is also notable that after the re-coding process, the number of cases containing 10 secondary diagnosis codes has increased to 9 (1.9%) cases. Interestingly, from these 9 cases, 8 (88.9%) of the cases were initially assigned to a lower number of secondary diagnosis codes before the commencement of this study.

After the evaluation by the Independent Senior Coder, the number of cases that were assigned to more than 10 secondary diagnosis codes has increased significantly. In total, the Independent Senior Coder has assigned 13 (2.8%) cases with more than 10 secondary diagnosis codes. The highest number of secondary diagnosis code assigned after the re-coding process was 18 codes with the total number of case assigned to 18 secondary diagnosis codes was 1 (0.2%) case.

In this study, a bivariate analysis using chi-square test was conducted to determine the association between the number of secondary diagnosis codes and coding errors. The association between the number of the secondary diagnosis code and coding error was proven to be statistically significant with a chi-square value of X^2 (4) = 15.191, p=0.003 (Table 4.9). This table shows that the highest coding errors (98.1%) were recorded in cases with four and above secondary diagnoses and followed by those with three secondary diagnoses (92.1%). These findings reflect that in-house coders were more likely to have difficulty to code cases with a higher number of the secondary diagnoses.

Table 4.7 Number of Secondary Diagnosis Codes Assigned Per Patient Before and After the Re-Coding Process

	Before Re-Coding					After Re-Coding			
	n = 464		n = *			n = 464	n = **		
No.	No. of Secondary Diagnosis Code	No. of Cases (%)*	No. of Cases with Similar No of Secondary Diagnosis Code After Re-Coding (%)	No. of Cases With Lower No of Secondary Diagnosis Code After Re-Coding (%)	No. of Cases With Higher No of Secondary Diagnosis Code After Re-Coding (%)	No. of Secondary Diagnosis Code	No. of Cases (%)**	No. of Cases with Similar No of Secondary Diagnosis Code After Re-Coding (%)	No. of Cases With Lower No of Secondary Diagnosis Code Before Re-Coding (%)	No. of Cases With Higher No of Secondary Diagnosis Code Before Re-Coding (%)
1.	0	115 (24.8)	39 (34.0)	0 (0.0)	76 (66.1)	0	43 (9.3)	39 (90.7)	0 (0.0)	4 (9.3)
2.	1	78 (16.8)	27 (34.6)	4 (5.1)	47 (60.3)	1	66 (14.2)	27 (40.9)	23 (34.8)	16 (24.2)
3.	2	87 (18.8)	21 (24.1)	6 (6.9)	60 (69.0)	2	72 (15.5)	21 (29.2)	41 (56.9)	10 (13.9)
4.	3	77 (16.6)	18 (23.4)	13 (16.9)	46 (59.7)	3	70 (15.1)	18 (25.7)	45 (64.3)	7 (10.0)
5.	4	43 (9.3)	9 (21.0)	7 (16.3)	27 (37.0)	4	65 (14.0)	9 (13.8)	47 (67.1)	9 (13.8)
6.	5	28 (9.3)	5 (17.9)	6 (21.4)	17 (60.7)	5	46 (9.9)	5 (10.9)	38 (58.5)	3 (6.5)
7.	6	16 (3.4)	1 (6.3)	10 (62.5)	5 (31.3)	6	29 (6.3)	1 (3.4)	26 (89.7)	2 (6.9)
8.	7	9 (1.9)	1 (11.1)	2 (22.2)	6 (66.7)	7	22 (4.7)	1 (4.5)	20 (90.9)	1 (4.5)
9.	8	6 (1.3)	1 (16.7)	3 (50.0)	2 (33.3)	8	16 (3.4)	1 (6.3)	15 (93.8)	0 (0.0)
10.	9	3 (0.6)	0 (0.0)	1 (33.3)	2 (66.7)	9	14 (3.0)	0 (0.0)	14 (100.0)	0 (0.0)
11.	10	2 (0.4)	1 (50.0)	0 (0.0)	1 (50.0)	10	9 (1.9)	1 (11.1)	8 (88.9)	0 (0.0)
12.	NIL	NIL	NIL	NIL	NIL	11 and more	13 (2.8)	0 (0.0)	13 (100.0)	0 (0.0)

Table 4.8 Distributions of Error Cases by Number of Secondary Diagnosis Code

No. of Secondary Diagnosis Code	Non Error Case	%	Error Case	%	Total	%
0	21	18.3	94	81.7	115	100
1	9	11.5	69	88.5	78	100
2	12	13.8	75	88.0	87	100
3	6	7.9	71	92.1	77	100
4 and above	2	1.9	105	98.1	107	100

$X^2 = 15.905$, df =4, p =0.003

b. Type of Coding Errors of Secondary Diagnosis Codes

Data analysis in the present study showed that the commonest type of errors in the assignment of secondary diagnosis code was under-coding. From the 1,782 secondary diagnosis codes reviewed by the Independent Senior Coder, 746 (41.9%) of the secondary diagnosis phrases were missed and not coded by the in-house coder. The second highest type of errors was the error at the second digit level in which in total there were 105 (5.9%) cases with this type of error. Coding error at the fourth digit level of the code was the third highest type of errors of which 104 (5.8%) cases were due to this type of coding errors. In the assignment of the secondary diagnosis code, the less common type of errors was the error at the fifth digit level of the code. There were only 2 (0.1%) cases reported with this type of error. Table 4.9 illustrates the type of coding errors which occurred in the assignment of the secondary diagnosis code.

Table 4.9 Type of Coding Errors of Secondary Diagnosis Code

Type of Errors	Nos of Error Cases	%
Under-coding	746	41.9
Error at Second Digit Level	105	5.9
Error at Fourth Digit Level	104	5.8
Wrong Selection of Secondary Diagnosis Code	93	5.2

Error at Third Digit Level	87	4.9
Up-coding	50	2.8
Error at Fifth Digit Level	2	0.1

c. Examples of Error Cases of Secondary Diagnosis Codes

Table 4.10 shows two examples of cases with an error in the assignment of secondary diagnosis code. Case 1 was selected among error cases without changes in the assignment of hospital tariff. In contrast, Case 2 was selected among error cases to demonstrate changes in the assignment of hospital tariff.

Case 1 is an example of the undercoding case. As apparent in Table 4.10, this case was assigned to an accurate primary diagnosis code (K35.8) and primary procedure code (47.09). After the re-coding process, the Independent Senior Coder has listed code J45.9 as the accurate secondary diagnosis code for this case. However, the accurate secondary diagnosis for this case was missed and not coded by the in-house coder. Even though there was undercoded code identified in this case, the code missed by the in-house coder does not reflect the accuracy of the MY-DRG® code. After the re-grouping, the MY-DRG® (K-1-13-1) code for this case was unchanged with the hospital tariff amounting to RM3,169.67.

On the other hand, Case 2 consisted of two types of errors in the assignment of its secondary diagnosis code namely, the error at the fourth digit level and undercoding. Likewise to Case 1, the primary diagnosis code and the primary procedure code for Case 2 was assigned accurately by the in-house coder. However, there were several issues in the assignment of its secondary diagnosis code. Firstly the number of secondary diagnosis code for this case has increased from 3 codes to 5. This indicates that there were two codes that were not coded by the in-house coder namely code E14.9 and Z86.3. Besides this error, there was one code that was wrongly assigned at the fourth digit level. According to the examination of the medical record, the accurate secondary diagnosis code listed by the independent senior coder was E78.8 but was codified as E78.5

by the in-house coder. Other than these codes, the remaining two codes namely I10 and E78.0 were codified accurately by the in-house coder. Although after the re-grouping process this case was assigned to the similar MY-DRG® group as before the re-coding process (L-1-50), the severity level of this case has increased from I (Mild) to II (Moderate). The increment of the severity level has subsequently led to the increment in the assignment of hospital tariff from RM4,529.91 to RM 11,278.66.

Table 4.10 Examples of Coding Errors Cases of Secondary Diagnosis Code

	Before	After
Case 1		
MRN	N194800	N194800
Admission Date	24/04/13	24/04/13
Discharge Date	26/04/13	26/04/13
Primary Diagnosis Code	K35.8 (Acute appendicitis, other and unspecified)	K35.8 (Acute appendicitis, other and unspecified)
Secondary Diagnosis Code	NIL	J45.9 (Asthma, unspecified)
Primary Procedure Code	47.09 (Other appendectomy)	47.09 (Other appendectomy)
Secondary Procedure Code	NIL	NIL
MY-DRG Group	K-1-13-I (Appendix Operation - Mild)	K-1-13-I (Appendix Operation - Mild)
Hospital Tariff	RM3,169.67	RM3,169.67
Type of Error in Secondary Diagnosis Code	Under-coding	
Case 2		
MRN	M788388	M788388
Admission Date	11/07/13	11/07/13
Discharge Date	12/07/13	12/07/13

Primary Diagnosis Code	D24 (Benign neoplasm of breast)	D24 (Benign neoplasm of breast)
Secondary Diagnosis Code	I10 ([Essential] Hypertension), E78.5 (Hyperlipidaemia, unspecified), E78.0 (Pure hypercholesterolaemia)	I10 ([Essential] Hypertension), E14.9 (Unspecified diabetes mellitus unspecified), E78.8 (Other disorder of lipoprotein metabolism), E78.0 (Pure hypercholesterolaemia), Z86.3 (Personal history of endocrine, nutritional and metabolic disease)
Primary Procedure Code	85.21 (Local excision of lesion of breast)	85.21 (Local excision of lesion of breast)
Secondary Procedure Code	NIL	NIL
MY-DRG Group	L-1-50-I (Breast operation – Mild)	L-1-50-II (Breast operation – Medium)
Hospital Tariff	RM4,529.91	RM11,278.66
Type of Error in Secondary Diagnosis Code	Error at fourth digit level, under-coding	

d. Top 10 Secondary Diagnosis Codes Assigned Before and After the Re-Coding Process

Table 4.11 shows the top 10 secondary diagnosis codes assigned before and after the re-coding process. It is notable that the most used secondary diagnosis code was similar both for before and after the re-coding process namely, code Z37.0 (Single live birth). The number of cases assigned to code Z37.0 was almost similar before and after the re-coding process with only 5 cases higher after the re-coding process (123 vs 118). It is also apparent in Table 4.11 that majority of the codes that were listed as the top 10 secondary diagnosis codes assigned before and after the re-coding process were among codes that are related to Chapter 15 (Pregnancy, childbirth and the puerperium) and Chapter 16 (Certain conditions originating in the perinatal period). Before the re-coding process, there were 3 (30.0%) listed codes that were unrelated to Chapter 15 and Chapter 16 namely codes I10 ([Essential] Hypertension), E11.9 (Type 2 diabetes mellitus without complication) and E78.5 (Hyperlipidaemia, unspecified). On the other hand, after the re-coding process, there were only 2 (20.0%) listed codes that were unrelated to Chapter 15 and Chapter 16, namely codes I10 and E11.9.

It is notable in Table 4.11 that from the 368 cases that were assigned to the top 10 secondary diagnosis codes before the re-coding process, 348 (94.6%) of the cases were assigned to at least one error secondary diagnosis codes in it. The highest coding errors rate in comparisons to the number of cases assigned to the code was among cases that contained code E78.5 (Hyperlipidaemia, unspecified), O24.4 (Diabetes mellitus arising in pregnancy) and O83.8 (Other specified assisted single delivery) as its secondary diagnosis code. All the cases that were assigned to these three codes as the secondary diagnosis codes were codified with at least one errors secondary diagnosis codes in it causing an errors rate of 100.0%. Interestingly, after the re-coding process, these three codes were unlisted as the top highest assigned secondary diagnosis codes.

Among the top 10 secondary diagnosis codes assigned after the re-coding process, the highest errors rate involves cases that were assigned to code Z87.5 (Personal history of complications of pregnancy, childbirth and the puerperium) and O70.0 (First degree perineal laceration during delivery). From Table 4.11, it is notable that none of the cases that contained either one of these codes as their secondary diagnosis code were codified correctly by the in-house coder. On the other hand, the lowest errors rate in the assignment of secondary diagnosis codes among the top 10 secondary diagnosis codes after the re-coding process were involving cases that were assigned to code P59.9. In total, after the re-coding process, there were 39 (2.2%) cases containing code P59.9 as its secondary diagnosis codes. Subsequently, among these

39 cases, 29 (74.4%) of the cases contained at least one wrong secondary diagnosis code before the re-coding process.

Another striking finding from Table 4.11 is involving the number of cases assigned to these top 10 highest frequency secondary diagnosis codes. The total number listed in the table has increased dramatically from 368 cases before the re-coding process to 534 cases after the audit. This increasing number of cases after the audit reflects the commonest type of errors in the assignment of the secondary diagnosis code, namely under-coding. This finding reflects that the in-house coder were more likely to miss the secondary diagnoses in most significant number of cases.

4.3.3 Coding Errors of Primary Procedure Code

Data analysis from the present study indicates an increment in the number of cases assigned to primary procedure code. Prior the re-coding process, there were 369 cases contained primary procedure code during their episode of care. Subsequently the re-coding process the number of cases with primary procedure code has increased to 451 cases.

In the first level of coding error calculation, 236 (50.9%) of cases were found to contain errors in the assignment of its primary procedure codes. In total, there were 451 codes reviewed by the Independent Senior Coder during the re-coding process. From these 451 codes, 236 (52.3%) of the codes were the error codes.

Table 4.11 Distributions of Top 10 Secondary Diagnosis Codes Assigned Before and After the Re-Coding Process

		Before Re-Coding Process				After Re-Coding Process			
		n = 1049	n = *			n = 1740	n = **		
No.	Codes	Description	Frequency (%)*	No. of Error Cases (%)	Codes	Description	Frequency (%)**	No. of Cases Without Coding Errors (%)
1.	Z37.0	Single live birth	123 (11.7)	117 (95.1)	Z37.0	Single live birth	118 (6.8)	6 (5.1)
2.	I10	Essential [primary] hypertension	51 (4.9)	45 (88.2)	I10	Essential [primary] hypertension	55 (3.2)	6 (10.9)
3.	E11.9	Type 2 diabetes mellitus without complications	38 (3.6)	35 (92.1)	O80.0	Spontaneous vertex delivery	54 (3.1)	2 (3.7)
4.	O82.1	Delivery by emergency caesarean section	38 (3.6)	36 (94.7)	O82.1	Delivery by emergency caesarean section	40 (2.3)	1 (2.5)
5.	E78.5	Hyperlipidaemia, unspecified	22 (2.1)	22 (100.0)	P59.9	Neonatal jaundice, unspecified	39 (2.2)	10 (25.6)
6.	P59.9	Neonatal jaundice, unspecified	22 (2.1)	21 (95.5)	E11.9	Type 2 diabetes mellitus without complications	30 (1.7)	1 (3.3)
7.	O80.0	Spontaneous vertex delivery	21 (2.0)	20 (95.2)	P59.8	Neonatal jaundice from other specified causes	30 (1.7)	1 (3.3)
8.	O24.4	Diabetes mellitus arising in pregnancy	19 (1.8)	19 (100.0)	Z87.5	Personal history of complications of pregnancy, childbirth and the puerperium	26 (1.5)	0 (0.0)
9.	O83.8	Other specified assisted single delivery	18 (1.7)	18 (100.0)	O34.2	Maternal care due to uterine scar from previous surgery	25 (1.4)	1 (4.0)
10.	P92.9	Feeding problem of newborn, unspecified	16 (1.5)	15 (93.8)	O70.0	First Degree Perineal Laceration during Delivery	23 (5.0)	0 (0.0)

a. Type of Coding Errors among Primary Procedure Codes

In the assignment of the primary procedure code, quite frequently the in-house coders did not detect the primary procedures which lead to under-coding of 80 (17.7%). The second highest type of errors was the wrong selection of primary procedure code covering 75 (16.6%) of the error cases. The third highest type of coding errors was due to the up-coding covering 33 (7.3%) of the error cases. The fourth highest type of errors was an error at the second digit level of the code with 30 (6.7%) number of error cases. The error at the fourth digit level of the code was the fifth highest comprising 20 (4.4%) of the error cases. Following this, 19 (4.2%) of the error cases were due to the wrong assignment of the code at the third digit of the code. The less common type of errors found in the assignment of primary procedure code was due to the incorrect sequence of the primary procedure code whereby 17 (3.8%) cases were with this type of coding errors, respectively. Table 4.12 shows the distributions of the type of coding errors occurred within the assignment of primary procedure codes.

Table 4.12 Distributions of the Type of Coding Errors within Primary Procedure Codes

Type of Error	No. of Error Cases	%
Under-coding	80	17.7
Wrong Selection of Primary Procedure Code	75	16.6
Up-coding	33	7.3
Error at Second Digit Level	30	6.7
Error at Fourth Digit Level	20	4.4
Error at Third Digit Level	19	4.2
Principal Procedure Incorrectly Sequenced	17	3.8

b. Examples of Error Cases in the Assignment of Primary Procedure Codes

Table 4.13 shows two examples of cases with an error in the assignment of primary procedure code. Case 1 was selected among error cases without changes in the assignment of hospital tariff. In contrast, Case 2 was selected among error cases to demonstrate changes in the assignment of hospital tariff.

In Case 1, the primary procedure code was not coded by the in-house coder causing the issue of under-coding. This case was assigned to the accurate primary diagnosis code namely P59.9 (Neonatal jaundice, unspecified). Both coders agreed that the assignment of the secondary diagnosis code was unnecessary for this case. However, the Independent Senior Coder has listed code 99.83 (Other phototherapy) as the primary procedure code for this case whereas there was no procedure code listed by the in-house coder for this case. Although there was a coding error issue, in this case, the error unaffected the assignment of MY-DRG® code (P-8-17-I) before and after the re-coding process.

Table 4.13 Examples of Error Cases in the Assignment of Primary Procedure Codes

	Before	After
Case 1		
MRN	N527770	N527770
Admission Date	10/09/13	10/09/13
Discharge Date	11/09/13	11/09/13
Primary Diagnosis Code	P59.9 (Neonatal jaundice, unspecified)	P59.9 (Neonatal jaundice, unspecified)
Secondary Diagnosis Code	NIL	NIL
Primary Procedure Code	NIL	99.83 (Other phototherapy)
Secondary Procedure Code	NIL	NIL
MY-DRG Group	P-8-17-I (Neonate, birthweight more than 2499 grams without complex operation)	P-8-17-I (Neonate, birthweight more than 2499 grams without complex operation)

Hospital Tariff	RM1,412.48	RM1,412.48
Type of Error in Primary Procedure Code	Under-coding	
Case 2		
MRN	M479783	M479783
Admission Date	25/04/13	25/04/13
Discharge Date	02/05/13	02/05/13
Primary Diagnosis Code	S82.81 (Torus fracture of upper end of fibula)	S82.81 (Torus fracture of upper end of fibula)
Secondary Diagnosis Code	T13.1 (Open wound of lower limb, level unspecified), E11.9 (Non-insulin diabetes mellitus without complication), I10 ([Essential] hypertension), L40.9 (Psoriasis, unspecified), E78.5 (Hyperlipidaemia, unspecified),	S91.10 (Unspecified open wound of toe without damage to nail), I10 ([Essential] hypertension), E11.9 (Non insulin diabetes mellitus without complication), E78.8 (Other inappropriate of lipoprotein metabolism), L40.9 (Psoriasis, unspecified),
Primary Procedure Code	79.1 (Closed reduction of fracture with internal fixation)	93.44 (Other skeletal traction)
Secondary Procedure Code	87.44 (Routine chest x-ray, so described), 86.22 (Excisional debridement of wound, infection or burn)	86.28 (Non-excisional debridement of wound, infection or burn)
MY-DRG Group	M-1-60-I (Other operation of musculoskeletal system & connective tissue –Minor)	M-4-12-II (Fracture or dislocation excluding femur & pelvis – Moderate)
Hospital Tariff	RM4,877.96	RM4,099.83
Type of Error in Primary Procedure Code	Wrong selection of Primary Procedure Code	

On the other hand, Case 2 is an example of error case where the in-house coder wrongly selected the primary procedure code. Before the re-coding process, this case was assigned to code 79.1 (Close reduction of fracture with internal fixation). However, after the re-coding process, the Independent Senior Coder has assigned code 93.44 (Other skeletal traction) as the accurate primary procedure code for this case. In addition to this error, there were also two other errors in the assignment of the secondary diagnosis code namely, error at fourth digit level (E78.5 [wrong code, E78.8 [accurate code]) and a wrong selection of secondary diagnosis code (T13.1 [wrong code], S91.10 [accurate code]). Despite the errors in the assignment of primary procedure code and secondary diagnosis code, this case was assigned to the accurate primary diagnosis code. The errors identified in this case specifically in the assignment of primary procedure code have affected the assignment of the case-type of the code. Before the re-coding process, due to the assignment of code 79.1, this case was assigned to a surgical case with the MY-DRG® code M-1-60-I. However, after the re-coding process, the accurate MY-DRG® code identified for this case was M-4-12-II. Although the severity of this case increased from severity I (mild) to severity II (moderate), the amount of hospital tariff has decreased from RM 4,877.96 to RM 4,099.83. The decreased in the tariff was due to the change in the type of the case from surgical case to medical case.

c. **Top 10 Primary Procedure Code Assigned Before and After the Re-Coding Process**

The findings of this study revealed that the disparity in the assignment of primary procedure code is higher than the assignment of primary diagnosis code (k=0.159 vs k =.0.495). Table 4.14 shows the top 10 primary procedure codes assigned to a patient before and after the re-coding process. As can be seen in the table, codes 74.1 (Low cervical caesarean section), 99.83 (Other phototherapy), 87.44 (Routine chest x-ray, so described), 99.25 (Injection or infusion of cancer chemotherapeutic substance) and 87.03 (Computerized axial tomography of head) were among the highest frequency of primary procedure codes that were assigned before and after the re-coding process. It is also apparent in Table 4.14 that, from the 205 cases assigned to the top 10 primary procedure codes before the re-coding process, 158 (77.1%)

of the cases were assigned to wrong primary procedure codes by the in-house coders.

From Table 4.14, it is notable that before the re-coding process, the highest coding errors rate was involving cases containing code 93.9 (Respiratory therapy), 89.52 (Electrocardiogram) and 87.03 (Computerized axial tomography of head) as its primary procedure code. Observation from the data analysis revealed that all of the cases that were assigned to these two codes were assigned to a wrong procedure code. For this reason, codes 93.9 and 89.52 were unlisted as the top 10 highest frequency primary procedure codes after the re-coding process. On the contrary, before the re-coding process, among the top 10 primary procedure codes, the lowest coding errors rate involved the assignment of code 99.83 (Other phototherapy). From 33 (8.9%) cases that were assigned to code 99.83 as their primary procedure code before the re-coding process, only 16 (48.5%) of the cases were assigned with a wrong primary procedure code.

On the other hand, among the top 10 primary procedure codes after the re-coding process, the coding errors rate was the highest among the assignment of code 88.38 (Other computerized axial tomography), 88.72 (Diagnostic ultrasound of heart) and 87.03 (Computerized axial tomography of head). As apparent in Table 4.12, none of the cases that were assigned to code 88.38, 88.72 and 87.03 was assigned with the similar primary procedure code as before the re-coding process. In comparison with the number of case assigned to the code, the lowest coding errors rate among the top 10 primary procedure codes assigned after the re-coding process was involving the assignment of code 74.1. From the 57 (13.7%) cases that were assigned to code 74.1 as its primary procedure code after the re-coding process, 35 (61.4%) of the cases were assigned to a wrong primary procedure code before the re-coding process.

Table 4.14 Top 10 Code Assigned as Primary Procedure Code Before and After the Re-Coding Process

	Before Re-Coding Process				After Re-Coding Process		
		n = 369	n =*			n =417	n =**
No.	Primary Procedure Code	Description	n* (%)	No. of Cases with Coding Error (%)	Primary Procedure Code	Description	n** (%)	No. of Cases with Similar Primary Diagnosis Code Before Audit (%)
1.	74.1	Low cervical caesarean section	55 (14.9)	33 (60.0)	99.83	Other phototherapy	69 (16.5)	17 (24.6)
2.	99.83	Other phototherapy	33 (8.9)	16 (48.5)	74.1	Low cervical caesarean section	57 (13.7)	22 (38.6)
3.	87.44	Routine chest x-ray, so described	29 (7.9)	27 (93.1)	88.38	Other computerized axial tomography	29 (7.0)	0 (0.0)
4.	75.69	Repair of other current obstetric laceration	25 (6.8)	22 (88.0)	75.69	Repair of other current obstetric laceration	19 (4.6)	3 (15.8)
5.	73.6	Episiotomy	20 (5.4)	19 (95.0)	87.44	Routine chest x-ray, so described	13 (3.1)	2 (15.4)
6.	93.9	Respiratory therapy	11 (3.0)	11 (100.0)	88.72	Diagnostic ultrasound of heart	9 (2.2)	1 (11.1)
7.	89.52	Electrocardiogram	9 (2.4)	9 (100.0)	72.7	Vacuum extraction	8 (1.9)	0 (0.0)
8.	69.02	Dilation and curettage following delivery or abortion	8 (2.2)	7 (87.5)	87.03	Computerized axial tomography of head	8 (1.9)	0 (0.0)
9.	99.25	Injection or infusion of cancer chemotherapeutic substance	8 (2.2)	7 (87.5)	13.41	Phacoemulsification and aspiration of cataract	7 (1.7)	2 (28.6)
10.	87.03	Computerized axial tomography of head	7 (1.9)	7 (100.0)	99.25	Injection or infusion of cancer chemotherapeutic substance	7 (1.7)	1 (14.3)

Kappa value = 0.159, $p < 0.001$

To sum it up, the agreement between Independent Senior Coder and the in-house coder in the assignment of primary procedure code was poor. The bivariate analysis using the Cohen Kappa Test showed a kappa value of 0.159 indicating a poor agreement between both of the coders in the assignment of primary procedure code. Moreover, the number of cases that were listed as the top 10 codes showed a slight increment from 205 cases before the re-coding process to 226 cases after the re-coding process. The increasing pattern of the cases in Table 4.14 before and after the audit is linked to the commonest type of coding errors in the assignment of primary procedure code namely undercoding.

d. Changes in Top 10 Primary Procedure Codes Due to Coding Errors

Table 4.15 shows the changes occurred among the top 10 primary procedure codes after the re-coding process by the Independent Senior Coder. From the 205 cases assigned to the top 10 primary procedure codes, 158 (77.1%) of the cases were assigned to a wrong primary procedure code by the in-house coder.

As apparent in the table, among the cases that were assigned to the top 10 primary procedure codes before this study, none of the cases were codified with a wrong primary procedure code at the fourth digit level of the code. The commonest type of errors among the cases that were assigned to these top 10 primary procedure codes before the re-coding process was a wrong selection of primary procedure code indicating errors at the first digit level of the code. The number of error cases with a wrong selection of primary procedure code was 78 (49.4%) cases. Most of these 78 error cases were wrongly assigned to code 87.44 (Routine chest x-ray, so described) before the audit. As shown in Table 4.15, mostly the assignment of primary procedure code was unnecessary among the cases that were assigned to code 87.44 before the re-coding process. In addition, cases that were assigned to code 87.44

before the re-coding process were commonly re-assigned to code 99.83 (Other phototherapy) after the re-coding process.

To sum it up most of the cases that were assigned to the top 10 primary procedure codes before the re-coding process were assigned to a wrong primary procedure code with the errors rate of 77.1%. Mostly these error cases were assigned to a wrong primary procedure codes. On the contrary, among these cases, there was no error case detected with a wrong assignment at the third digit level of the code.

Table 4.15 Changes in Top 10 Code Assigned as Primary Procedure Code Due to Coding Error

No.	Before Re-Coding Process			After Re-Coding Process		
	n = 369			Cases With New Primary Procedure Code due to Coding Error		
	Original Primary Procedure Code	Description	No. of Cases (%)	No. of Cases with Unchanged Primary Procedure Code (%)	New Primary Procedure Code	Description	No. of Cases (%)
1.	74.1	Low cervical caesarean section	55 (14.9)	22 (40.0)	75.69	Repair of other current obstetric laceration	12 (21.8)
					88.38	Other computerized axial tomography	9 (16.4)
					72.7	Vacuum extraction	2 (3.6)
					72.79	Other vacuum extraction	2 (3.6)
					88.78	Diagnostic ultrasound of gravid uterus	2 (3.6)
					None	None	2 (3.6)
					73.4	Medical induction of labour	1 (1.8)
					73.59	Other manually assisted delivery	1 (1.8)
					74.9	Caesarean section of unspecified type	1 (1.8)
					75.4	Manual removal of retained placenta	1 (1.8)
2.	99.83	Other phototherapy	33 (8.9)	17 (51.5)	None	None	8 (24.2)
					87.44	Routine chest x-ray, so described	2 (6.1)
					18.11	Otoscopy	1 (3.0)
					39.95	Haemodialysis	1 (3.0)

					88.01	Computerized axial tomography of abdomen	1 (3.0)
					88.71	Diagnostic ultrasound of head and neck	1 (3.0)
					88.72	Diagnostic ultrasound of heart	1 (3.0)
					99.04	Transfusion of packed cells	1 (3.0)
					None	None	8 (27.6)
3.	87.44	Routine chest x-ray, so described	29 (7.9)	2 (6.9)	99.83	Other phototherapy	7 (24.1)
					99.25	Injection or infusion of cancer chemotherapeutic substance	3 (10.3)
					88.72	Diagnostic ultrasound of heart	2 (6.9)
					23.09	Extraction of other tooth	1 (3.4)
					34.04	Insertion of intercostal catheter for drainage	1 (3.4)
					51.11	Endoscopic retrograde cholangiography [ERC]	1 (3.4)
					54.98	Peritoneal dialysis	1 (3.4)
					74.1	Low cervical caesarean section	1 (3.4)
					96.33	Gastric lavage	1 (3.4)
					99.29	Injection or infusion of other therapeutic or prophylactic substance	1 (3.4)
4.	75.69	Repair of other current obstetric laceration	25 (6.8)	3 (12.0)	74.1	Low cervical caesarean section	9 (36.0)
					88.38	Other computerized axial tomography	5 (20.0)
					72.7	Vacuum extraction	2 (8.0)
					11.64	Other penetrating keratoplasty	1 (4.0)
					49.01	Incision of perianal abscess	1 (4.0)

No.	Code	Procedure	N (%)	Associated Code	Associated Procedure	N (%)
5.	73.6	Episiotomy	20 (5.4)	1 (5.0)		
				72.1	Low forceps operation with episiotomy	1 (4.0)
				86.04	Other incision with drainage of skin and subcutaneous tissue	1 (4.0)
				88.78	Diagnostic ultrasound of gravid uterus	1 (4.0)
				96.48	Irrigation of other indwelling urinary catheter	1 (4.0)
				74.1	Low cervical caesarean section	8 (40.0)
				88.38	Other computerized axial tomography	7 (35.0)
				75.69	Repair of other current obstetric laceration	3 (15.0)
				72.7	Vacuum extraction	1 (5.0)
6.	93.9	Respiratory therapy	11 (3.0)	0 (0.0)		
				99.83	Other phototherapy	5 (45.5)
				None	None	2 (18.2)
				31.42	Laryngoscopy and other tracheoscopy	1 (9.1)
				87.17	Other x-ray of skull	1 (9.1)
				87.44	Routine chest x-ray, so described	1 (9.1)
				88.71	Diagnostic ultrasound of head and neck	1 (9.1)
7.	89.52	Electrocardiogram	9 (2.4)	0 (0.0)		
				None	None	3 (33.4)
				18.11	Otoscopy	1 (11.1)
				55.02	Nephrostomy	1 (11.1)
				75.69	Repair of other current obstetric laceration	1 (11.1)
				87.03	Computerized axial tomography of head	1 (11.1)
				88.72	Diagnostic ultrasound of heart	1 (11.1)
				96.26	Manual reduction of rectal prolapse	1 (11.1)
8.	69.02	Dilation and curettage following delivery or abortion	8 (2.2)	1 (12.5)		
				86.22	Excisional debridement of wound, infection, or burn	2 (25.0)

				10.1	Other incision of conjunctiva	1 (12.5)
				47.09	Other appendectomy	1 (12.5)
				53.05	Repair of inguinal hernia with graft or prosthesis, not otherwise specified	1 (12.5)
				86.04	Other incision with drainage of skin and subcutaneous tissue	1 (12.5)
				88.67	Phlebography of other specified sites using contrast material	1 (12.5)
				None	None	3 (37.5)
				34.9	Other operations on thorax	1 (12.5)
				51.1	Diagnostic procedures on biliary tract	1 (12.5)
				87.44	Routine chest x-ray, so described	1 (12.5)
				88.72	Diagnostic ultrasound of heart	1 (12.5)
9.	99.25	Injection or infusion of cancer chemotherapeutic substance	8 (2.2)	1 (12.5)	None	None	2 (28.5)
				18.11	Otoscopy	1 (14.3)
				51.85	Endoscopic sphincterotomy and papillotomy	1 (14.3)
				77.4	Biopsy of bone	1 (14.3)
				87.44	Routine chest x-ray, so described	1 (14.3)
10.	87.03	Computerized axial tomography of head	7 (1.9)	0 (0.0)	99.83	Other phototherapy	1 (14.3)

4.3.4 Coding Errors of Secondary Procedure Code

In the first level of coding error calculation within secondary procedure codes, coding errors occurred in 270 (58.2%) of the selected cases. In total, there were 652 secondary procedure codes reviewed by the Independent Senior Coder. These reviewed codes were inclusive all the up-coding and under-coding codes. From these 652 reviewed codes, 566 (86.8%) of the codes were considered as error codes.

Before the re-coding process, the total number of secondary diagnosis codes assigned to the entire case was 361 codes and has grossly increased to 550 codes after the re-coding process. The maximum number of secondary procedure codes assigned to the patient was 7 with the mean of 0.78 (SD 1.04). After the re-coding process, the maximum number of secondary procedure code increased to 10 codes with the mean of 1.19 (1.66). The level of agreement between the in-house coder and the Independent Senior Coder in the number of secondary diagnosis code assigned per patient was fair with the kappa value of 0.210 (Table 4.16).

Table 4.16 Distributions of Total Number of Secondary Procedure Code Assigned to Patient Before and After the Re-Coding Process

No. of Secondary Procedure Code	Before	After	Kappa value	p value
			0.210	<0.001
Total Nos of Code	361	550		
Max. Codes	7	10		
Mean (SD)	0.78 (1.04)	1.19 (1.66)		

a. Comparison of Number of Secondary Procedure Code Before and After the Re-Coding Process

In this study, a bivariate analysis using chi-square test was conducted to determine the association between the number of secondary procedure codes and coding errors. The association between the number of the secondary procedure codes and coding errors was proven to be statistically insignificant with a chi-square value of X^2 (3) = 7.552, p=0.057 (Table 4.17). This table show that the highest coding errors (95.8%) were in cases with three and above secondary procedures. These findings reflect that in-house coders were more likely to having difficulty to code cases with a higher number of the secondary procedures.

Table 4.17 Distributions of Coding Error Cases by Number of Secondary Procedure Code

No. of Secondary Procedure Code	No. of Non Error Case	%	No. of Error Case	%	Total	%
0	33	14.0	196	85.6	229	100.0
1	10	6.5	144	93.6	154	100.0
2	5	8.7	52	91.3	57	100.0
3 and above	1	4.2	23	95.8	24	100.0

X^2 = 7.522, df =3, p =0.057

Before the re-coding process, there were a total of 229 (49.4%) cases with no secondary procedure code. Data analysis showed that, after the re-coding process, from these 229 cases, 68 (29.7%) of the cases were re-assigned to at least one secondary procedure code. The highest number of secondary procedure code before the audit was seven codes per patient. However, there was only 1 (0.2%) case that was assigned to 7 secondary procedure codes before the audit. Interestingly, after the re-coding process, the number of cases assigned to 7 secondary procedure codes has increased to 3 (0.6%) cases. This reflecting that the in-house coders tend to under-code cases with a higher number of secondary procedures.

After the re-coding process, there were 6 (1.3%) cases that were assigned to more than 7 secondary procedure codes. In total, there were 2 (0.4%) cases that were assigned to 8 secondary procedure codes and 3 (0.6%) cases that were assigned to 9 secondary procedure codes. The maximum number of secondary procedure code assigned to a patient after the re-coding process was ten codes with 1 (0.2%) case was assigned with this maximum number of secondary procedure code after the re-coding process. The number of cases that were unassigned to any secondary procedure codes showed a slight decrement from 229 cases to 225 cases. Table 4.18 shows the comparison of the distributions of the total number of secondary procedure code assigned to a patient before and after the evaluation conducted by this study.

Table 4.18 Comparisons of Number of Secondary Procedure Code Assigned per Patient Before and After the Re-Coding Process

No.	Before Re-Coding Process					After Audit				
	n = 464		n = *			n = 464		n = **		
	No. of Secondary Procedure Code	No. of Cases (%) *	No. of Cases Without Coding Errors (%)	No. of Errors Cases with Lower No of Secondary Procedure Code After Audit (%)	No. of Errors Cases with Higher No of Secondary Procedure Code After Audit (%)	No. of Secondary Procedure Code	No. of Cases (%) **	No. of Cases without Coding Errors (%)	No. of Errors Cases with Lower No of Secondary Procedure Code Before Audit (%)	No. of Errors Cases with Higher No of Secondary Procedure Code Before Audit (%)
1.	0	229 (49.4)	161 (70.3)	0 (0.0)	68 (29.7)	0	225 (48.5)	161 (71.6)	0 (0.0)	58 (25.7)
2.	1	156 (33.7)	46 (29.5)	57 (36.5)	53 (34.0)	1	97 (20.9)	44 (45.4)	33 (34.0)	20 (20.6)
3.	2	57 (12.3)	10 (17.5)	25 (43.9)	22 (38.6)	2	45 (9.7)	10 (22.2)	31 (68.9)	4 (8.9)
4.	3	12 (2.6)	1 (8.3)	9 (75.0)	2 (16.7)	3	55 (11.9)	2 (3.6)	51 (92.7)	2 (3.6)
5.	4	6 (1.3)	0 (0.0)	2 (33.3)	4 (66.7)	4	22 (4.7)	0 (0.0)	21 (95.5)	1 (4.5)
6.	5	2 (0.4)	0 (0.0)	1 (50.0)	1 (50.0)	5	6 (1.3)	0 (0.0)	6 (100.0)	0 (0.0)
7.	6	1 (0.2)	0 (0.0)	1 (100.0)	0 (0.0)	6	1 (0.2)	0 (0.0)	0 (0.0)	1 (100.0)
8.	7	1 (0.2)	1 (100.0)	0 (0.0)	0 (0.0)	7	3 (0.6)	1 (100.0)	2 (28.7)	0 (0.0)
9.	8	N/A	N/A	N/A	N/A	8 and above	6 (1.3)	0 (0.0)	6 (100.0)	0 (0.0)

Kappa value = 0.210, $p < 0.001$

b. Type of Coding Errors in Secondary Procedure Code

Data analysis in the present study showed that the commonest type of error in the assignment of secondary procedure code was under-coding. From the 652 secondary procedure codes reviewed by the Independent Senior Coder 297 (45.6%) of the codes was under-coded by the in-house coder. The second highest type of errors found within the secondary procedure codes was the wrong selection of secondary procedure code reaching 111 error cases (17.0%). The up-coding was the third highest type error in which 95 (14.6%) of error cases were due to this type of coding errors. In the assignment of secondary procedure code, the less common type of errors was error at the fourth digit level of the code covering 10 (1.5%) of the error cases. The details on the type of coding errors in the assignment of secondary procedure code are illustrates in Table 4.19.

Table 4.19 Distributions of Type of Coding Errors in Secondary Procedure Code

Type of Error	No. of Error Cases	%
Under-coding	297	45.6
Wrong Selection of Secondary Procedure Code	111	17.0
Up-coding	95	14.6
Error at Second Digit Level	32	4.9
Error at Third Digit Level	21	3.2
Error at Fourth Digit Level	10	1.5

c. Examples of Error Cases in the Assignment of Secondary Procedure Code

Table 4.20 shows two examples of error cases in the assignment of secondary procedure code. These two cases were selected among cases containing the error in the assignment of its secondary procedure code.

Case 1 is an example of error case where this case containing an undercoding issue in the assignment of its secondary procedure code.

As apparent in the Table 4.20, this case was assigned to an accurate primary diagnosis code (P36.9), accurate secondary diagnosis code (P70.4) and accurate primary procedure code (99.83). Before the re-coding process, this case was assigned to code 88.72 as its secondary procedure code. Although the assignment of code 88.72 was accurate for this case, the in-house coder has not code another relevant secondary procedure code for this case namely 89.52. However, despite the error in the assignment of secondary procedure code, the assignment of the MY-DRG® code after the re-grouping process was unchanged. This case was remained assigned to code P-8-16-II (Neonate birthweight >2499 grams with congenital sepsis- Moderate) with the hospital tariff amounting to RM3,383.85.

Table 4.20 Example of Error Cases in the Assignment of Secondary Procedure Code

	Before	After
Case 1		
MRN	N420889	N420889
Admission Date	02/01/13	02/01/13
Discharge Date	04/01/13	04/01/13
Primary Diagnosis Code	P36.9 (Bacteria Sepsis of newborn, unspecified)	P36.9 (Bacteria Sepsis of newborn, unspecified)
Secondary Diagnosis Code	P70.4 (Other neonatal hypoglycaemia)	P70.4 (Other neonatal hypoglycaemia)
Primary Procedure Code	99.83 (Other phototherapy)	99.83 (Other phototherapy)
Secondary Procedure Code	88.72 (Diagnostic ultrasound of heart)	88.72 (Diagnostic ultrasound of heart), 89.52 (Electrocardiogram)
MY-DRG Group	P-8-16-II (Neonate birthweight >2499 grams with congenital sepsis- Moderate)	P-8-16-II (Neonate birthweight >2499 grams with congenital sepsis- Moderate)
Hospital Tariff	RM 3,383.85	RM 3,383.85
Type of Error in Secondary Procedure Code	Under-coding	

Case 2

MRN	N206787	N206787
Admission Date	27/05/13	27/05/13
Discharge Date	30/05/13	30/05/13
Primary Diagnosis Code	N49.2 (Inflammatory disorders of scrotum)	N49.2 (Inflammatory disorders of scrotum)
Secondary Diagnosis Code	I10 ([Essential] hypertension), E11.9 (Non-insulin dependent diabetes mellitus without complications), I51.9 (Heart disease unspecified)	I10 ([Essential] hypertension), E11.9 (Non-insulin dependent diabetes mellitus without complications), I25.9 (Chronic ischaemic unspecified)
Primary Procedure Code	61.0 (Incision and drainage of scrotum and tunica vaginalis)	61.0 (Incision and drainage of scrotum and tunica vaginalis)
Secondary Procedure Code	89.52 (Electrocardiogram)	88.72 (Diagnostic ultrasound of heart)
MY-DRG Group	V-1-13-I (Simple prostate & scrotal operation –Minor)	V-1-13-I (Simple prostate & scrotal operation –Minor)
Hospital Tariff	RM 3,210.27	RM 3,210.27
Type of Error in Secondary Procedure Code	Error at second digit level	

On the other hand, Case 2 is an example of error case where the secondary procedure code was assigned wrongly at the second digit level. Before the re-coding process, this case was assigned to code 89.52 as its secondary procedure code but, the accurate secondary procedure code for this case was 88.72. In addition to the wrong assignment of the secondary procedure code at the second digit level of the code, this case is also containing one error code in the assignment of secondary diagnosis code (I51.9 (Wrong code), I25.9 (Accurate Code). However, the primary diagnosis code for this case namely N49.2 was assigned accurately by the in-house coder. Similar to Case 1, although there were coding errors identified in this case, this case was assigned to the same MY-DRG® code before and after the re-coding process; V-1-13-I (Simple prostate & scrotal operation –Minor).

d. Top 10 Code Assigned as Secondary Procedure Before and After the Re-Coding Process

Coding errors occurred among the secondary procedure codes has caused changes in the distribution of the frequency of codes. Table 4.21 shows the distributions of top 10 secondary procedure codes assigned before and after the re-coding process. The number of cases listed in Table 4.21 has increased dramatically from 219 cases before the re-coding process to 334 cases after the re-coding process. It is visible on the Table 4.23 that the highest coding errors rate among the top 10 secondary procedure code assigned before the re-coding process were among codes 99.04 and 39.95. The cases that were assigned to code 99.04 or 39.95 as their secondary procedure code before the re-coding process were assigned to at least one error secondary procedure code by the in-house coder. In contra, the lowest coding errors rate among the top 10 secondary procedure codes were among cases that were assigned to code 73.3 and 88.72. As apparent in Table 4.23 all cases that were assigned to code 73.3 and 88.72 before the audit were assigned with accurate secondary procedure codes.

Among the top 10 highest secondary procedure codes after the re-coding process, the highest coding errors were involving the assignment of codes 99.04, 39.95 and 75.69 (Repair of other current obstetric laceration). Data analysis revealed that cases that were assigned to these three codes after the process was originally assigned with at least one error secondary procedure code before the re-coding process. On the contrary, the lowest coding errors rate among the top 10 highest secondary procedure code after the process were involving the assignment of 88.72. From the 15 cases that were assigned to this code after the re-coding process, 7 (46.7%) of the cases were assigned with the similar secondary procedure codes as before the re-coding process.

Table 4.21 Top 10 Code Assigned as Secondary Procedure Code Before and After the Re-Coding Process

		Before Re-Coding Process			After Re-Coding Process			
			n = 361	n = *			n = 550	n = **
No.	Codes	Description	Frequency (%)*	No. of Error Cases (%)	Codes	Description	Frequency (%)**	No. of Cases Without Coding Errors (%)
1.	75.34	Other fetal monitoring	84 (23.3)	79 (94.0)	57.94	Insertion of indwelling urinary catheter	84 (15.3)	1 (1.2)
2.	87.44	Routine chest x-ray, so described	42 (11.6)	39 (92.9)	88.38	Other computerized axial tomography	75 (13.6)	2 (2.7)
3.	89.52	Electrocardiogram	23 (6.4)	20 (87.0)	97.64	Removal of other urinary drainage device	73 (13.3)	1 (1.4)
4.	73.4	Medical induction of labour	19 (5.3)	17 (89.5)	99.04	Transfusion of packed cells	27 (4.9)	0 (0.0)
5.	99.04	Transfusion of packed cells	15 (4.2)	15 (100.0)	87.44	Routine chest x-ray, so described	15 (2.7)	3 (20.0)
6.	93.9	Respiratory Therapy	9 (2.5)	7 (77.8)	88.72	Diagnostic ultrasound of heart	15 (2.7)	7 (46.7)
7.	73.3	Failed Forceps	8 (2.2)	0 (0.0)	88.79	Other diagnostic ultrasound	13 (2.4)	0 (0.0)
8.	88.72	Diagnostic ultrasound of heart	7 (1.9)	0 (0.0)	89.52	Electrocardiogram	13 (2.4)	3 (23.1)
9.	13.71	Insertion of intraocular lens prosthesis at time of cataract extraction, one-stage	6 (1.7)	4 (66.7)	39.95	Haemodialysis	10 (1.8)	0 (0.0)
10.	39.95	Haemodialysis	6 (1.7)	6 (100.0)	75.69	Repair of other current obstetric laceration	9 (1.6)	0 (0.0)

4.4 Coding Erros by Case-Type

As this study employed a stratified sampling method, all types of cases were stratified equally according to the sample requirement. In total, there were 116 cases per case-type that were analysed in this study. After the re-coding process was performed by the Independent Senior Coder, the highest coding error cases was found within O&G cases, covering up to 110 (94.8%) cases. Next, medical cases recorded the second highest error cases type with 107 (92.2%) coding error cases. This is followed by paediatric cases with 102 (87.9%) error cases and surgical cases with 96 (94.8%) error cases respectively. A chi-square test was conducted to evaluate the association between MY-DRG® type of cases and the coding errors. The result was proven to be statistically significant with X^2 (3) = 11.518, p = 0.009. Table 4.22 shows the distribution of error cases by the type of cases.

Table 4.22 Distributions of Coding Errors by MY-DRG® Case-Type

Type of Case	No. of Case without Coding Error	%	No of Case with Coding Error/s	%	Total Reviewed Case	%
O&G	6	5.2	110	94.8	116	100.0
Medical	9	7.8	107	92.2	116	100.0
Paediatric	4	3.4	102	87.9	116	100.0
Surgical	20	17.8	96	82.8	116	100.0

X^2 = 11.518, df = 3, p = 0.009

The coding errors identified in this study have affected the distributions of the assignment of case-type in MY-DRG® code of the selected cases. As illustrates in Table 4.23, 69 of the error cases showed changes in the assignment of their case-type in MY-DRG® code after the re-coding process. After the re-coding process, the number of medical cases has increased to 130 cases. Meanwhile, for surgical cases, the number of cases has decreased to 100 cases. Similar with medical case-type, O&G cases also showed increment from 116 cases to 119 cases. Lastly, for paediatric case, due to the ungroupable cases, the number of cases has decreased to 108 cases (Table 4.23). However, in this study, coding errors has not caused changes in the case-type in the assignment of MY-DRG code. Most of the cases remained in the same case-type even with coding errors since the kappa value showed a good agreement of the distribution of case-type before and after the audit value of 0.814.

Table 4.23 Distributions of Cases by MY-DRG® Case-Type After Audit

		Type of Case After Re-Coding					
		Medical	Surgical	O&G	Paediatric	Ungroupable	Total
Type of Case before Re-Coding	Medical	97	15	2	2	0	116
	Surgical	25	83	6	2	0	116
	O&G	3	2	111	0	0	116
	Paediatric	4	0	0	104	8	116
	Total	130	100	119	108	8	464

Kappa Value = 0.814, $p < 0.001$

Even though the percentage of error cases in O&G case was the highest among, the number of error cases with changes in their case-type after the re-coding process was the lowest among O&G case-type. There were only 5 (4.3%) O&G cases that have being re-assigned to other case-type after the re-coding process. From these 5 cases, 3 (60.0%) of the cases were re-assigned to medical case-type and 2 (40.0%) of the cases were re-assigned to surgical case-type after the re-coding process.

On the contrary, the percentage of coding error was the lowest among surgical cases but the number of cases with changes in the case-type within surgical cases was the highest, reaching 33 cases. Out of these 33 cases, 25 (75.8%) of the cases were re-assigned to medical case-type and the remaining 6 (18.2%) cases were re-assigned to O&G case-type.

Another important finding in the assignment of case-type after the re-coding process was the ungroupable cases. After the re-coding process, 8 of the cases that were originally assigned as paediatric cases have been detected by the grouper as the ungroupable cases. Further analysis revealed that these ungroupable cases were due to the missing information of the birth weight of the patients. All these ungroupable cases were also were codified with a wrong primary diagnosis code before the re-coding process.

To sum it up, coding errors were the highest among O&G cases with 110 (94.8%) error cases. However, coding errors detected within O&G cases were mainly a minor error as the number of error cases that were re-assigned to other case-type was the lowest comprising only 5 (4.3%) cases. On the other hand, among these four case-types, coding error cases were less found among surgical cases in which the numbers of error cases were only 96 (82.8%) cases. Overall, the coding errors detected in this study has not caused changes in the case-type in the assignment of MY-DRG® code. Most of the cases remained in the same case-type even with coding errors since the kappa value showed a good agreement of the distribution of case-type before and after the audit value of 0.814.

4.4.1 Coding Errors of Medical Case-Type

Coding error cases detected within medical case-type was the second highest among the other case-type, in which the number of error cases has reached 107 (92.2%) cases. In this case-type, the coding errors were mostly high in the assignment of its secondary diagnosis code covering 98 (84.5%) cases. Fewer errors were found in the assignment of primary diagnosis code where the numbers of error cases were only 65 (44.0%) cases. Table 4.24 summarised the distributions of coding error cases among medical cases by the coding item.

Table 4.24 Distributions of Coding Error Cases by Coding Item in Medical Case-Type

Coding Items	Total Case Reviewed	No. of Case without Coding Error (%)	No. of Case with Coding Error/s(%)	Kappa Value	p value
Primary Diagnosis	116	51 (44.0)	65 (56.0)	0.441	<0.001
Secondary Diagnosis	116	18 (15.5)	98 (84.5)	0.180	<0.001
Primary Procedure	116	50 (43.1)	66 (56.9)	0.010	<0.001
Secondary Procedure	116	49 (42.2)	67 (57.8)	0.176	<0.001

Cohen's Kappa Test was conducted to determine the level of agreement between the in-house coder and Independent Senior Coder in the assignment of codes among medical cases. For primary diagnosis and primary procedure code, the test was conducted by comparing the code assigned to the episode of care before and after the audit. The output of the kappa test showed that among the medical cases, the assignment of primary procedure code was more prone to error compared to the primary diagnosis code (kappa value 0.010 vs. 0.441). On the other hand, for secondary diagnosis and secondary procedure code, the kappa test was conducted by comparing the total number of codes assigned to the episode of care before and after the audit. The output of the test showed that, among cases that were assigned to medical case-type, although the number of error cases is higher among secondary diagnosis code than secondary procedure code (84.5% vs. 57.8%), the number of secondary procedure code was most likely to be codified wrongly by the in-house coder compared to the number of secondary diagnosis code assigned per episode of care (kappa value: 0.176 vs. 0.180).

a. **Coding Errors of Primary Diagnosis within Medical Case-Type**

At the first level of coding error calculation within the primary diagnosis codes of cases assigned to medical case-type, coding errors occurred in 65 (56.0%) of the selected cases. The second level of coding error calculation within the primary diagnosis codes also showed the same percentage of errors; 56.0% in respect to the similar number of the denominator in both level of calculations (n=464).

i. Type of Coding Errors in Primary Diagnosis Within Medical Case-Type

In the assignment of the primary diagnosis code, most of the codes were codified wrongly at the fourth digit level of the code, which comprised of 21 (18.1%) error cases. The second highest type of error was the wrong selection of primary diagnosis code covering 20 (17.2%) of error cases. The third highest type of coding error was the error at the third digit level of the code reaching 12 (10.3%) of the error cases. Following this, the Independent Senior Coder has identified 9 (7.8%) cases with the error at the second digit level of the code. There were 2 (1.7%) cases with error at the assignment of the fifth digit of the code. In addition to this, there was one (0.9%) case where the primary diagnosis code was incorrectly sequenced by the in-house coder (Table 4.25).

Table 4.25 Distribution of Type of Coding Errors Among Primary Diagnosis Code in Medical Case-Type

Type of Error	No. of Error Cases	%
Error at Fourth Digit Level	21	18.1
Wrong Selection of Primary Diagnosis Code	20	17.2
Error at Third Digit Level	12	10.3
Error at Second Digit Level	9	7.8
Error at Fifth Digit Level	2	1.7
Primary Diagnosis Code Incorrectly Sequenced	1	0.9

ii. Top 10 Primary Diagnosis Code Assigned Before and After the Re- Coding Process within Medical Case-Type

The coding errors occurred in the assignment of the primary diagnosis codes in medical case-type have affected the distributions of the frequency of codes assigned as the primary diagnosis code. Table 4.26 shows the distributions of the top 10 highest frequencies of primary procedure codes before and after the evaluation carried out by the Independent Senior Coder. As illustrates in Table 4.26, there were 5 common codes that were listed in the list of top 10 primary diagnosis codes assigned before and after the re-coding process namely A41.9 (Septicaemia, unspecified), A90 (Dengue fever [classical dengue]), A08.0 (Rotaviral enteritis), E87.1 (Hypo-osmolality and hyponatraemia) and I12.0 (Unstable angina). A bivariate analysis using Cohen Kappa Test showed that the level of agreement between the Independent Senior Coder and in-house coder was moderate with kappa values of 0.441.

From Table 4.26, it is notable that the highest coding errors rate among the top 10 primary diagnosis code assigned before the re-coding process were involving cases that were assigned to code D64.9 (Anaemia, unspecified), G40.9 (Epilepsy, unspecified) and H25.9 (Senile cataract, unspecified). All the cases that were assigned to these three codes before the re-coding process was assigned to a wrong primary diagnosis code by the in-house coder. On the contrary, the lowest coding error rates among the top 10 primary diagnosis code assigned before the re-coding process were involving cases that were assigned to codes A90, A80.0, I12.0 and J44.1 (Chronic obstructive pulmonary disease with acute exacerbation unspecified). Apparently, from Table 4.26 all cases that were assigned to these four codes were assigned to the accurate primary diagnosis codes before the re-coding process.

On the other hand, among the top 10 primary diagnosis codes assigned after the re-coding process, the coding errors rate was the highest in the assignment of code A09.9 (Rotaviral enteritis), A41.0 (Sepsis due to staphylococcus), H26.9 (Cataract, unspecified), I20.0 (Unstable angina) and I74.3 (Embolism and thrombosis of arteries of lower extremities). It was revealed that none of the cases that were assigned to these five codes after the re-coding process was assigned to accurate primary diagnosis code by the Independent Senior Coder. On the contrary the lowest coding errors rate among cases were among the top 10 primary diagnosis code after the re-coding process were involving the assignment of codes A90, A08.0 and A41.9. As presented in Table 4.26, all of the cases that were assigned to these three codes were assigned to the accurate primary diagnosis code before the re-coding process.

From Table 4.26 it can be concluded that the majority of cases that were assigned to the top 10 primary diagnosis code before the re-coding process was assigned to an accurate primary diagnosis code by the Independent Senior Coder. The top 10 primary diagnosis codes assigned after the re-coding process consisted of 5 primary diagnosis codes without any coding error cases. Accordingly, Table 4.27 shows the changes which occurred among the remaining 5 codes with coding error cases after the re-coding process.

From Table 4.27 it is notable that there were 24 cases that were assigned to the top 10 highest primary diagnosis frequency primary diagnosis code before the re-coding process. From these 24 cases, 10 (41.7%) of the cases were assigned to the wrong primary diagnosis code. The commonest type of errors among these 10 error cases was the wrong selection of primary diagnosis code which consisted 4 (40.0%) of error cases. The remaining 6 (60.0%) error cases were assigned wrongly at the third digit level of the code and fourth digit level of the code with 3 error cases per type of coding error.

In conclusion, coding errors in the assignment of primary diagnosis code among medical cases were moderate. This is proven by the moderate agreement between the Independent Senior Coder and in-house coders in the assignment of primary diagnosis code within medical cases (k=0.441). This implies that the skill of the in-house coders in assigning primary diagnosis code within medical cases was moderate.

Table 4.26 Primary Diagnosis Code Assigned Before and After Audit within Medical Case-Type

No.	Before Re-Coding Process				After Re-Coding Process			
	Codes	Description	Frequency (%)* n = 116	No. of Error Cases (%) n =*	Codes	Description	Frequency (%)** n = 116	No. of Cases With Unchanged Primary Diagnosis Code (%) n =**
1.	A41.9	Septicaemia, unspecified	3 (2.6)	1 (33.3)	A90	Dengue fever [classical dengue]	3 (2.6)	3 (100.0)
2.	A90	Dengue fever [classical dengue]	3 (2.6)	0 (0.0)	A08.0	Rotaviral enteritis	2 (1.7)	2 (100.0)
3.	D64.9	Anaemia, unspecified	3 (2.6)	3 (100.0)	A09.9	Gastroenteritis and colitis of unspecified origin	2 (1.7)	0 (0.0)
4.	I20.0	Unstable angina	3 (2.6)	2 (66.7)	A41.0	Sepsis due to Staphylococcus aureus	2 (1.7)	0 (0.0)
5.	A08.0	Rotaviral enteritis	2 (1.7)	0 (0.0)	A41.9	Septicaemia, unspecified	2 (1.7)	2 (100.0)
6.	E87.1	Hypo-osmolality and hyponatraemia	2 (1.7)	0 (0.0)	E87.1	Hypo-osmolality and hyponatraemia	2 (1.7)	2 (100.0)
7.	G40.9	Epilepsy, unspecified	2 (1.7)	2 (100.0)	H26.9	Cataract, unspecified	2 (1.7)	0 (0.0)
8.	H25.9	Senile Cataract, Unspecified	2 (1.7)	2 (100.0)	I20.0	Unstable angina	2 (1.7)	2 (100.0)
9.	I12.0	Unstable angina	2 (1.7)	0 (0.0)	I63.9	Cerebral infarction, unspecified	2 (1.7)	2 (100.0)
10.	J44.1	Chronic obstructive pulmonary disease with acute exacerbation, unspecified	2 (1.7)	0 (0.0)	I74.3	Embolism and thrombosis of arteries of lower extremities	2 (1.7)	0 (0.0)

Kappa Value = 0.441, p <0.001

Table 4.27 Changes in the Assignment of Top 10 Primary Procedure Code within Medical Case-Type

		Before Re-Coding Process n = 116		After Re-Coding Process n = *		
				Cases With New Primary Diagnosis Code due to Coding Error		
No.	Original Primary Diagnosis Code	No. of Cases* (%)	No. of Cases with Unchanged Primary Diagnosis Code (%)	New Primary Diagnosis Code	Description	No. Cases (%)
1.	A41.9 (Septicaemia, unspecified)	3 (2.6)	2 (66.7)	A41.5	Sepsis due to other Gram-negative organisms	1 (33.3)
2.	A90 (Dengue fever [classical dengue])	3 (2.6)	3 (100.0)	NIL	NIL	NIL
3.	D64.9 (Anaemia, unspecified)	3 (2.6)	0 (0.0)	A09.9	Gastroenteritis and colitis of unspecified origin	1 (33.3)
				D61.9	Aplastic anaemia, unspecified	1 (33.3)
				N60.1	Diffuse cystic mastopathy	1 (33.3)
4.	I20.0 (Unstable angina)	3 (2.6)	1 (33.3)	Z40.8	Other prophylactic surgery	1 (33.3)
				Z49.2	Other dialysis	1 (33.3)
5.	A08.0 (Rotaviral enteritis)	2 (1.7)	2 (33.3)	NIL	NIL	NIL
6.	E87.1 (Hypo-osmolality and hyponatraemia)	2 (1.7)	2 (33.3)	NIL	NIL	NIL
7.	G40.9 (Epilepsy, unspecified)	2 (1.7)	0 (0.0)	G40.1	Localization-related (focal)(partial) symptomatic epilepsy and epileptic syndromes with simple partial seizures	1 (50.0)
				G40.3	Generalized idiopathic epilepsy and epileptic syndromes	1 (50.0)
8.	H25.9 (Senile Cataract, Unspecified)	2 (1.7)	0 (0.0)	H26.9	Cataract, unspecified	2 (100.0)
9.	I12.0 (Unstable angina)	2 (1.7)	2 (100.0)	NIL	NIL	NIL
10.	J44.1 (Chronic obstructive pulmonary disease with acute exacerbation, unspecified)	2 (1.7)	2 (100.0)	NIL	NIL	NIL

b. Coding Errors of Secondary Diagnosis Code Within Medical Case-Type

Before the re-coding process, 99 of medical case-types were assigned to at least one secondary diagnosis code. After the re-coding process, the number of cases that were assigned to at least one secondary diagnosis code has increased to 103 cases. During the first level of coding error calculation within the secondary diagnosis codes, coding errors occurred in 98 (84.5%) of the selected cases. In total, there were 539 secondary diagnosis codes reviewed by the Independent Senior Coder during the audit within medical cases. From these 539 codes, 377 (69.9%) of the codes were considered as error codes by the Independent Senior Coder.

Before the audit, the total numbers of codes assigned as secondary diagnosis code in medical case-type were 323 codes and have grossly increased to 517 codes after the re-coding process. Before the re-coding process, the maximum number of codes assigned per patient was 10 codes with the mean of 2.76 (SD: 2.28). After the audit, the maximum number of codes assigned per patient has increased dramatically to 16 codes with the mean of 3.98 (SD: 3.07). The level of agreement between the Independent Senior Coder and in-house coder on the number of secondary diagnosis code assigned per patient was tested using Cohen's Kappa test and the result showed poor agreement with kappa value of 0.180 (Table 4.28).

Table 4.28 Distributions of the Number of Secondary Diagnosis Codes Assigned Before and After the Re-Coding Process within Medical Case-Type

No. of Secondary Diagnosis Code	Before	After	Kappa value	p value
			0.180	<0.001
Total No. of Code	323	517		
Max. Codes	10	16		
Mean (SD)	2.76 (2.28)	3.98 (3.07)		

i. **Comparisons of Number of Secondary Diagnosis Code Assigned per Patient Before and After the Re-Coding Process**

As illustrated in Table 4.29, there were 16 (13.8%) medical case-type cases that were unassigned to any secondary diagnosis code before the re-coding process. After the re-coding process, the number of cases without any secondary diagnosis code has declined to 11 (8.5%) cases. From these 11 cases, 10 (90.9%) of the cases were originally unassigned to any secondary diagnosis code even before the re-coding process. The remaining one (9.1%) case was originally assigned to one secondary diagnosis code before the evaluation performed by the Independent Senior Coder.

From the data, before the re-coding process was performed, the highest number of secondary diagnosis assigned to medical case-type patients was 10 codes per patient. In total, there was 1 (0.9%) case that was assigned to 10 secondary diagnosis codes before the re-coding process. Data analysis after the re-coding process revealed that the number of cases that were assigned to 10 secondary diagnosis codes has reached 5 (3.8%) cases. From these 5 cases, one of the cases was originally assigned to the same number of secondary diagnosis code and the remaining 4 cases were assigned to a lower number of secondary diagnosis code in which, 1 case was assigned to 7 secondary diagnosis codes, 1 case was assigned 6 secondary diagnosis codes and 2 cases were assigned to 2 secondary diagnosis codes.

From Table 4.29, it was also notable that after the re-coding process was performed by the Independent Senior Coder; there were 5 (3.8%) cases that were assigned to more than 10 secondary diagnosis codes. The highest number of secondary diagnosis code assigned to medical case-type patients was 16 codes. In total, there was 1 (0.8%) case that was assigned to 16 secondary diagnosis codes after the re-coding process. This case was originally assigned to 9 secondary diagnosis codes before the re-coding process.

Table 4.34 below shows the distribution of coding error cases by the number of secondary diagnosis codes. From the table, it could be derived that coding errors were likely to occur among cases with 4 and above secondary diagnoses (97.1%) and cases with 3 secondary diagnoses (95.8%). This implies that the in-house coders have difficulties to code cases with a higher number of secondary diagnosis code. A chi-square test was run to determine the association between the number of the secondary diagnosis code and the coding errors. The result was statistically insignificant with $X^2 (4) = 4.328$, p>0.05.

Table 4.29 Comparisons of Number of Secondary Diagnosis Code Assigned per Patient Before and After the Re-Coding Process in Medical Case-Type

No.	Before Re-Coding Process						After Re-Coding Process			
	n =116		n = *			n = 130		n = **		
	No. of Secondary Diagnosis Code	No. of Cases (%) *	No. of Cases with Similar No of Secondary Diagnosis Code After (%)	No. of Cases With Lower No of Secondary Diagnosis Code After (%)	No. of Cases With Higher No of Secondary Diagnosis Code After (%)	No. of Secondary Diagnosis Code	No. of Cases (%) **	No. of Cases with Similar No of Secondary Diagnosis Code Before (%)	No. of Cases With Lower No of Secondary Diagnosis Code Before (%)	No. of Cases With Higher No of Secondary Diagnosis Code Before (%)
1.	0	16 (13.8)	5 (31.3)	0 (0.0)	11 (68.8)	0	11 (8.5)	10 (90.9)	1 (9.1)	0 (0.0)
2.	1	24 (20.7)	5 (20.8)	1 (4.2)	18 (75.0)	1	13 (10.0)	4 (30.8)	4 (30.8)	5 (38.5)
3.	2	18 (15.5)	6 (33.3)	2 (11.1)	10 (55.6)	2	25 (19.2)	8 (32.0)	12 (48.0)	5 (20.0)
4.	3	24 (20.7)	8 (33.3)	6 (25.0)	10 (41.7)	3	20 (15.4)	8 (40.0)	11 (55.0)	1 (5.0)
5.	4	14 (12.1)	3 (21.4)	2 (14.3)	9 (64.3)	4	15 (11.5)	3 (20.0)	9 (60.0)	3 (20.0)
6.	5	6 (5.2)	2 (33.3)	0 (0.0)	4 (66.7)	5	17 (13.1)	2 (11.8)	14 (82.4)	1 (5.9)
7.	6	4 (3.4)	0 (0.0)	1 (25.0)	3 (75.0)	6	6 (4.6)	1 (16.7)	2 (33.3)	3 (50.0)
8.	7	4 (3.4)	0 (0.0)	1 (25.0)	3 (75.0)	7	8 (6.2)	0 (0.0)	8 (100.0)	0 (0.0)
9.	8	2 (1.7)	1 (50.0)	0 (0.0)	1 (50.0)	8	2 (1.5)	1 (50.0)	1 (50.0)	0 (0.0)
10.	9	3 (2.6)	0 (0.0)	1 (33.3)	2 (66.7)	9	3 (2.3)	0 (0.0)	3 (100.0)	0 (0.0)
11.	10	1 (0.9)	1 (100.0)	0 (0.0)	0 (0.0)	10	5 (3.8)	1 (20.0)	4 (80.0)	0 (0.0)
12.	N/A	N/A	N/A	N/A	N/A	11 and above	5 (3.8)	0 (0.0)	5 (100.0)	0 (0.0)

Table 4.30 Distributions of Coding Error Cases by Number of Secondary Diagnosis Codes

No. of Secondary Diagnosis Code	No. of Case without Coding Error	%	No. of Case with Coding Error/s	%	Total	%
0	3	18.8	13	81.2	16	100.0
1	2	8.3	22	91.7	24	100.0
2	1	5.6	17	94.4	18	100.0
3	1	4.2	23	95.8	24	100.0
4 and above	1	2.9	33	97.1	34	100.0

$X^2 = 4.328$, df = 4, p = 0.363

ii. Type of Coding Errors in the Assignment of Secondary Diagnosis Code within Medical Case-Type

Data analysis in the present study shows that the commonest type of error in the assignment of secondary diagnosis code within medical case-type was under-coding. From the 539 secondary diagnosis codes reviewed by the Independent Senior Coder, 224 (41.6%) of the codes were not coded by the in-house coder. The second highest type of errors found within the secondary diagnosis codes was the wrong selection of primary diagnosis code covering 52 (9.6%) of error cases. The coding errors at the fourth digit level of the code were the third highest error with 31 (5.8%) cases. During the assignment of the secondary diagnosis code, the less common type of errors was an error at the fifth digit level of the code. Only 1 (0.2%) cases that was reported contained this type of error in their assignment of secondary diagnosis code. The details on the type of coding errors in the assignment of secondary diagnosis code within the cases that were assigned to medical case-type are illustrated in Table 4.31.

Table 4.31 Distributions of Type of Coding Errors in Secondary Diagnosis Code within Medical Case-Type

Type of Error	No. of Error Cases	%
Under-coding	224	41.6
Wrong Selection of Primary Diagnosis Code	52	9.6
Error at Fourth Digit Level	31	5.8
Error at Second Digit Level	27	5.0
Error at Third Digit Level	25	4.6
Up-coding	17	3.2
Error at Fifth Digit Level	1	0.2

iii. Comparisons of Top 10 Secondary Diagnosis Code Assigned Before and After the Re-Coding Process within Medical Case-Type

Table 4.32 shows the comparison of the top 10 secondary diagnosis codes within medical cases assigned before and after the re-coding process. The code assigned as secondary diagnosis code was I10 ([Essential] Hypertension). It is also worth mentioning that the total number of cases listed before the re-coding process was higher compared to the number of cases listed after the re-coding process (91 vs 60, respectively). A lower number of cases listed in the list after the audit reflects a more various type of secondary diagnosis codes assigned by the Independent Senior Coder after the re-coding process.

From Table 4.32 it is also observable that before the re-coding process, 84 (92.3%) out of 91 cases listed in the Table 4.32 consisted of at least one error code in the assignment of their secondary diagnosis codes. The highest error rate was among the cases that were assigned to code E78.5 (Hyperlipidaemia, unspecified), I25.9 (Chronic ischaemic heart disease, unspecified), N18.0 (End-stage renal disease), Z53.8 (Procedure not carried out for other reason) and I25.1 (Atherosclerotic heart disease). Evidently, from Table 4.32, none of the cases that were assigned to these 5 codes was assigned to an accurate secondary diagnosis code. On the contrary, in comparison to the number of cases assigned to the code, the lowest coding errors rate was among cases that were assigned to code Z51.1(Chemotherapy session for neoplasm). As notable in Table 4.37, the coding error rate among cases containing code Z51.1 as its secondary diagnosis code was only 66.7%.

It is also apparent in Table 4.32, from the 60 cases listed with the top 10 secondary diagnosis codes assigned after the re-coding process, 54 (90.0%) of the cases consisted of at least of one error secondary diagnosis codes. The highest coding error rate was among cases that contained code I12.0 (Hypertensive renal disease with renal failure), A41.9 (Sepsis, unspecified organism), I11.9 (Hypertensive heart disease without heart failure, J18.9 (Pneumonia, unspecified organism) and N17.9 (Acute kidney failure, unspecified) as its secondary diagnosis code. As it can be seen in the table, none of the cases that were assigned to these 5 codes was assigned to an accurate secondary diagnosis code.

Table 4.32 Comparisons of Top 10 Secondary Diagnosis Code Assigned within Medical Case-Type

No.	Before Re-Coding					After Re-Coding			
			n = 323	n = *			n = 517	n = **
	Codes	Description	Frequency (%)*	No. of Error Cases (%)	Codes	Description	Frequency (%)**	No. of Cases Without Coding Errors (%)
1.	I10	Essential [primary] hypertension	24 (7.4)	22 (91.7)	I10	Essential [primary] hypertension	24 (4.6)	1 (4.2)
2.	E11.9	Type 2 diabetes mellitus without complications	18 (5.6)	17 (94.4)	E11.9	Type 2 diabetes mellitus without complications	9 (1.7)	1 (11.1)
3.	E78.5	Hyperlipidaemia, unspecified	13 (4.0)	13 (100.0)	I12.0	Hypertensive renal disease with renal failure	6 (1.2)	0 (0.0)
4.	I25.9	Chronic ischaemic heart disease, unspecified	6 (1.9)	6 (100.0)	A41.9	Sepsis, unspecified organism	3 (0.6)	0 (0.0)
5.	Z51.1	Chemotherapy session for neoplasm	6 (1.9)	4 (66.7)	E86	Volume depletion	3 (0.6)	1 (33.3)
6.	E86	Volume depletion	5 (1.5)	4 (80.0)	I11.9	Hypertensive heart disease without heart failure	3 (0.6)	0 (0.0)
7.	I48	Atrial fibrillation and flutter	5 (1.5)	4 (80.0)	J18.9	Pneumonia, unspecified organism	3 (0.6)	0 (0.0)
8.	N18.0	End-stage renal disease	5 (1.5)	5 (100.0)	N17.9	Acute kidney failure, unspecified	3 (0.6)	0 (0.0
9.	Z53.8	Procedure not carried out for other reasons	5 (1.5)	5 (100.0)	T88.7	Unspecified adverse effect of drug or medicament	3 (0.6)	1 (33.3)
10.	I25.1	Atherosclerotic heart disease	4 (1.2)	4 (100.0)	Z51.1	Chemotherapy session for neoplasm	3 (0.6)	2 (66.7)

c. Coding Errors of Primary Procedure Code within Medical Case-Type

Data analysis from the present study indicates an increment in the number of cases assigned to primary procedure code within medical case-type. Prior the re-coding process by the Independent Senior Coder, there were 88 cases contained primary procedure code during their episode of care. Subsequently to the re-coding process, the number of cases that contained primary procedure code has increased to 95 cases.

In the first level of coding errors calculation, 65 (56.0%) of cases were found containing errors in the assignment of its primary procedure codes. In total, there were 112 codes reviewed by the Independent Senior Coder during the audit. From these 112 codes, 62 (77.7%) of the codes were the error codes.

i. Type of Coding Errors in the Assignment of Primary Procedure Code within Medical Case-Type

In the assignment of the primary procedure code, from the 112 codes reviewed by the Independent Senior Coder, 17 (15.2%) of the cases were being assigned to a wrong primary procedure code. The second highest type of errors was up-coding, whereby 15 (13.4%) of cases consisted of this type of coding error. The third highest type of coding error was due to under-coding, covering 11 (9.8%) of the error cases. Following this, the Independent Senior Coder has identified 7 (6.3%) of error cases with the error at the second digit level of the code. The error at the third and fourth digit level of the code was the fifth highest type of error, comprising of 12 (10.7%) of the error cases with 6 (5.4%) cases for each time of the error. The less common type of errors in the assignment of primary procedure code was due to the incorrect sequence of the primary procedure code, whereby 5 (4.5%) cases were found with this type of coding errors. Table 4.33 shows the distributions of the type of coding errors which occurred within the assignment of primary procedure codes among the medical type of cases.

Table 4.33 Distributions of the Type of Coding Errors within Primary Procedure Codes in Medical Case-Type

Type of Error	No. of Error Cases	%
Wrong Selection of Primary Procedure Code	17	15.2
Up-coding	15	13.4
Under-coding	11	9.8
Error at Second Digit Level	7	6.3
Error at Third Digit Level	6	5.4
Error at Fourth Digit Level	6	5.4
Principal Procedure Incorrectly Sequenced	5	4.5

ii. Comparisons of Top 10 Primary Procedure Code Assigned in Medical Case-Type Before and After the Re-Coding Process

Table 4.34 shows the comparisons of the top 10 primary procedure codes which were assigned to medical case-type before and after the re-coding process. As shown in Table 4.40, from the 10 listed codes before the audit, only 4 codes remained listed as the top 10 primary procedure codes assigned after the audit (87.44 (Routine chest x-ray so described, 87.03 (Computerized axial tomography of head), 99.25 (Injection or infusion of cancer chemotherapeutic substance) and 51.1 (Diagnostic procedure on biliary tract). This indicates a significant number of error cases in the assignment of primary procedure code among medical cases. This is proven by the bivariate analysis using the Cohen's Kappa test, where the level of agreement between the Independent Senior Coder and in-house coders in the assignment of primary procedure code among cases that were assigned to medical case-type was poor, with the kappa value of 0.010.

Among the cases that were assigned to medical case-type before the audit, 52 cases were assigned to the top 10 primary procedure codes. From these 52 cases, 35 (67.3%) of the cases were assigned to a wrong primary procedure code before the audit. The highest coding error rates involved cases that were assigned to codes 88.79 (Other diagnostic ultrasound) and 99.04 (Transfusion of packed cells). As apparent in Table 4.40, all of the cases that were assigned to code 88.79 and 99.04 before the audit were assigned to a wrong primary procedure code by the in-house coders.

Table 4.34 Comparisons of Top 10 Primary Procedure Code Assigned Before and After the Audit within Medical Case-Type

	Before Re-Coding Process				After Re-Coding Process			
			n = 88	n = *			n = 95	n = **
No.	Codes	Description	Frequency (%)*	No. of Error Cases (%)	Codes	Description	Frequency (%)**	No. of Cases Without Coding Errors (%)
1.	87.44	Routine chest x-ray, so described	12 (12.1)	9 (75.0)	87.03	Computerized axial tomography of head	7 (6.8)	6 (85.7)
2.	89.52	Electrocardiogram	9 (9.1)	7 (77.8)	99.25	Injection or infusion of cancer chemotherapeutic substance	7 (6.8)	4 (57.1)
3.	87.03	Computerized axial tomography of head	7 (7.1)	1 (14.3)	87.44	Routine chest x-ray, so described	5 (4.9)	2 (40.0)
4.	99.25	Injection or infusion of cancer chemotherapeutic substance	7 (7.1)	7 (85.7)	88.72	Diagnostic ultrasound of heart	4 (3.9)	1 (25.0)
5.	51.1	Diagnostic procedures on biliary tract	4 (4.0)	2 (50.0)	18.11	Otoscopy	3 (2.9)	0 (0.0)
6.	45.13	Other endoscopy of small intestine	3 (3.0)	1 (33.3)	51.1	Diagnostic procedures on biliary tract	3 (2.9)	2 (66.7)
7.	88.79	Other diagnostic ultrasound	3 (3.0)	3 (100.0)	86.04	Other incision with drainage of skin and subcutaneous tissue	3 (2.9)	1 (33.3)
8.	99.04	Transfusion of packed cells	3 (3.0)	3 (100.0)	88.78	Diagnostic ultrasound of gravid uterus	3 (2.9)	0 (0.0)
9.	86.22	Excisional debridement of wound, infection, or burn	2 (2.0)	1 (50.0)	97.64	Removal of other urinary drainage device	3 (2.9)	0 (0.0)
10.	88.01	Computerized axial tomography of abdomen	2 (2.0)	1 (50.0)	17.24	Laparoscopic bilateral repair of inguinal hernia with graft or prosthesis, not otherwise specified	2 (1.9)	0 (0.0)

k = 0.010 (p<0.001)

From Table 4.34, it is also revealed that, after the re-coding process, the number of cases listed in the top 10 primary procedure code has shown to have a decreasing pattern. From 53 cases before the re-coding process, the number was reduced to 40 cases after the re-coding process. Despite the decreasing number of cases listed in Table 4.34 after the re-coding process, the number of cases which consisted of primary procedure code increased from 88 cases to 95 cases. This reflects the Independent Senior Coder's higher knowledge than the in-house coder, where the Independent Senior Coder does not only use the common codes to codify the primary procedure phrase of the patients. It is also notable in Table 4.40, from the 40 cases that were assigned to the top 10 primary procedure codes assigned after the re-coding process, 24 (60.0%) of the cases were of the error cases, indicating a poor accuracy in the assignment of primary procedure code among medical cases.

As the result of the coding errors in the assignment of primary procedure code, Table 4.35 illustrates the changes which occurred among the error cases that were assigned to the top 10 primary procedure code assigned before the re-coding process. As apparent in the table, the commonest type of errors among the cases that were assigned to the top 10 primary procedure codes assigned before the re-coding process was the error at the fourth digit level of the code. From the 35 error cases, 11 (31.4%) of the error cases were assigned with a wrong selection of primary procedure code. Among these 11 cases, 3 (38.5%) of the cases were originally assigned to code 87.44 by the in-house coder. After the audit, these 3 cases were re-assigned to code 18.11 (Otoscopy), 58.5 (Release of urethral stricture) and 99.25 (Injection or infusion of cancer chemotherapeutic).

To sum it up, the quality of coding in the assignment of primary procedure code within the medical type of case was poor, with the kappa value of 0.010. From the 53 cases assigned to the top 10 primary procedure code assigned before the re-coding process, 35 (67.3%) of the cases were assigned to the wrong primary procedure code. Mostly these error cases were assigned to a wrong selection of primary procedure code. On the other hand, after the re-coding process, the number of cases assigned to the top 10 code has decreased to only 40 cases. More varieties of codes were assigned by the Independent Senior Coder proved a higher coding knowledge among the Independent Senior Coder than the in-house coder.

Table 4.35 Changes in the Assignment of Top 10 Highest Frequency Primary Procedure Code before the Audit within Medical Case-Type

No.	Before Re-Coding Process n =99			After Re-Coding Process n = *		
	Original Primary Procedure Code	No. of Cases* (%)	No. of Cases with Unchanged Primary Procedure Code (%)	Cases With New Primary Procedure Code due to Coding Error		
				New Primary Procedure Code	Description	No. Cases (%)
1.	87.44 (Routine chest x-ray, so described)	12 (12.1)	3 (25.0)	None	None	4 (3.3)
				18.11	Otoscopy	1 (8.3)
				58.5	Release of urethral stricture	1 (8.3)
				88.72	Diagnostic ultrasound of heart	1 (8.3)
				99.25	Injection or infusion of cancer chemotherapeutic	2 (16.7)
2.	89.52 (Electrocardiogram)	9 (9.1)	2 (22.2)	None	None	4 (44.4)
				87.44	Routine chest x-ray, so described	1 (11.1)
				88.72	Diagnostic ultrasound of heart	1 (11.1)
				99.04	Transfusion of packed cells	1 (11.1)
3.	87.03 (Computerized axial tomography of head)	7 (7.1)	6 (85.7)	57.94	Insertion of indwelling urinary catheter	1 (14.3)

#	Procedure	n (%)	Code	Sub-procedure	n (%)
4.	99.25 (Injection or infusion of cancer chemotherapeutic substance)	7 (7.1)	18.11	Otoscopy	1 (14.3)
			99.04	Transfusion of packed cells	1 (14.3)
			99.24	Injection of other hormone	4 (57.1)
			99.29	Injection or infusion of other therapeutic or prophylactic substance	1 (14.3)
5.	51.1 (Diagnostic procedures on biliary tract)	4 (4.0)	2 (50.0)	51.11	Endoscopic retrograde cholangiography [ERC]	1 (25.0)
			51.85	Endoscopic sphincterotomy and papillotomy	1 (25.0)
6.	45.13 (Other endoscopy of small intestine)	3 (3.0)	2 (66.7)	88.93	Magnetic resonance imaging of spinal canal	1 (33.3)
7.	88.79 (Other diagnostic ultrasound)	3 (3.0)	0 (0.0)	34.91	Thoracentesis	1 (33.3)
			57.94	Insertion of indwelling urinary catheter	1 (33.3)
			83.96	Injection of therapeutic substance into bursa	1 (33.3)
8.	99.04 (Transfusion of packed cells)	3 (3.0)	0 (0.0)	None	None	1 (33.3)
			87.41	Computerized axial tomography of thorax	1 (33.3)
			99.25	Injection or infusion of cancer chemotherapeutic	1 (33.3)
9.	86.22 (Excisional debridement of wound, infection, or burn)	2 (2.0)	1 (50.0)	86.28	Non-excisional debridement of wound, infection or burn	1 (50.0)
10.	88.01 (Computerized axial tomography of abdomen)	2 (2.0)	1 (50.0)	51.1	Otoscopy	1 (50.0)

d. Coding Errors in the Assignment of Secondary Procedure Code within Medical Case-Type

In the first level of coding error calculation within the secondary procedure codes, coding errors occurred in 67 (57.8%) of the selected cases. In total, there were 159 secondary procedure codes which were reviewed by the Independent Senior Coder. These reviewed codes were inclusive of all of the up-coding and under-coding codes. From these 159 reviewed codes, 131 (82.4%) of the codes were considered as error codes.

Before the re-coding process, the total number of secondary diagnosis codes assigned to the entire case was 81 codes and has grossly increased to 102 codes after the audit by the Independent Senior Coder. The maximum number of secondary procedure codes assigned to the patient was 4 codes, with the mean of 0.69 (SD 0.99). After the re-coding process, the maximum number of secondary procedure codes increased to 9 codes, with the mean of 0.78 (01.27). The level of agreement between the in-house coder and the Independent Senior Coder in the number of secondary procedure code assigned per patient was poor, with the kappa value of 0.176 (Table 4.36).

Table 4.36 Distributions of Total Number of Secondary Procedure Code Assigned to Patient Before and After the Re-Coding Process within Medical Case-Type

No. of Secondary Procedure Code	Before	After	Kappa value	p value
			0.176	<0.001
Total Nos of Code	81	102		
Max. Codes	4	9		
Mean (SD)	0.69 (0.99)	0.78 (1.27)		

i. Comparisons of Number of Secondary Procedure Code Before and After the Audit

From the 116 cases assigned under medical case type, 65 of the cases were unassigned to any secondary procedure code. From these 65 cases, 21 (18.1%) of the cases were identified as coding error cases. The coding error cases were the highest among cases with 3 and above secondary procedure codes, in which the percentage of error cases has reached 85.7%. A chi-square test was conducted to determine all the association between the number of secondary procedure codes and coding errors. The result was proven to be statistically insignificant, with the chi-square value of 3.709 and p value of 0.295 (Table 4.37).

Table 4.37 Distributions of Coding Errors Cases by Number of Secondary Procedure Code within Medical Case-Type

No. of Secondary Procedure Code	No. of Case without Coding Error	%	No. of Case with Coding Error/s	%	Total	%
0	43	67.2	21	32.8	64	100.0
1	10	29.4	24	70.6	34	100.0
2	2	18.2	9	81.8	11	100.0
3 and above	1	14.3	6	85.7	7	100.0

$X^2 = 3.709$, df $=3$, p $=0.295$

Table 4.38 shows the distributions of the number of secondary procedure codes assigned to a patient before and after the re-coding process. It is worth noting that due to the changes in the case-type of the case, cases listed before the re-coding process were not the same as after the audit. Thus the distribution of cases with or without coding errors was not necessary to be mutual before and after the audit.

Before the re-coding process was performed by the Independent Senior Coder, there were 64 (56.0%) cases that were unassigned to any secondary procedure codes. However after the re-coding process, from these 64 cases, only 43 (9.2%) of the cases remained to be unassigned to any secondary procedure codes after the re-coding process. From Table 4.38, it is notable that the maximum number of secondary procedure codes assigned to cases under the medical case-type was 4 codes. In total, there were 4 (3.4%) cases that were assigned to 4 secondary procedure codes before the re-coding process. However, interestingly, after the re-coding process, none of these 4 cases were assigned with the similar number of secondary procedure codes, in which 2 (50.0%) of the cases were assigned to a higher number of secondary procedure code and another 2 (50.0%) of the cases were assigned to a lower number of secondary procedure code.

On the contrary, after the re-coding process, the number of cases that were unassigned to any secondary procedure code has increased to 75 (57.7%) cases. From these 75 cases, 51 (68.0%) of the cases were originally unassigned to any secondary procedure and 24 (32.0%) of the cases were assigned to at least one secondary procedure code before the re-coding process. Among these 51 cases that were unassigned to any secondary procedure code after the audit, 43 (84.3%) of the cases were assigned to the similar case type as prior to the re-coding process, whereas 8 (15.7%) of the cases were assigned to a different case type prior the audit. It is also apparent from Table 4.38, that the highest number of secondary procedure codes assigned in cases assigned to medical case-type was 9 codes, covering 1 (0.8%) case. This 1 case was originally assigned to 4 secondary procedures prior the re-coding process.

Table 4.38 Comparison of Number of Secondary Procedure Code Assigned per Patient Before and After the Re-Coding Process within Medical Case-Type

		Before Re-Coding Process				After Re-Coding Process			
		n =116		n = *		n =130		n =**	
No	No. of Secondary Procedure Code	No. of Cases (%) *	No. of Cases Without Coding Errors (%)	No. of Errors Cases with Lower No of Secondary Procedure Code After Re-Coding Process (%)	No. of Errors Cases with Higher No of Secondary Procedure Code After Re-Coding Process (%)	No. of Secondary Procedure Code	No. of Cases (%)**	No. of Cases without Coding Errors (%)	No. of Errors Cases with Lower No of Secondary Procedure Code Before Re-Coding Process (%)	No. of Errors Cases with Higher No of Secondary Procedure Code Before Re-Coding Process (%)
1.	0	64 (56.0)	43 (9.2)	0 (0.0)	21 (32.8)	0	75 (57.7)	51 (68.0)	0 (0.0)	24 (32.0)
2.	1	34 (29.3)	10 (29.4)	17 (50.0)	7 (20.5)	1	30 (23.1)	10 (33.3)	16 (53.3)	4 (13.3)
3.	2	11 (9.5)	2 (18.2)	3 (27.3)	6 (54.5)	2	12 (9.2)	2 (16.7)	9 (75.0)	1 (8.3)
4.	3	3 (2.6)	1 (33.3)	1 (33.3)	1 (33.3)	3	9 (6.9)	1 (11.1)	7 (77.8)	1 (11.1)
5.	4	4 (3.4)	0 (0.0)	2 (50.0)	2 (50.0)	4	3 (2.3)	0 (0.0)	3 (100.0)	0 (0.0)
6.	9	N/A	N/A	N/A	N/A	9	1 (0.8)	0 (0.0)	1 (100.0)	0 (0.0)

Kappa value = 0.176, p <0.001

ii. Type of Coding Errors in the Assignment of Secondary Procedure Code within Medical Case-Type

Data analysis in the present study shows that the commonest type of error in the assignment of secondary procedure code within the medical type of case was under-coding. From the 159 secondary procedure codes reviewed by the Independent Senior Coder, 70 (44.0%) of the codes was under-coded by the in-house coder. The second highest type of errors found within the secondary procedure codes was up-coding. It was revealed that in the assignment of secondary procedure code, the number of up-coding cases has reached 23 (14.5%). The wrong selection of secondary procedure code was the third highest type of error, in which 17 (10.7%) of error cases were due to this type of coding error. The fourth highest type of error in the assignment of secondary procedure within the medical type of case was the error at the third digit level, in which 5 (3.1%) cases were reported with this type of error. In the assignment of the secondary procedure code within the medical type of case, the less common type of errors was the error at the fourth digit level of the code. There were only 3 (1.9%) cases reported which contained this type of error in their assignment of secondary procedure code. The details on the types of coding errors in the assignment of the secondary procedure code are as illustrated in Table 4.39.

Table 4.39 Distributions of Type of Coding Errors in Secondary Procedure Code within Medical Case-Type

Type of Error	No. of Error Cases	%
Under-coding	70	44.0
Up-coding	23	14.5
Wrong Selection of Secondary Procedure Code	17	10.7
Error at Second Digit Level	13	8.2
Error at Third Digit Level	5	3.1
Error at Fourth Digit Level	3	1.9

iii. Comparisons of Top 10 Secondary Procedure Code Assigned Before and After the Re-Coding Process within Medical Case-Type

Table 4.40 shows the comparisons of the top 10 secondary procedure codes assigned before and after the re-coding process for medical type cases. From the table it was understood that in total there were four codes that were listed before the re-coding process that remained listed even after the re-coding process, namely codes 89.52 (Electrocardiogram), 99.04 (Transfusion of packed cells), 88.72 (Diagnostic ultrasound of heart) and 39.95 (Haemodialysis).

As presented in Table 4.40, prior to the re-coding process, there were 52 cases listed in the table. Among these 52 cases, 47 (90.4%) of the cases contained at least one error code in the assignment of its secondary procedure code. It is also notable in Table 4.48 that the highest errors rate involved cases that contain the codes 87.03 (Computerized axial tomography of head), 88.72, 93.9 (Other physical therapy), 75.34 (Other fetal monitoring), 88.01 (Computerized axial tomography of abdomen) and 88.19 (Other x-ray abdomen) as its secondary procedure codes. Apparently, none of the cases contained these codes as its secondary procedure code and was assigned to accurate secondary procedure codes by the in-house coder.

On the other hand, after the re-coding process, the number of cases assigned to the top 10 secondary procedure codes after the re-coding process has increased to 62 cases. However, the coding error cases among these 62 cases were exceptionally high covering up to 57 (91.9%) cases. The highest number of coding error cases involved cases that contained code 57.94 (Insertion of indwelling urinary catheter) as its secondary procedure code. It is apparent in Table 4.48, all of these 12 cases that were assigned to code 57.94 as its secondary procedure code after the re-coding process contained at least one error for its secondary diagnosis codes. Besides that, cases that were assigned to the codes 97.64 (Removal of other urinary drainage device), 88.72, 88.79 (Other diagnostic ultrasound), 88.75 (Diagnostic ultrasound of urinary system) and also 88.74 (Diagnostic ultrasound of digestive system) also contained at least one error for its secondary diagnosis code.

Table 4.40 Comparisons of Top Secondary Procedure Code Assigned within Medical Case-Type

		Before Re-Coding Process				After Re-Coding Process		
		n = 81	n =*			n = 102	n =**	
No.	Codes	Description	Frequency (%)*	No. of Error Cases (%)	Codes	Description	Frequency (%)**	No. of Cases Without Coding Errors (%)
1.	87.44	Routine chest x-ray, so described	17 (21.0)	16 (94.1)	57.94	Insertion of indwelling urinary catheter	12 (11.8)	0 (0.0)
2.	89.52	Electrocardiogram	9 (11.1)	7 (77.8)	99.04	Transfusion of packed cells	12 (11.8)	1 (8.3)
3.	99.04	Transfusion of packed cells	7 (8.6)	6 (85.7)	97.64	Removal of other urinary drainage device	9 (8.8)	0 (0.0)
4.	87.03	Computerized axial tomography of head	4 (4.9)	4 (100.0)	39.95	Haemodialysis	5 (4.9)	1 (20.0)
5.	88.72	Diagnostic ultrasound of heart	4 (4.9)	4 (100.0)	88.72	Diagnostic ultrasound of heart	5 (4.9)	0 (0.0)
6.	93.39	Other physical therapy	3 (3.7)	3 (100.0)	88.79	Other diagnostic ultrasound	5 (4.9)	0 (0.0)
7.	39.95	Haemodialysis	2 (2.5)	1 (50.0)	89.52	Electrocardiogram	5 (4.9)	2 (40.0)
8.	75.34	Other fetal monitoring	2 (2.5)	2 (100.0)	88.75	Diagnostic ultrasound of urinary system	4 (3.9)	0 (0.0)
9.	88.01	Computerized axial tomography of abdomen	2 (2.5)	2 (100.0)	88.74	Diagnostic ultrasound of digestive system	3 (2.9)	0 (0.0)
10.	88.19	Other x-ray of abdomen	2 (2.5)	2 (100.0)	51.87	Endoscopic insertion of stent (tube) into bile duct	2 (2.0)	1 (50.0)

4.4.2 Coding Errors of Surgical Case-Type

Coding errors cases detected within surgical case-type was the lowest among the other case-types in which the number of error cases was 96 (82.8%) cases. Among the surgical cases, the coding errors were mostly high in the assignment of its secondary diagnosis code covering up to 87 (75.0%) cases. Fewer errors were found in the assignment of the primary diagnosis code, where the numbers of error cases were only 47 (40.5%) cases. Table 4.491 summarised the distributions of the coding error cases that were assigned to the surgical case type by the coding item.

Table 4.41 Distributions of Coding Error Cases by Coding Item in Surgical Case-Type

Coding Items	Total Case Reviewed	No. of Cases without Coding Error (%)	No of Cases with Coding Error/s (%)	Kappa Value	p value
Primary Diagnosis	116	69 (59.6)	47 (40.5)	0.581	<0.001
Secondary Diagnosis	116	29 (25.0)	87 (75.0)	0.171	<0.001
Primary Procedure	116	58 (50.0)	58 (50.0)	0.022	<0.001
Secondary Procedure	116	40 (24.5)	76 (65.5)	0.145	<0.001

Cohen's Kappa Test was conducted to determine the level of agreement between the in-house coder and Independent Senior Coder in the assignment of codes among the cases assigned to surgical case-type. The output of the kappa test showed that among the surgical cases, the assignment of primary procedure code was more likely to be an error-prone process compared to the primary diagnosis code (kappa value 0.022 vs. 0.581). On the other hand, for secondary diagnosis code and secondary procedure code, although the number of error cases is higher among secondary diagnosis code than the secondary procedure code (75.0% vs. 65.5%), the number of secondary procedure code was most likely to be codified wrongly by the in-house coder compared to the number of secondary diagnosis code assigned per episode of care (kappa value: 0.145 vs. 0.171).

a. **Coding Errors of Primary Diagnosis Code within Surgical Case-Type**

In surgical case-type, at the first level of coding error calculation within the primary diagnosis codes, the coding errors occurred in 47 (40.5%) of the selected cases. The second level of coding error calculation within the primary diagnosis codes were also showed to have the same percentage of errors; 40.5% in respect to the similar number of the denominator in both levels of calculations (n=116).

i. **Type of Coding Errors of Primary Diagnosis within Surgical Case-Type**

In the assignment of the primary diagnosis code, most of the codes were assigned to a wrong selection of primary diagnosis code comprising of 17 (14.7%) of the error cases. The second highest type of errors was the error at the third digit level of the code, in which 11 (9.5%) of cases contained this type of coding errors. The third highest type of coding errors was the error at the fourth digit level of the code covering 10 (8.6%) of the error cases. In addition to that, the Independent Senior Coder has identified 5 (4.3%) cases which consisted of the error at the second digit level of the code. The less common type of error detected in the surgical type of case in the assignment of primary diagnosis code was primary diagnosis being incorrectly sequenced, in which 4 (3.4%) of cases were found with this type of error (Table 4.42).

Table 4.42 Distribution of Type of Coding Errors Among Primary Diagnosis Code in Surgical Case-Type

Type of Error	No. of Error Cases	%
Wrong Selection of Primary Diagnosis Code	17	14.7
Error at Third Digit Level	11	9.5
Error at Fourth Digit Level	10	8.6
Error at Second Digit Level	5	4.3
Primary Diagnosis Code Incorrectly Sequenced	4	3.4

ii. Top 10 Primary Diagnosis Codes Assigned Before and After The Re-Coding Process within Surgical Case-Type

Table 4.43 shows the comparisons of the top 10 primary diagnosis codes assigned before and after the re-coding process in surgical cases. It is notable in Table 4.43 that the code with the highest frequency assigned before and after the re-coding process is associated with Cataract. As it is also apparent in Table 4.43, from the 10 codes listed before the re-coding process, there were 6 codes that still remained listed after the re-coding process, namely codes K35.0 (Acute appendicitis with generalized peritonitis), K35.9 (Acute appendicitis, unspecified), O03.4 (Incomplete spontaneous abortion without complication), H27.0 (Aphakia), N20.0 (Calculus of Kidney) and D25.9 (Leiomyoma of uterus, unspecified). This implies a moderate agreement between the Independent Senior Coder and the in-house coder in the assignment of primary diagnosis code for surgical cases. This is proven by the bivariate analysis using Cohen's Kappa test, with a kappa value of 0.581.

As notable in Table 4.43, prior to the re-coding process performed by the Independent Senior Coder, there were 35 cases assigned to the top 10 highest primary diagnosis codes. From these 35 cases, 15 (42.9%) of the cases consisted a wrong primary diagnosis code. The highest coding errors rate were involving cases that were assigned to codes H25.9 (Senile Cataract, unspecified) and C20 (Malignant neoplasm of rectum) prior to the re-coding process. Apparently, all of the cases that were assigned to this two codes before the commencement of this study were assigned wrongly by the in-house coder.

After the re-coding process, it is apparent as shown in Table 4.43 that the number of cases listed in the top 10 primary diagnosis codes has decreased from 35 cases to 31 cases. The decreasing number of cases listed in Table 4.43 after the re-coding process due to the decrement of the total number of cases assigned to surgical case-type after the re-coding process. It is also notable from Table

4.43 that from the 31 cases listed after the re-coding process, 13 (41.9%) of the cases were originally assigned to a wrong primary diagnosis code. The highest coding errors rate was involving cases that were assigned to codes K35.0 (Acute appendicitis with generalized peritonitis), O034 (Incomplete spontaneous abortion without complication), D25.9 (Leimyomama of uterus, unspecified) and H27.0 (Aphakia) in which the coding errors rate for this cases were 100.0%.

On the other hand, Table 4.44 shows the consequences of the coding errors in the distributions of primary diagnosis code in cases that were assigned to surgical case-type. It is notable from the table that the commonest type of coding errors among these cases was errors at the third digit level of the code. From the 15 error cases, 5 (33.3%) of the cases were assigned with a wrong primary diagnosis code at the third digit level of the codes. Most of the error cases at the third digit level of the code were originally assigned to code H25.9 (Senile Cataract, unspecified). After the re-coding process, 4 (80.0%) out of 5 cases that were assigned to code H25.9 before the audit were re-assigned to codes H26.9 (Cataract, unspecified) and H28.0 (Diabetic cataract) with 2 cases for each code.

Table 4.43 Top Primary Diagnosis Code Assigned Before and After Re-Coding Process within Surgical Case-Type

		Before Re-Coding Process			After Re-Coding Process			
			n = 116	n = *			n = 100	n = **
No.	Codes	Description	Frequency (%)*	No. of Error Cases (%)	Codes	Description	Frequency (%)**	No. of Cases With Unchanged Primary Diagnosis Code (%)
1.	H25.9	Senile Cataract, Unspecified	5 (4.3)	5 (100.0)	H26.9	Cataract, unspecified	5 (5.0)	1 (20.0)
2.	K35.0	Acute appendicitis with generalized peritonitis	4 (3.4)	3 (75.0)	K35.9	Acute appendicitis, unspecified	5 (3.0)	4 (80.0)
3.	K35.9	Acute appendicitis, unspecified	4 (3.4)	0 (0.0)	C19	Malignant neoplasm of rectosigmoid junction	3 (3.0)	1 (33.3)
4.	N40	Hyperplasia of prostate	4 (3.4)	1 (25.0)	I25.1	Atherosclerotic heart disease	3 (3.0)	2 (66.7)
5.	O03.4	Incomplete spontaneous abortion without complication	4 (3.4)	0 (0.0)	K35.0	Acute appendicitis with generalized peritonitis	3 (3.0)	3 (100.0)
6.	O34.2	Maternal care due to uterine scar from previous surgery	4 (3.4)	2 (50.0)	N20.0	Calculus of Kidney	3 (3.0)	1 (33.3)
7.	H27.0	Aphakia	3 (2.6)	1 (33.3)	O03.4	Incomplete spontaneous abortion without complication	3 (3.0)	3 (100.0)
8.	N20.0	Calculus of Kidney	3 (2.6)	1 (33.3)	A41.0	Septicaemia due to staphylococcus aureus	2 (2.0)	0 (0.0)
9.	C20	Malignant neoplasm of rectum	2 (1.7)	2 (100.0)	D25.9	Leiomyoma of uterus, unspecified	2 (2.0)	2 (100.0)
10.	D25.9	Leiomyoma of uterus, unspecified	2 (1.7)	0 (0.0)	H27.0	Aphakia	2 (2.0)	2 (100.0)

Kappa Value = 0.581, p <0.001

Table 4.44 Changes in the Top 10 Primary Diagnosis Code Assigned Before the Re-Coding Process in Surgical Case-Type

No.	Before Re-Coding Process n =116			After Re-Coding Process n = *		
	Original Primary Diagnosis Code	No. of Cases* (%)	No. of Cases with Unchanged Primary Diagnosis Code (%)	Cases With New Primary Diagnosis Code due to Coding Error		
				New Primary Diagnosis Code	Description	No. Cases of (%)
1.	H25.9 (Senile Cataract, Unspecified)	5 (4.3)	0 (0.0)	H26.9	Cataract, unspecified	2 (40.0)
				H28.0	Diabetic cataract	2 (40.0)
				N20.0	Calculus of kidney	1 (20.0)
2.	K35.0 (Acute appendicitis with generalized peritonitis)	4 (3.4)	1 (25.0)	K35.9	Acute appendicitis, unspecified	3 (75.0)
3.	K35.9 (Acute appendicitis, unspecified)	4 (3.4)	4 (100.)	NIL	NIL	NIL
4.	N40 (Hyperplasia of prostate)	4 (3.4)	3 (75.0)	Z43.5	Attention to cystostomy	1 (25.0)
5.	O03.4 (Incomplete spontaneous abortion without complication)	4 (3.4)	4 (100.0)	NIL	NIL	NIL
6.	O34.2 (Maternal care due to uterine scar from previous surgery)	4 (3.4)	2 (50.0)	O75.7	Vaginal delivery following previous caesarean section	2 (50.0)
7.	H27.0 (Aphakia)	3 (2.6)	2 (66.3)	H27.1	Dislocation of lens	1 (33.3)
8.	N20.0 (Calculus of Kidney)	3 (2.6)	2 (66.3)	H28.0	Diabetic cataract	1 (33.3)
9.	C20 (Malignant neoplasm of rectum)	2 (1.7)	0 (0.0)	C19	Malignant neoplasm of rectosigmoid junction	1 (33.3)
				K63.1	Perforation of intestine (nontraumatic)	1 (33.3)
10.	D25.9 (Leiomyoma of uterus, unspecified)	2 (1.7)	2 (100.0)	NIL	NIL	NIL

b. Coding Errors in Secondary Diagnosis Code Within Surgical Case-Type

For surgical cases, prior to the re-coding process, there were 74 cases that were assigned to at least one secondary diagnosis code. After the re-coding process, despite the decreasing number of cases assigned to the surgical case-type, the number of cases with secondary diagnosis code has increased to 90 cases. During the first level of coding error calculation within the secondary diagnosis codes, coding errors occurred in 87 (75.0%) of the selected cases. In total, there were 371 secondary diagnosis codes reviewed by the Independent Senior Coder during the audit within surgical cases. From these 371 codes, 267 (72.0%) of the codes were considered as error codes by the Independent Senior Coder.

Prior to the re-coding process, the total number of codes assigned as secondary diagnosis code among the surgical case-type were 202 codes and have grossly increased to 367 codes after the re-coding process. Before the re-coding process, the maximum number of codes assigned per patient was 10 codes, with the mean of 1.74 (SD: 1.98). After the audit, the maximum number of codes assigned per patient has increased dramatically to 18 codes, with the mean of 3.67 (SD: 3.22). The level of agreement between the Independent Senior Coder and in-house coder on the number of secondary diagnosis code assigned per patient was tested using Cohen's Kappa test and the result showed poor agreement with the kappa value of 0.171 (Table 4.45).

Table 4.45 Distributions of the Number of Secondary Diagnosis Codes Assigned Before and After the Re-Coding Process within Surgical Case-Type

No. of Secondary Diagnosis Code	Before	After	Kappa value	p value
			0.171	<0.001
Total No. of Code	202	367		
Max. Codes	10	18		
Mean (SD)	1.74 (1.98)	3.67 (3.22)		

i. **Comparisons of Number of Secondary Diagnosis Code Assigned per Patient Before and After the Re-Coding Process in Surgical Case-Type**

Table 4.46 shows the comparisons of the number of secondary diagnosis codes assigned per patient before and after the re-coding process was performed by the Independent Senior Coder for the surgical type of cases.

As seen in Table 4.46, in total there were 42 (36.2%) cases that were unassigned to any secondary diagnosis code before the audit. After the re-coding process, from these 42 cases, only 13 (31.0%) of the cases remained unassigned to any secondary diagnosis code. The remaining 29 cases (69.0%) were re-assigned to at least one secondary diagnosis codes after the audit. On the other hand, after the re-coding process, in total there were only 10 (1.0%) cases that were unassigned to any secondary diagnosis code. Data analysis showed that all of these 10 cases were also originally unassigned to any secondary diagnosis code before the re-coding process was performed by the Independent Senior Coder.

Before the re-coding process, the maximum number of secondary diagnosis codes assigned to patients in surgical case type was 10 codes with the number of the case was 1 (0.9%). However, after the audit, this case was re-assigned to a higher number of secondary diagnosis codes by the Independent Senior Coder. As illustrated in Table 4.46, after the audit, in total there were 6 (6.0%) cases that were assigned to 10 and more secondary diagnosis codes. The maximum number of secondary diagnosis codes assigned to the surgical patient after the re-coding process was 18 codes.

Table 4.47 shows the distribution of coding error cases by the number of secondary diagnosis codes. From the table, it could be derived that the percentage of coding error is the highest among cases with 4 and above secondary diagnosis codes (100.0%). A chi-square test was run to determine the association between the number of the secondary diagnosis code and coding errors. The result was statistically insignificant with $X^2 (4) = 6.470$, $p > 0.05$.

Table 4.46 Comparisons of Number of Secondary Diagnosis Code Assigned per Patient Before and After the Re-Coding Process in Surgical Case-Type

No.	Nos of Secondary Diagnosis Code	Before Re-Coding Process				After Re-Coding Process			
		n =116	n = *			n = 100	n = **		
		Nos of Cases (%) *	Nos of Cases with Similar No of Secondary Diagnosis Code After Re-Coding Process (%)	Nos of Cases With Lower No of Secondary Diagnosis Code After Re-Coding Process (%)	Nos of Cases With Higher No of Secondary Diagnosis Code After Re-Coding Process (%)	Nos of Cases (%) **	Nos of Cases with Similar No of Secondary Diagnosis Code After Re-Coding Process (%)	Nos of Cases With Lower No of Secondary Diagnosis Code Before Re-Coding Process (%)	Nos of Cases With Higher No of Secondary Diagnosis Code Before Re-Coding Process (%)
1.	0	42 (36.2)	13 (31.0)	0 (0.0)	29 (69.0)	10 (1.0)	10 (100.0)	0 (0.0)	0 (0.0)
2.	1	21 (18.1)	9 (42.9)	0 (0.0)	12 (57.1)	17 (17.0)	9 (52.9)	6 (35.3)	2 (11.8)
3.	2	20 (17.2)	9 (45.0)	2 (10.0)	9 (45.0)	16 (16.0)	7 (43.8)	9 (56.2)	0 (0.0)
4.	3	14 (12.1)	5 (35.7)	0 (0.0)	9 (64.3)	15 (15.0)	4 (26.6)	10 (66.7)	1 (6.7)
5.	4	8 (6.9)	2 (25.0)	2 (25.0)	4 (50.0)	12 (12.0)	1 (8.3)	9 (75.0)	2 (16.7)
6.	5	6 (5.2)	3 (50.0)	2 (33.3)	1 (16.7)	9 (9.0)	2 (22.2)	7 (77.8)	0 (0.0)
7.	6	2 (1.7)	1 (50.0)	1 (50.0)	0 (0.0)	7 (7.0)	0 (0.0)	7 (100.0)	0 (0.0)
8.	7	1 (0.9)	0 (0.0)	1 (100)	0 (0.0)	4 (4.0)	0 (0.0)	1 (100.0)	0 (0.0)
9.	8	1 (0.9)	0 (0.0)	0 (0.0)	1 (50.0)	1 (1.0)	0 (0.0)	1 (100.0)	0 (0.0)
10.	10	1 (0.9)	0 (0.0)	0 (0.0)	1 (100.0)	3 (3.0)	0 (0.0)	3 (100.0)	0 (0.0)
11.	10 and above	N/A	N/A	N/A	N/A	6 (6.0)	0 (0.0)	6 (100.0)	0 (0.0)

k= 0.171, p < 0.001

Table 4.47 Distributions of Coding Errors Cases by Number of Secondary Diagnosis Codes in Surgical Case-Type

No. of Secondary Diagnosis Code	No. of Case without Coding Error	%	No. of Case with Coding Error/s	%	Total	%
0	7	16.7	35	83.3	42	100.0
1	4	19.0	17	81.0	21	100.0
2	6	30.0	14	70.0	20	100.0
3	3	21.4	11	78.6	14	100.0
4 and above	0	0.0	19	100.0	19	100.0

$X^2 = 6.470$, df =4, p =0.167

ii. Type of Coding Errors in the Assignment of Secondary Procedure Code within Surgical Case-Type

Data analysis in the present study shows that the commonest type of error in the assignment of the secondary procedure code within the surgical type of cases was under-coding. From the 371 secondary procedure codes reviewed by the Independent Senior Coder, 174 (46.9%) of the codes was being undercoded by the in-house coder. The second highest type of errors found within the secondary procedure codes was the error at the first digit level, with the number of error code of 24 (6.5%) codes. The error at the third digit level was the third highest type of error in which 23 (6.2%) of error codes were due to this type of error. The fourth highest type of error in the assignment of the secondary procedure within surgical case type was the error at the fourth digit level in which 21 (5.7%) error codes were reported with this type of error. Following this, in total there were 13 (3.5%) up-coded codes identified in the assignment of the secondary diagnosis in cases that were assigned to surgical case type. Lastly, the less common type of errors was the error at the second digit level of the code. There were only 12 (3.2%) codes reported with this type of error in their assignment of secondary procedure code. The details of the type of coding errors of the secondary procedure code among the surgical type of cases are illustrated in Table 4.48.

Table 4.48 Distributions of Type of Coding Errors in Secondary Procedure Code within Surgical Case-Type

Type of Error	No. of Error Cases	%
Under-coding	174	46.9
Wrong Selection of Secondary Procedure Code	24	6.5
Error at Third Digit Level	23	6.2
Error at Fourth Digit Level	21	5.7
Up-coding	13	3.5
Error at Second Digit Level	12	3.2

iii. Comparisons of Top 10 Secondary Diagnosis Code Assigned Before and After the Re-Coding Process within Surgical Case-Type

Table 4.60 shows the comparison of the top 10 secondary diagnosis codes assigned before and after the re-coding process. From Table 4.60, it is apparent that the highest frequency for secondary diagnosis code before and after the re-coding process was for the code I10 (Essential [primary] hypertension). It is also worth noting that from the 10 codes listed before the re-coding process, there were only four codes that remained listed after the re-coding process namely codes I10 (Essential [primary] hypertension), E11.9 (Type 2 diabetes mellitus without complications), E78.5 (Hyperlipidaemia, unspecified) and D64.9 (Anaemia, unspecified). This implies a poor coding quality in the assignment of secondary diagnosis codes among the surgical cases.

From Table 4.60, it is notable that in total there were 72 cases which consists the top 10 secondary diagnosis codes assigned before the re-coding process. Subsequently, from these 72 cases, 60 (83.3%) of the cases contained at least one error for the secondary diagnosis code in it. The highest coding errors rate was among cases containing the codes Z37.0 (Single live birth), O82.0 (Delivery by elective caesarean section), Z30.2 (Sterilization), A41.9 (Sepsis, unspecified organism) and G47.3 (Sleep apnoea) as its secondary diagnosis code. The coding errors rate among these cases which contained these five codes were 100.0%, in which none of the cases was codified with the accurate secondary diagnosis codes.

On the other hand, after the re-coding process there were 71 cases in total that were listed in the top 10 secondary diagnosis codes. From these 71 cases, 59 (83.0%) of the cases contained at least one error for its secondary diagnosis code. The highest coding errors rate involved cases that contain the codes Z86.7 (Personal history of diseases of the circulatory system) and I12.0 (Hypertensive renal disease with renal failure) in the assignment of its secondary diagnosis code after the re-coding process. It is apparent from Table 4.60 that none of the cases contained these two codes was codified with accurate secondary diagnosis code by the in-house coder before the re-coding process was performed by the Independent Senior Coder.

It is also notable that the code E11.9 was found to be the second highest frequency for the secondary diagnosis code, both for before and after the re-coding process. Before the re-coding process, there were 14 (6.9%) cases that were assigned to the code E11.9 as its secondary diagnosis code. Among these 14 cases, 12 (85.7%) of the cases were among the error cases. Even though code E11.9 remained as the second highest frequency secondary diagnosis code, the number of cases that were assigned to this code has decreased to 11 (3.0%) after the re-coding process performed by the Independent Senior Coder. Among these 11 cases assigned to code E11.9 as its secondary diagnosis code, only 2 (18.9%) of the cases were codified without any coding errors.

Even though the total number of cases assigned to surgical case type has decreased after the re-coding process, the total number of secondary diagnosis code has increased dramatically from 202 codes before the re-coding process to 367 codes after the re-coding process. The increasing pattern of the number of secondary diagnosis codes assigned to cases for the surgical cases is parallel with the most common type of errors identified within this case type namely undercoding.

Table 4.49 Comparisons of Top 10 Secondary Diagnosis Code within Surgical Case-Type

		Before Re-Coding Process			After Re-Coding Process			
			n = 202	n = *			n = 367	n = **
No.	Codes	Description	Frequency (%) *	No. of Error Cases (%)	Codes	Description	Frequency (%) **	No. of Cases Without Coding Errors (%)
1.	I10	Essential [primary] hypertension	24 (11.9)	19 (79.2)	I10	Essential [primary] hypertension	27 (7.4)	4 (14.8)
2.	E11.9	Type 2 diabetes mellitus without complications	14 (6.9)	12 (85.7)	E11.9	Type 2 diabetes mellitus without complications	11 (3.0)	2 (18.2)
3.	Z37.0	Single live birth	9 (4.5)	9 (100.0)	E78.8	Other disorders of lipoprotein metabolism	9 (2.5)	1 (11.1)
4.	E78.5	Hyperlipidaemia, unspecified	7 (3.5)	4 (57.1)	I25.9	Chronic ischemic heart disease, unspecified	6 (1.6)	1 (11.1)
5.	O82.0	Delivery by elective caesarean section	4 (2.0)	4 (100.0)	D64.9	Anaemia, unspecified	5 (1.4)	1 (20.0)
6.	Z30.2	Sterilization	4 (2.0)	4 (100.0)	Z86.7	Personal history of diseases of the circulatory system	5 (1.4)	0 (0.0)
7.	D64.9	Anaemia, unspecified	3 (1.5)	2 (66.7)	E14.9	Unspecified diabetes mellitus without complications	4 (1.1)	1 (25.0)
8.	N40	Hyperplasia of prostate	3 (1.5)	2 (66.7)	E78.5	Hyperlipidaemia, unspecified	4 (1.1)	1 (25.0)
9.	A41.9	Sepsis, unspecified organism	2 (1.0)	2 (100.0)	I12.0	Hypertensive renal disease with renal failure	4 (1.1)	0 (25.0)
10.	G47.3	Sleep apnoea	2 (1.0)	2 (100.0)	J45.9	Asthma, unspecified	4 (1.1)	1 (25.0)

c. Coding Errors of Primary Procedure Code within Surgical Case-Type

Prior to the re-coding process performed by the Independent Senior Coder, from the 116 cases assigned to the surgical cases type, 114 (98.3%) of the cases contained a primary procedure code. After the re-coding process, from the 100 cases assigned to surgical case type, all of the cases consisted of a primary procedure code.

In the first level of the calculation of coding errors in the assignment of the primary procedure within the surgical cases, 58 (50.0%) of the cases were identified as error cases. In total, there were 114 primary procedure codes reviewed by the Independent Senior Coder during the re-coding process. From these 114 codes, 58 (50.9%) of the codes were considered as error codes by the Independent Senior Coder.

i. Type of Coding Errors in the Assignment of Primary Procedure Code within Surgical Case-Type

In the assignment of the primary procedure code within the surgical type of cases, the highest type of errors was of the wrong selection of the primary procedure code, covering 24 (21.1%) of the error cases. The second highest type of errors was the error at the third digit level of the code in which the numbers of error cases have reached 10 (8.8%) cases. The numbers of cases with the error in the assignment of the second and third digit level of the code were mutual, with 9 (7.9%) error cases per each time of coding errors. The fifth highest type of error was wrong sequenced of primary procedure code comprising, 5 (4.4%) error cases. The least common type of errors in the assignment of primary procedure code was up-coding cases, with only 1 (0.9%) case that was found with this type of coding errors. Table 4.50 shows the distributions of the type of coding errors which occurred within the assignment of the primary procedure codes for the surgical type of case. As seen in the table, there are no under-coding cases identified during the assignment of primary procedure code within the surgical type of case.

Table 4.50 Distributions of the Type of Coding Errors within Primary Procedure Codes in Surgical Case-Type

Type of Error	No. of Error Cases	%
Wrong Selection of Primary Procedure Code	24	21.1
Error at Third Digit Level	10	8.8
Error at Second Digit Level	9	7.9
Error at Fourth Digit Level	9	7.9
Primary Procedure Code Incorrectly Sequenced	5	4.4
Up-coding	1	0.9

ii. Comparisons of Top 10 Primary Procedure Code in Surgical Case-Type Before and After the Re-Coding Process

Table 4.51 shows the comparisons of the top 10 primary procedure codes assigned before and after the re-coding process for the surgical type of cases. As shown in the table, from the 10 listed codes before the re-coding process, there were six codes that remained listed after the re-coding process was performed. The six codes are 69.02 (Dilation and curettage following delivery or abortion), 13.41 (Phacoemulsification and aspiration of cataract), 47.01 (Laparoscopic appendectomy), 47.09 (Other appendectomy), 75.69 (Repair of other current obstetric laceration) and 74.1 (Low cervical caesarean section). The level of agreement between the Independent Senior Coder and in-house coder in the assignment of primary procedure code was poor with the kappa value of 0.022.

From Table 4.51, it is notable that in total there were 39 cases listed in the top 10 primary procedure codes assigned before the re-coding process. Among these 39 cases, 37 (94.9%) of the cases were codified to a wrong primary procedure code before the re-coding process. From the 10 listed primary procedure codes, only two codes namely code 69.02 and 47.09 contained cases with accurate primary procedure code, whereas all the cases that were assigned to the remaining eight codes were codified to a wrong primary procedure code by the in-house coder.

On the other hand, after the re-coding process, in total there were 29 cases listed in the table for the top 10 for primary procedure codes assigned after the re-coding process. The lower number of cases listed in Table 4.51 after the re-coding process compared to the before the re-coding process was due to the decreasing of the number of cases assigned to the surgical case type in MY-DRG code. It is also notable from Table 4.51 that from the 29 listed cases after the re-coding process, 28 (96.6%) of the cases were codified with a wrong primary procedure code before the re-coding process.

Subsequent to the coding errors, Table 4.52 shows the changes in the assignment of primary procedure code of cases that were assigned to the top 10 for primary procedure code assigned before the re-coding process. As apparent in Table 4.52, the commonest type of coding errors identified among the error cases listed in the table was the wrong selection of primary procedure code. It is apparent from the table that, from the 37 error cases, 36 (97.3%) of the cases were assigned to a wrong selection of primary procedure code indicating an error at the first digit level of the code. The highest error was recorded among cases that were assigned to the code 69.02 (Dilation and curettage following delivery or abortion). From the 7 cases that were assigned to this code before the re-coding process, 6 (85.7%) of the cases were assigned to a wrong primary procedure code by the in-house coder.

Table 4.51 Comparisons of Top 10 Highest Frequency Primary Procedure Code Before and After the Re-Coding Process within Surgical Case-Type

		Before Re-Coding Process				After Re-Coding Process		
			n = 114	n =*			n = 100	n =**
No.	Codes	Description	Frequency (%) *	No. of Error Cases (%)	Codes	Description	Frequency (%) **	No. of Cases Without Coding Errors (%)
1.	69.02	Dilation and curettage following delivery or abortion	7 (6.1)	6 (85.7)	13.41	Phacoemulsification and aspiration of cataract	5 (5.0)	0 (0.0)
2.	13.41	Phacoemulsification and aspiration of cataract	5 (4.4)	5 (100.0)	47.09	Other appendectomy	5 (5.0)	1 (20.0)
3.	47.01	Laparoscopic appendectomy	4 (3.5)	4 (100.0)	47.01	Laparoscopic appendectomy	3 (3.0)	0 (0.0)
4.	47.09	Other appendectomy	4 (3.5)	3 (75.0)	69.02	Dilation and curettage following delivery or abortion	3 (3.0)	0 (0.0)
5.	60.18	Other diagnostic procedures on prostate and periprostatic tissue	4 (3.5)	4 (100.0)	74.1	Low cervical caesarean section	3 (3.0)	0 (0.0)
6.	75.69	Repair of other current obstetric laceration	4 (3.5)	4 (100.0)	49.01	Incision of perianal abscess	2 (2.0)	0 (0.0)
7.	74.1	Low cervical caesarean section	4 (3.5)	4 (100.0)	55.03	Percutaneous nephrostomy without fragmentation	2 (2.0)	0 (0.0)
8.	86.22	Excisional debridement of wound, infection, or burn	3 (2.6)	3 (100.0)	68.49	Other and unspecified total abdominal hysterectomy	2 (2.0)	0 (0.0)
9.	08.2	Excision or destruction of lesion or tissue of eyelid	2 (1.8)	2 (100.0)	69.52	Aspiration curettage following delivery or abortion	2 (2.0)	0 (0.0)
10.	13.71	Insertion of intraocular lens prosthesis at time of cataract extract	2 (1.8)	2 (100.0)	75.69	Repair of other current obstetric laceration	2 (2.0)	0 (0.0)

Kappa value = 0.022 p <0.001

Table 4.52 Changes Among the Top 10 Primary Procedure Code Assigned Among Surgical Case-Type due to Coding Errors

No.	Before Re-Coding Process n =116			After Re-Coding Process n = *		
	Original Primary Procedure Code	Nos of Cases* (%)	Nos of Cases with Unchanged Primary Procedure Code (%)	Cases With New Primary Procedure Code due to Coding Error		
				New Primary Procedure Code	Description	Nos Cases (%)
1.	69.02 (Dilation and curettage following delivery or abortion)	7 (6.0)	1 (16.7)	10.2	Diagnostic Procedures On Conjunctiva	1 (16.7)
				47.1	Incidental appendectomy	1 (16.7)
				53.1	Other bilateral repair of inguinal hernia	1 (16.7)
				86.04	Other incision with drainage of skin and subcutaneous tissue	1 (16.7)
				86.22	Excisional debridement of wound, infection, or burn	1 (16.7)
				88.67	Phlebography of other specified sites using contrast material	1 (16.7)
2.	13.41 (Phacoemulsification and aspiration of cataract)	5 (4.4)	0 (0.0)	55.04	Percutaneous nephrostomy with fragmentation	2 (40.0)

#	Code	Procedure	n (%)	n (%)	Sub-code	Sub-procedure	n (%)
					69.02	Dilation and curettage following delivery or abortion	2 (40.0)
					88.38	Other computerized axial tomography	1 (20.0)
3.	47.01	(Laparoscopic appendectomy)	4 (3.5)	0 (0.0)	49.39	Other local excision or destruction of lesion or tissue of anus	1 (25.0)
					55.87	Correction of ureteropelvic junction	1 (25.0)
					88.38	Other computerized axial tomography	1 (25.0)
					97.64	Removal of other urinary drainage device	1 (25.0)
4.	47.09	(Other appendectomy)	4 (3.5)	1 (25.0)	38.6	Other excision of vessel	2 (50.0)
					69.02	Dilation and curettage following delivery or abortion	1 (25.0)
5.	60.18	(Other diagnostic procedures on prostate and periprostatic tissue)	4 (3.5)	0 (0.0)	17.13	Laparoscopic repair of inguinal hernia with graft or prosthesis, not otherwise specified	1 (25.0)
					47.01	Laparoscopic appendectomy	1 (25.0)
					57.33	Closed [transurethral] biopsy of bladder	1 (25.0)
					86.3	Other local excision or destruction of lesion or tissue of skin and subcutaneous tissue	1 (25.0)
6.	75.69	(Repair of other current obstetric laceration)	4 (3.5)	0 (0.0)	11.64	Other penetrating keratoplasty	1 (25.0)
					49.01	Incision of perianal abscess	1 (25.0)

7.	74.1 (Low cervical caesarean section)	4 (3.5)	0 (0.0)	86.04	Other incision with drainage of skin and subcutaneous tissue	1 (25.0)
				96.48	Irrigation of other indwelling urinary catheter	1 (25.0)
				13.7	Insertion of prosthetic lens [pseudophakia]	2 (50.0)
				1.39	Other incision of brain	1 (25.0)
				13.6	Other cataract extraction	1 (25.0)
8.	86.22 (Excisional debridement of wound, infection, or burn)	3 (2.6)	0 (0.0)	42.7	Esophagomyotomy	2 (66.7)
				69.52	Aspiration curettage following delivery or abortion	1 (33.3)
9.	08.2 (Excision or destruction of lesion or tissue of eyelid)	2 (1.8)	0 (0.0)	84.01	Amputation and disarticulation of finger	1 (50.0)
				85.21	Local excision of lesion of breast	1 (50.0)
10.	13.71 (Insertion of intraocular lens prosthesis at time of cataract extract)	2 (1.8)	0 (0.0)	74.1	Low cervical caesarean section	1 (50.0)
				97.64	Removal or other urinary drainage device	1 (50.0)

d. Coding Errors in the Assignment of Secondary Procedure Code within Surgical Case-Type

In the first level of coding error calculation within the secondary procedure codes in the surgical type of cases, coding errors occurred in 76 (65.5%) of the selected cases. In total, there were 216 secondary procedure codes reviewed by the Independent Senior Coder. These reviewed codes were inclusive of all of the upcoding and undercoding codes. From these 216 reviewed codes, 176 (81.5%) of the codes were considered as error codes.

Prior to the re-coding process, the total number of secondary diagnosis codes assigned to the entire case were 133 codes and has grossly increased to 213 codes after the re-coding process was performed by the Independent Senior Coder. The maximum number of secondary procedure codes assigned to the patient was 7, with the mean of 1.15 (SD 01.40). After the re-coding process, the maximum number of secondary procedure codes increased to 10 codes, with the mean of 2.13 (2.28). The level of agreement between the in-house coder and the Independent Senior Coder in the number of secondary procedure code assigned per patient was poor with the kappa value of 0.145 (Table 4.66).

Table 4.53 Distributions of Total Number of Secondary Procedure Code Assigned to Patient Before and After the Re-Coding Process within Surgical Case-Type

No. of Secondary Procedure Code	Before	After	Kappa value	p value
			0.145	<0.001
Total No. of Code	133	213		
Max. Codes	7	10		
Mean (SD)	1.15 (1.40)	2.13 (2.28)		

i. Comparison of Number of Secondary Procedure Code Before and After the Re-coding process

From the 116 cases selected under the surgical type of cases, 43 of the cases were unassigned to any secondary procedure code before the re-coding process was performed. From these 43 cases, 32 (74.4%) of the cases were identified as coding error cases. The coding error cases were the highest among cases with 3 and above secondary procedure code (91.7%). A chi-square test was conducted to determine the association between the number of secondary procedure code and the coding errors. The result was proven to be statistically insignificant with the $X^2(3) = 3.630$, p > 0.05 (Table 4.54).

Table 4.54 Distributions of Coding Errors Cases by Number of Secondary Procedure Code within Surgical Case-Type

No. of Secondary Procedure Code	No. of Case without Coding Error	%	No. of Case with Coding Error/s	%	Total	%
0	11	25.6	32	74.4	43	100.0
1	5	11.9	37	88.1	42	100.0
2	3	15.8	16	84.2	19	100.0
3 and above	1	8.3	11	91.7	12	100.0

$X^2 = 3.630$, df =3 p =0.304

Table 4.55 shows the distributions of cases that were assigned to the surgical case-type by the number of secondary procedure code assigned to the patient before and after the re-coding process. Before the re-coding process, there were 43 (37.1%) cases that were unassigned to any secondary procedure code. From these 43 cases, only 26 (9.2%) cases remained unassigned to any secondary procedure code after the re-coding process. The remaining 17 (39.5%) cases were re-assigned to at least one secondary procedure code after the audit.

From Table 4.55, it is also notable that before the re-coding process, the maximum number of secondary procedure code assigned to cases surgical cases was 7 codes. In total, there were 2 (1.7 %) cases that were assigned to 7 secondary procedure codes before the re-coding process. After the re-coding process from these 2 cases, only 1 (50.0%) case remained assigned to the 7 secondary procedures codes but this case has then been re-assigned to another case type after the re-coding process was performed by the Independent Senior Coder.

After the re-coding process, the number of cases that were unassigned to any secondary procedure code has decreased to 26 (26.0%) cases. From Table 4.55, the highest number of secondary procedure codes assigned among surgical cases was 10 codes. There was 1 (1.0%) case that was assigned to 10 secondary procedure codes after the re-coding process. Interestingly, this case was assigned to only 1 secondary procedure code before the re-coding process was performed by the Independent Senior Coder.

Table 4.55 Comparison of Number of Secondary Procedure Code Assigned per Patient Before and After the Re-Coding Process within Surgical Case-Type

No.	No. of Secondary Procedure Code	n =116 No. of Cases (%)*	Before Re-Coding Process			No. of Secondary Procedure Code	n =100 No. of Cases (%)**	After Re-Coding Process		
			No. of Cases Without Errors in the number of Secondary Procedure Code (%)	n = * No. of Errors Cases with Lower No of Secondary Procedure Code After Re-Coding Process (%)	No. of Errors Cases with Higher No of Secondary Procedure Code After Re-Coding Process (%)			No. of Cases Without Errors in the number of Secondary Procedure Code (%)	n = ** No. of Errors Cases with Lower No of Secondary Procedure Code Before Re-Coding Process (%)	No. of Errors Cases with Higher No of Secondary Procedure Code Before Re-Coding Process (%)
1.	0	43 (37.1)	26 (60.5)	0 (0.0)	17 (39.5)	0	26 (26.0)	21 (80.8)	0 (0.0)	5 (19.2)
2.	1	42 (36.2)	15 (35.7)	10 (23.8)	17 (40.5)	1	26 (26.0)	13 (50.0)	10 (38.5)	3 (11.5)
3.	2	19 (16.4)	5 (26.2)	7 (36.9)	7 (36.9)	2	17 (17.0)	5 (29.4)	11 (64.7)	1 (5.9)
4.	3	5 (4.3)	0 (0.0)	4 (80.0)	1 (20.0)	3	8 (8.0)	0 (0.0)	7 (87.5)	1 (12.5)
5.	4	2 (1.7)	0 (0.0)	0 (0.0)	2 (100.0)	4	9 (9.0)	0 (0.0)	8 (88.9)	1 (11.1)
6.	5	2 (1.7)	0 (0.0)	1 (50.0)	1 (50.0)	5	6 (6.0)	0 (0.0)	0 (0.0)	6 (100.0)
7.	6	1 (0.9)	0 (0.0)	1 (100.0)	0 (0.0)	6	1 (1.0)	0 (0.0)	0 (0.0)	1 (100.0)
8.	7	2 (1.7)	1 (50.0)	1 (50.0)	0 (0.0)	7	3 (3.0)	0 (0.0)	0 (0.0)	3 (100.0)
9.	8	N/A	N/A	N/A	N/A	8 and more	4 (4.0)	0 (0.0)	4 (100.0)	0 (0.0)

Kappa value = 0.145, p <0.001

To sum it up, among the surgical type of cases, the level of agreement between the in-house coder and the Independent Senior Coder in the assignment of the number of the secondary procedure code per patient was poor with the kappa value of 0.145. However, the chi-square result showed an insignificant relationship between the number of secondary procedure code assigned to the patient and coding errors with X^2 = 3.630, p >0.05. The highest number of secondary procedure assigned to a patient before the re-coding process was 7 codes. On the contrary, after the re-coding process was performed by the Independent Senior Coder, the number of cases assigned to 7 and more secondary procedure codes has increased to 7 cases, with 10 codes as the maximum number of secondary procedure codes assigned to a patient.

ii. Type of Coding Errors of Secondary Procedure Code within Surgical Case-Type

Data analysis in this study showed that the commonest type of error in the assignment of the secondary procedure code within cases that were assigned to surgical cases type was under-coding. From the 216 secondary procedure codes reviewed by the Independent Senior Coder, 93 (43.1%) of the codes were under-coded by the in-house coder. The second highest type of errors found within the secondary procedure codes was up-coding and wrong selection of the secondary procedure code covering 28 (13.0%) error cases for each type of errors. The error at the second digit level was the third highest type of error in which 14 (6.5%) of the error cases were due to these type errors. The fourth highest type of error in the assignment of secondary procedure within surgical cases was error at the fourth digit level, in which 7 (3.2%) cases were identified with this type of error. Lastly, the less common type of errors was the error at the third digit level of the code. There were only 6 (2.8%) cases reported which contained this type of error in their assignment of secondary procedure code.

The details on the types of coding errors in the assignment of secondary procedure code are illustrated in Table 4.69.

Table 4.56 Distributions of Type of Coding Errors in Secondary Procedure Code within Surgical Case-Type

Type of Error	No. of Error Cases	%
Under-coding	93	43.1
Up-coding	28	13.0
Wrong Selection of Secondary Procedure Code	28	13.0
Error at Second Digit Level	14	6.5
Error at Fourth Digit Level	7	3.2
Error at Third Digit Level	6	2.8

iii. Comparisons of Top 10 Secondary Procedure Code Assigned Before and After the Re-Coding Process within Surgical Case-Type

Table 4.57 below, shows the comparisons of the top 10 codes assigned as secondary procedure code before and after the re-coding process for the surgical type of cases. From the table, it was notable from the 10 listed codes before the re-coding process, there were 5 codes that remained listed after the re-coding process namely code 87.44 (Routine chest x-ray, so described), 89.2 (Electrodiagram), 13.71 (Insertion of intraocular lens prosthesis at time of cataract extraction, one stage), 39.95 (Haemodialysis) and 99.04 (Transfusion of packed cells. It is also apparent as shown in Table 4.57; the total number of secondary procedure codes has increased rapidly from 133 codes before the re-coding process to 213 codes after the re-coding process.

From Table 4.57, the total number of cases containing the top 10 secondary procedure was 62 cases before the re-coding process was carried out. Out of these 62 cases, 54 (87.1%) cases consisted of at least one error for the secondary procedure code. The highest coding errors rate was involving cases that contain the codes 66.39 (Other bilateral destruction or occlusion of fallopian tubes),

88.19 (Other x-ray abdomen), 90.99 (Microscopic examination of specimen from lower gastrointestinal tract and of stool, other microscopic examination) and 99.04 (Transfusion of packed cells). The error rates of cases containing these four secondary procedure codes were 100.0%.

Table 4.57 Comparisons of Top 10 Secondary Procedure Code Assigned within Surgical Case-Type

		Before Re-Coding Process				After Re-Coding Process		
		n = 133		n = *		n = 213		n = **
No.	Codes	Description	Frequency (%)*	No. of Error Cases (%)	Codes	Description	Frequency (%)**	No. of Cases Without Coding Errors (%)
1.	87.44	Routine chest x-ray, so described	13 (9.8)	12 (92.3)	57.94	Insertion of indwelling urinary catheter	16 (7.5)	0 (0.0)
2.	89.52	Electrocardiogram	12 (9.0)	11 (91.7)	97.64	Removal of other urinary drainage device	12 (5.6)	0 (0.0)
3.	75.34	Other fetal monitoring	7 (5.3)	6 (85.7)	99.04	Transfusion of packed cells	9 (4.2)	0 (0.0)
4.	13.71	Insertion of intraocular lens prosthesis at time of cataract extraction, one stage	6 (4.5)	2 (33.3)	88.79	Other diagnostic ultrasound	8 (3.8)	0 (0.0)
5.	66.39	Other bilateral destruction or occlusion of fallopian tubes	5 (3.8)	5 (100.0)	87.44	Routine chest x-ray, so described	7 (3.3)	1 (14.3)
6.	39.95	Haemodialysis	4 (3.0)	3 (75.0)	89.52	Electrocardiogram	7 (3.3)	1 (14.3)
7.	88.19	Other x-ray of abdomen	4 (3.0)	4 (100.0)	13.71	Insertion of intraocular lens prosthesis at time of cataract extract	6 (2.8)	3 (50.0)
8.	90.99	Microscopic examination of specimen from lower gastrointestinal tract and of stool, other microscopic examination	4 (3.0)	4 (100.0)	54.59	Other lysis of peritoneal adhesions	6 (2.8)	0 (0.0)
9.	99.04	Transfusion of packed cells	4 (3.0)	4 (100.0)	39.95	Haemodialysis	5 (2.3)	1 (20.0)
10.	69.09	Other dilation and curettage	3 (2.3)	3 (66.7)	88.72	Diagnostic ultrasound of heart	4 (1.9)	0 (0.0)

On the contrary, after the re-coding process, the number of cases listed on the top 10 highest frequency for the secondary procedure codes was 80 cases. From these 80 cases, 74 (92.5%) of the cases contained at least one error in its secondary procedure code. It is notable, as shown in Table 4.57, that only cases that contained codes 87.44, 89.52, 13.71 and 39.95 (Haemodialysis) as its secondary procedure code after the re-coding process was codified accurately by the in-house coder.

4.4.3 Coding Errors of O&G Case-Type

Coding error cases detected among O&G case-type was the highest among other case types, covering 110 (94.8%) error cases. In this case-type, the coding errors were mostly high in the assignment of its secondary diagnosis code, which covers 108 (93.1%) cases. Fewer errors were found in the assignment of the secondary procedure code, where the numbers of error cases were only 51 (44.0%) cases. Table 4.72 summarised the distributions of coding error cases among cases that were assigned to O&G case type by the coding item.

Table 4.58 Distributions of Coding Error Cases by Coding Item in O&G Case-Type

Coding Items	Total Case Reviewed	No. of Case without Coding Error (%)	No. of Case with Coding Error/s (%)	Kappa Value	p value
Primary Diagnosis	116	55 (47.4)	61 (52.6)	0.444	<0.001
Secondary Diagnosis	116	8 (6.9)	108 (93.1)	0.038	<0.001
Primary Procedure	116	65 (56.0)	51 (44.0)	0.023	<0.001
Secondary Procedure	116	18 (15.5)	98 (84.5)	0.052	<0.001

Cohen's Kappa Test was conducted to determine the level of agreement between the in-house coder and the Independent Senior Coder in the assignment of the codes for O&G type of cases. The output of the kappa test showed that the level of agreement in the assignment of the primary diagnosis code is higher than the primary procedure code (kappa value of 0.444 vs. 0.023, respectively). On the other hand, for secondary diagnosis and secondary procedure code, the output of the test showed that, in O&G case-type, the number of secondary diagnosis code was most likely to be codified wrongly by the in-house coder when compared to the number of secondary procedure code assigned per episode of care (kappa value of 0.038 vs. 0.052).

a. Coding Errors of Primary Diagnosis Code within O&G Case-Type

In O&G case type, at the first level of coding error calculation within the primary diagnosis codes, coding errors occurred in 61 (52.6%) of the selected cases. The second level of coding error calculation within the primary diagnosis codes also showed the same percentage of errors; 52.6% in respect to the similar number of the denominator used in both level of calculations (n=116).

i. Type of Coding Errors of Primary Diagnosis Code Within O&G Case-Type

In the assignment of primary diagnosis code for O&G cases, all of the cases were coded accurately for the first digit level of the code, showing 0.0% of case with a wrong selection of primary diagnosis code. The highest type of error in the assignment of primary diagnosis among O&G cases was the error at the second digit level of the code, which comprises of 24 (20.7%) error cases. The second highest type of errors was primary diagnosis code incorrectly sequenced with the number of error cases of 14 (12.1%) cases. The third highest type of coding errors was the error at the fourth digit level of the code covering 12 (10.3%) of the error cases. Following this, the Independent Senior Coder has identified 11 (9.5%) cases with the error at the third digit level of the code.

Table 4.59 shows the distributions of types of coding errors in the assignment of the primary diagnosis codes among O&G cases.

Table 4.59 Distribution of Type of Coding Errors of Primary Diagnosis Code in O&G Case-Type

Type of Error	No. of Error Cases	%
Error at Second Digit Level	24	20.7
Primary Diagnosis Code Incorrectly Sequenced	14	12.1
Error at Fourth Digit Level	12	10.3
Error at Third Digit Level	11	9.5

ii. Top 10 Highest Frequency Primary Diagnosis Codes Before and After The Re-Coding Process within O&G Case-Type

Table 4.60 shows the comparisons of the top 10 primary diagnosis codes assigned before and after the re-coding process of O&G type of cases. As seen in the table, the primary diagnosis code with the highest frequency assigned before and after the re-coding process was code for O70.0 (First degree perineal laceration during delivery). In total, from the 10 codes listed before the re-coding process, there were 6 codes that remained listed as the top 10 primary diagnosis code assigned. The codes were O70.0 (First degree perineal laceration during delivery), O34.2 (Maternal care due to uterine scare from previous surgery), O80.0 (Spontaneous vertex delivery), O32.1 (Maternal care for breech presentation), O42.1 (Premature rapture of membranes, onset on labour after 24 hours Excludes: with labour delayed by therapy) and O32.2 (Maternal care for transverse and oblique lie). Subsequently, according to the bivariate analysis using Cohen's Kappa test, the level of agreement between the Independent Senior Coder and the in-house coders in the assignment of primary diagnosis code for O&G cases was moderate with the kappa value of 0.444.

From Table 4.60, it is notable that in O&G case-type, there were 76 cases that were assigned to the top 10 primary diagnosis codes before the re-coding process. Among these 76 cases, 63 (82.9%) of the cases were among the coding error cases. The highest errors rate involved cases that were assigned to codes O68.9 (Labour and delivery complicated by fetal stress, unspecified), O68.0 (Labour and delivery complicated by fetal heart rate anomaly) and O42.0 (Premature, rupture of membranes, onset of labour within 24 hours). Subsequently, all of the cases that were assigned to these codes as their primary diagnosis code before the re-coding process were codified wrongly by the in-house coder.

On the other hand, after the re-coding process was performed by the Independent Senior Coder, there were 77 cases assigned to the top 10 primary diagnosis codes after the re-coding process. Among these 77 cases, 65 (83.1%) of the cases were coding error cases. Apparently from Table 4.75, among the top 10 codes assigned after the re-coding process the highest coding errors rate after the re-coding process involved the assignment of the codes O36.3 (Maternal care for signs of fetal hypoxia), O68.8 (Labour and delivery complicated by other evidence of fetal stress) and O66.4 (Failed trial labour, unspecified). Findings from this study show that none of the cases that were assigned to these 3 codes after the re-coding process were codified with the accurate primary diagnosis code before the audit.

Table 4.61 shows the changes which occurred in the assignment of the primary diagnosis code after the re-coding process among the cases that were assigned to the top 10 primary diagnosis codes before the re-coding process. As apparent in the table, the most common type of errors among these cases listed in Table 4.61 was error involving the second digit level. From the 63 error cases, 47 (74.6%) of the cases were assigned wrongly for its second digit level of the code. It is also notable that, among O&G cases, none of the cases that were assigned to the top 10 primary diagnosis codes were codified wrongly at the first digit level of the code. This implies that all the O&G cases were assigned to the correct ICD chapter.

Table 4.60 Top 10 Primary Diagnosis Code Assigned Before and After Re-Coding Process within O&G Case-Type

No.	Before Re-Coding Process				After Re-Coding Process			
			n = 116	n =*			n = 119	n =**
	Codes	Description	Frequency (%)*	No. of Error Cases (%)	Codes	Description	Frequency (%)**	No. of Cases With Unchanged Primary Diagnosis Code (%)
1.	O70.0	First degree perineal laceration during delivery	16 (13.8)	10 (62.5)	O70.0	First degree perinea laceration during delivery	17 (14.3)	12 (70.6)
2.	O34.2	Maternal care due to uterine scare from previous surgery	8 (6.9)	7 (87.5)	O36.3	Maternal care for signs of fetal hypoxia	10 (8.4)	0 (0.0)
3.	O68.9	Labour and delivery complicated by fetal stress, unspecified	8 (6.9)	8 (100.0)	O80.0	Spontaneous vertex delivery	9 (7.6)	4 (44.4)
4.	O80.0	Spontaneous vertex delivery	7 (6.0)	6 (85.7)	O34.2	Maternal care due to uterine scare from previous surgery	8 (6.7)	4 (50.0)
5.	O83.8	Other specified assisted single delivery	7 (6.0)	6 (85.7)	O32.1	Maternal care for breech presentation	7 (5.9)	6 (85.7)
6.	O68.0	Labour and delivery complicated by fetal heart rate anomaly	6 (5.2)	6 (100.0)	O75.7	Vaginal delivery following previous caesarean section	7 (5.9)	1 (14.3)
7.	O32.1	Maternal care for breech presentation	5 (4.3)	4 (80.0)	O68.8	Labour and delivery complicated by other evidence of fetal stress	6 (5.0)	0 (0.0)
8.	O42.0	Premature rupture of membranes, onset of labour within 24 hours	5 (4.3)	5 (100.0)	O66.4	Failed trial labour, unspecified	5 (4.2)	0 (0.0)
9.	O42.1	Premature rapture of membranes, onset on labour after 24 hours Excludes: with labour delayed by therapy	4 (3.4)	3 (75.0)	O32.2	Maternal care for transverse and oblique lie	4 (3.4)	4 (100.0)
10.	O32.2	Maternal care for transverse and oblique lie	4 (3.4)	2 (50.0)	O42.1	Premature rapture of membranes, onset on labour after 24 hours Excludes: with labour delayed by therapy	4 (3.4)	2 (50.0)

Kappa Value = 0.444, $p < 0.001$

Table 4.61 Changes in the Top 10 Primary Diagnosis Code Assigned Before the Re-Coding Process in O&G Case-Type due to Coding Errors

No.	Before Re-Coding Process (n = 116)			After Re-Coding Process (n = *)		
	Original Primary Diagnosis Code	No. of Cases* (%)	No. of Cases with Similar Primary Diagnosis Code (%)	Cases With New Primary Diagnosis Code due to Coding Error		
				New Primary Diagnosis Code	Description	No. Cases (%)
1.	O70.0 (First degree perineal laceration during delivery)	16 (13.8)	6 (37.5)	O36.3	Maternal care for signs of fetal hypoxia	3 (18.8)
				O68.8	Labour and delivery complicated by other evidence of fetal stress	2 (12.5)
				O14.1	Severe pre-eclampsia	1 (6.3)
				O42.0	Premature rupture of membranes, onset of labour within 24 hours	1 (6.3)
				O70.1	Second degree perineal laceration during delivery	1 (6.3)
				O70.9	Perineal laceration during delivery, unspecified	1 (6.3)
				O80.0	Spontaneous vertex delivery	1 (6.3)
2.	O34.2 (Maternal care due to uterine scare from previous surgery)	8 (6.9)	1 (7.1)	O82.1	Delivery by emergency caesarean section	6 (42.9)

			O32.1	Maternal care for breech presentation	1 (7.1)
			O32.2	Maternal care for transverse and oblique lie	1 (7.1)
			O36.3	Maternal care for signs of fetal hypoxia	1 (7.1)
			O61.0	Failed medical induction of labour	1 (7.1)
			O62.0	Primary inadequate contractions	1 (7.1)
			O66.4	Failed trial of labour, unspecified	1 (7.1)
			O80.0	Spontaneous vertex delivery	1 (7.1)
3.	O68.9 (Labour and delivery complicated by fetal stress, unspecified)	8 (6.9)	O36.3	Maternal care for signs of fetal hypoxia	2 (25.0)
		0 (0.0)	O32.3	Maternal care for face, brow and chin presentation	1 (12.5)
			O42.1	Premature rupture of membranes, onset of labour after 24 hours	1 (12.5)
			O66.4	Failed trial of labour, unspecified	1 (12.5)
			O68.8	Labour and delivery complicated by other evidence of fetal stress	1 (12.5)
			O70.0	First degree perineal laceration during delivery	1 (12.5)
			O80.0	Spontaneous vertex delivery	1 (12.5)
4.	O80.0 (Spontaneous vertex delivery)	7 (6.0)	O62.0	Primary inadequate contractions	3 (42.9)
		1 (14.3)	O75.7	Vaginal delivery following previous caesarean section	2 (28.6)
			O70.0	First degree perineal laceration during delivery	1 (14.3)

5.	O83.8 (Other specified assisted single delivery)	7 (6.0)	1 (14.3)	O32.1	Maternal care for breech presentation	1 (14.3)
				O24.1	Diabetes mellitus in pregnancy: Pre-existing diabetes mellitus, non-insulin-dependent	1 (14.3)
				O33.0	Maternal care for disproportion due to deformity of maternal pelvic bones	1 (14.3)
				O62.1	Secondary uterine inertia	1 (14.3)
				O82.1	Delivery by emergency caesarean section	1 (14.3)
				O83.9	Assisted single delivery, unspecified	1 (14.3)
6.	O68.0 (Labour and delivery complicated by fetal heart rate anomaly)	6 (5.2)	0 (0.0)	O68.8	Labour and delivery complicated by other evidence of fetal stress	2 (33.3)
				O32.1	Maternal care for breech presentation	1 (16.7)
				O36.3	Maternal care for signs of fetal hypoxia	1 (16.7)
				O63.1	Prolonged second stage (of labour)	1 (16.7)
				O70.0	First degree perineal laceration during delivery	1 (16.7)
7.	O32.1 (Maternal care for breech presentation)	5 (4.3)	1 (20.0)	O34.2	Maternal care due to uterine scar from previous surgery	1 (20.0)
				O68.8	Labour and delivery complicated by other evidence of fetal stress	1 (20.0)
				O70.0	First degree perineal laceration during delivery	1 (20.0)
				O72.2	Delayed and secondary postpartum haemorrhage	1 (20.0)

8.	O42.0 (Premature rupture of membranes, onset of labour within 24 hours)	5 (4.3)	0 (0.0)	O36.3	Maternal care for signs of fetal hypoxia	1 (20.0)
				O42.1	Premature rupture of membranes, onset of labour after 24 hours	1 (20.0)
				O66.4	Failed trial of labour, unspecified	1 (20.0)
				O69.0	Labour and delivery complicated by prolapse of cord	1 (20.0)
				O70.9	Perineal laceration during delivery, unspecified	1 (20.0)
9.	O42.1 (Premature rapture of membranes, onset on labour after 24 hours Excludes: with labor delayed by therapy)	4 (3.4)	1 (25.0)	O34.2	Maternal care due to uterine scar from previous surgery	1 (25.0)
				O42.0	Premature rupture of membranes, onset of labour within 24 hours	1 (25.0)
				O63.1	Prolonged second stage (of labour)	1 (25.0)
10.	O32.2 (Maternal care for transverse and oblique lie)	4 (3.4)	2 (50.0)	O36.3	Maternal care for signs of fetal hypoxia	1 (25.0)
				O42.1	Premature rupture of membranes, onset of labour after 24 hours	1 (25.0)

b. **Coding Errors of Secondary Diagnosis Code Within O&G Case-type**

In the O&G type of cases, before the re-coding process, there were 115 cases that were assigned to at least one secondary diagnosis code. However, after the re-coding process by the Independent Senior Coder, all cases grouped under the O&G case-type was assigned to at least one secondary diagnosis code by the Independent Senior Coder. At the first level of coding errors calculation within secondary diagnosis codes, coding errors occurred in 108 (93.1%) of the selected cases. In total there were 626 secondary diagnosis codes reviewed by the Independent Senior Coder during the re-coding process within O&G type of cases. From these 626 codes, 350 (55.9%) of the codes were considered as error codes by the Independent Senior Coder.

Prior to the re-coding process the total numbers of codes assigned as secondary diagnosis code across O&G cases were 397 codes and have grossly increased to 632 codes after the re-coding process was performed. Before the re-coding process, the maximum number of code assigned per patient was 8 codes, with the mean of 3.42 (SD: 1.72). On the other hand, the maximum number of code assigned per patient has increased to 14 codes, with the mean of 5.31 (SD: 2.35) after the re-coding process. The level of agreement between the Independent Senior Coder and in-house coder on the number of secondary diagnosis code assigned per patient was tested using Cohen's Kappa test and the result showed a very poor agreement with kappa value of 0.038 (Table 4.62).

Table 4.62 Distributions of the Number of Secondary Diagnosis Codes Assigned Before and After the Re-Coding Process within O&G Case-Type

No. of Secondary Diagnosis Code	Before	After	Kappa value	p value
			0.038	<0.001
Total No. of Code	397	632		
Max. Codes	8	14		
Mean (SD)	3.42 (1.72)	5.31 (2.35)		

i. Comparisons of Number of Secondary Diagnosis Code Assigned per Patient Before and After the Re-Coding Process in O&G Case-Type

Table 4.63 shows the comparisons of the number of secondary diagnosis codes assigned per patient before and after the re-coding process was performed by the Independent Senior Coder for O&G case-type.

As seen in Table 4.63, in total there was 1 (0.9%) case that was unassigned to any secondary diagnosis code before the re-coding process. However, after the re-coding process all of the cases were assigned to O&G case type in MY-DRG group and was assigned to at least one secondary diagnosis code. Subsequently, after the re-coding process, the minimum number of secondary diagnosis code assigned to the patient of O&G type of case was 1. In total there were 3 (2.5%) cases that were assigned to this minimum number of secondary diagnosis code after the audit.

Before the re-coding process, the maximum number of secondary diagnosis codes assigned to the patient of O&G type of case was 8 codes with the total of 3 (2.6%) cases. However, after the re-coding process 2 (66.7%) out of these 3 cases was re-assigned to a lower number of secondary diagnosis codes and remaining 1 (33.3) case was re-assigned to a higher number of secondary diagnosis code. As illustrated in Table 4.63, after the re-coding process was performed by the Independent Senior Coder, in total there were 13 (10.9%) cases that were assigned to 8 secondary diagnosis codes. Data analysis of this study reveals that all of these 13 cases were originally assigned to a lower number of secondary diagnosis code before the re-coding process was done.

After the re-coding process there were total of 11 (9.2%) cases that were assigned to 9 and more secondary diagnosis codes. The highest number of secondary diagnosis code assigned to the patient of O&G type of case after the re-coding process was 14 codes. Data analysis showed that there was 1 (0.8%) case that was assigned to 14 secondary diagnosis codes after the re-coding process. This case was originally assigned to 8 secondary diagnosis codes before the re-coding process performed by the Independent Senior Coder. This implies that the in-house coders have a higher tendency to under-code cases with a higher number of secondary diagnoses.

Table 4.63 Comparisons of Number of Secondary Diagnosis Code Assigned per Patient Before and After the Re-Coding Process in O&G Case-Type

No	Before Re-Coding Process					After Re-Coding Process				
	n =116		n = *			n = 119		n = **		
	No. of Secondary Diagnosis Code	Nos of Cases (%) *	No. of Cases with Similar No of Secondary Diagnosis Code After Re-Coding Process (%)	No. of Cases With Lower No of Secondary Diagnosis Code After Re-Coding Process (%)	No. of Cases With Higher No of Secondary Diagnosis Code After Re-Coding Process (%)	No. of Secondary Diagnosis Code	No. of Cases (%)**	No. of Cases with Similar No of Secondary Diagnosis Code After Re-Coding Process (%)	No. of Cases With Lower No of Secondary Diagnosis Code Before Re-Coding Process (%)	No. of Cases With Higher No of Secondary Diagnosis Code Before Re-Coding Process (%)
1.	0	1 (0.9)	0 (0.0)	0 (0.0)	1 (100.0)	1	3 (2.5)	1 (33.3)	0 (0.0)	2 (66.7)
2.	1	7 (6.0)	1 (14.3)	0 (0.0)	6 (85.7)	2	4 (3.4)	2 (50.0)	1 (25.0)	1 (25.0)
3.	2	34 (29.3)	1 (2.9)	1 (2.9)	32 (94.1)	3	21 (17.6)	5 (23.8)	12 (57.1)	4 (19.1)
4.	3	29 (25.0)	3 (13.8)	2 (6.9)	24 (82.8)	4	25 (21.0)	2 (8.0)	19 (76.0)	4 (16.0)
5.	4	16 (13.8)	2 (12.5)	0 (0.0)	14 (87.5)	5	17 (14.3)	1 (5.9)	14 (82.4)	2 (11.7)
6.	5	13 (11.2)	0 (0.0)	1 (7.7)	12 (92.3)	6	15 (12.6)	0 (0.0)	15 (100.0)	0 (0.0)
7.	6	9 (7.8)	0 (0.0)	7 (77.8)	2 (22.2)	7	10 (8.4)	1 (10.0)	8 (80.0)	1 (10.0)
8.	7	4 (3.4)	1 (25.0)	1 (25.0)	4 (50.0)	8	13 (10.9)	0 (0.0)	13 (100.0)	0 (0.0)
9.	8	3 (2.6)	0 (0.0)	2 (66.7)	1 (33.3)	9 and above	11 (9.2)	0 (0.0)	11 (100.0)	0 (0.0)

k= 0.038, p < 0.001

Table 4.64 shows the distributions of coding error cases by number of the secondary diagnosis codes. From the table, it could be concluded that the highest coding error rate involves cases that were unassigned to any secondary diagnosis code (100.0%). The second highest coding error rate was among cases with 4 and above secondary diagnosis code (97.8%). A chi-square test was run to determine the association between the number of secondary diagnosis code and the coding errors. The result was statistically insignificant with X^2 (4) = 3.38, p >0.05.

Table 4.64 Distributions of Coding Errors Cases by Number of Secondary Diagnosis Codes in O&G Case-Type

No. of Secondary Diagnosis Code	No. of Case without Coding Error	%	No. of Case with Coding Error/s	%	Total	%
0	0	0.0	1	100.0	1	100.0
1	1	14.3	6	85.7	7	100.0
2	1	2.9	33	97.1	34	100.0
3	3	13.8	26	89.7	29	100.0
4 and above	1	2.2	44	97.8	45	100.0

X^2 = 3.38 df =4, p =0.535

ii. Type of Coding Errors of Secondary Diagnosis Code within O&G Case-Type

Data analysis of this study showed that the commonest type of error in the assignment of secondary procedure code among O&G cases was under-coding. From the 626 secondary procedure codes reviewed by the Independent Senior Coder, 235 (37.5%) of the codes were being undercoded by the in-house coder. The second highest type of errors found within the secondary procedure codes was the error at the second digit level with the number of error code of 36 (5.8%) codes. It was revealed that in the assignment of secondary procedure code, the error at the third digit level was the third highest type of error, in which 31 (5.0%) of error codes were due to this type of error. The fourth highest type of error in the assignment of secondary procedure within O&G cases was error at the fourth digit level, in which 28 (4.5%) of error codes were reported with this type of error. Following this, in total, there were 17 (2.7%) error cases due to the wrong selection of secondary diagnosis code. Lastly, the least common type of errors was error due to up-coding in which there were 3 (0.5%) cases which were reported with this type of errors. The details of the type of coding errors in the assignment of secondary procedure code among O&G type of cases are illustrated in Table 4.65.

Table 4.65 Distributions of Type of Coding Errors in Secondary Diagnosis Code within O&G Case-Type

Type of Error	No. of Error Cases	%
Under-coding	235	37.5
Error at Second Digit Level	36	5.8
Error at Third Digit Level	31	5.0
Error at Fourth Digit Level	28	4.5
Wrong Selection of Secondary Diagnosis Code	17	2.7
Up-coding	3	0.5

iii. Comparisons of Top 10 Secondary Diagnosis Code Assigned Before and After the Re-Coding Process within O&G Type of Case

Table 4.65 shows the comparison of the top 10 secondary diagnosis codes assigned before and after the re-coding process for O&G cases. As seen in the table, code Z37.0 (Single live birth) had the secondary diagnosis code among the O&G cases assigned before and after the re-coding process. It is also notable that from the 10 secondary diagnosis codes listed before the re-coding process, there were 7 common codes that were frequently assigned before and after the re-coding process. The codes were Z37.0 (Single live birth), O82.1 (Delivery by emergency caesarean section), O24.4 (Diabetes mellitus arising in pregnancy), O34.2 (Maternal care due to uterine scar from previous surgery), O82.0 (Delivery by elective caesarean section), and O99.0 (Anaemia complicating pregnancy, childbirth and the puerperium).

Prior to the re-coding process, there were 248 cases containing at least one of the top 10 secondary diagnosis codes were assigned by the Independent Senior Coder. From these 248 cases, 236 (95.2%) of the cases contained at least one error for the secondary diagnosis code. The highest coding errors rate (100.0%) was involving cases that contain codes O24.4, O83.8 (Other specified assisted single delivery), O81.4 (Vacuum extractor delivery) and O99.0 as its secondary diagnosis code.

On the other hand, after the re-coding process, there were 389 cases that were assigned to at least one of the top 10 secondary diagnosis codes assigned after the re-coding process by the Independent Senior Coder. From these 389 cases, 376 (97.4%) of the cases contained at least one error for its secondary diagnosis code. It is also notable that, cases consisted of the codes O24.4, Z87.5 (Personal history complications of pregnancy, childbirth and the puerperium), O99.8 (Other specified diseases and conditions complicating pregnancy, childbirth and the puerperium) and O99.0 (Anaemia complicating pregnancy, childbirth and the puerperium) as its secondary diagnosis code after the re-coding process were assigned to at least one error secondary diagnosis code before the re-coding process.

To sum it up, in comparison for the distributions of the top 10 of secondary diagnosis codes assigned before and after the re-coding process, O&G cases showed a higher similarity than the Medical and Surgical type of cases, in respect to the frequent secondary diagnosis code assigned by the in-house coders and the Independent Senior Coder. For the O&G cases, in total there were eight common codes listed as the top 10 secondary diagnosis code assigned before and after the re-coding process, whereas, for medical and surgical cases, the number of common codes were only four codes. This indicates that, in this study, the selection of secondary diagnosis codes to codify the types of illness among O&G's patient was not as vast as it is for other case types. However, interestingly, despite the higher similarity of frequently assigned secondary diagnosis code between the in-house coder and the Independent Senior Coder, the coding errors rate in the assignment of secondary diagnosis codes were the highest among the O&G cases. This implies that even though the frequently used secondary diagnosis codes were consistent among both coders, the possibility of the codes to be assigned to the same case before and after the re-coding process was low. Among plausible explanation of this incidence is, the high similarity of the disease treated among cases grouped under O&G case type, specifically among obstetric cases could highly contribute to confusion among coders in assigning accurate secondary diagnosis codes.

Table 4.66 Comparisons of Top 10 Secondary Diagnosis Code Assigned within O&G Case-Type

		Before Re-Coding Process				After Re-Coding Process		
			n = 397	n = *			n = 632	n = **
No.	Codes	Description	Frequency (%) *	No. of Error Cases (%)	Codes	Description	Frequency (%) **	No. of Cases Without Coding Errors (%)
1.	Z37.0	Single live birth	112 (28.2)	106 (94.6)	Z37.0	Single live birth	112 (17.7)	6 (5.4)
2.	O82.1	Delivery by emergency caesarean section	36 (9.1)	34 (94.4)	Z38.0	Singleton, born in hospital	103 (16.3)	3 (2.9)
3.	O80.0	Spontaneous vertex delivery	20 (5.0)	19 (95.0)	O80.0	Spontaneous vertex delivery	43 (6.8)	1 (2.3)
4.	O24.4	Diabetes mellitus arising in pregnancy	16 (4.0)	16 (100.0)	O82.1	Delivery by emergency caesarean section	36 (5.7)	1 (2.8)
5.	O83.8	Other specified assisted single delivery	14 (3.5)	14 (100.0)	O24.4	Diabetes mellitus arising in pregnancy	21 (3.3)	0 (0.0)
6.	O34.2	Maternal care due to uterine scar from previous surgery	12 (3.0)	11 (91.7)	Z87.5	Personal history complications of pregnancy, childbirth and the puerperium	20 (3.2)	0 (0.0)
7.	O81.4	Vacuum extractor delivery	11 (2.8)	11 (100.0)	O99.8	Other specified diseases and conditions complicating pregnancy, childbirth and the puerperium	18 (2.8)	0 (0.0)
8.	O82.0	Delivery by elective caesarean section	9 (2.3)	8 (88.9)	O34.2	Maternal care due to uterine scar from previous surgery	13 (2.1)	1 (7.7)
9.	O99.0	Anaemia complicating pregnancy, childbirth and the puerperium	9 (2.3)	9 (100.0)	O99.0	Anaemia complicating pregnancy, childbirth and the puerperium	12 (1.9)	0 (0.0)
10.	Z38.0	Singleton, born in hospital	9 (2.3)	8 (88.9)	O23.4	Unspecified infection of urinary tract in pregnancy	10 (1.6)	1 (9.1)

c. **Coding Errors of Primary Procedure Code within O&G Case-Type**

The coding errors of primary procedure code among O&G cases have caused an increment in the number of cases that contain primary procedure code after the re-coding process. Prior to the re-coding process, from the 116 cases assigned to O&G case type, 113 (97.4%) of the cases contained a primary procedure code. After the re-coding process was performed by the Independent Senior Coder, from the 119 cases assigned to O&G case type, 117 (98.3%) of the cases contained a primary procedure code. The number of cases with primary procedure code among O&G case type after the re-coding process showed an increment of 0.9%.

Due to changes in the number of the denominator, the percentage of coding errors of primary procedure code among O&G cases were different at the first level and second level of the coding errors calculation. At the first level of the calculation, the number of error cases was 51 (50.0%) cases. On the other hand, at the second level of the calculation, from the 120 primary procedure codes reviewed by the Independent Senior Coder, 55 (45.8%) of the codes were error codes.

i. **Type of Coding Errors of Primary Procedure Code In O&G Case-Type**

In the assignment of the primary procedure code within O&G type of cases, most of the cases were being under-coded covering 39 (32.5%) of error cases. The second highest type of errors was the wrong selection of the primary procedure code comprising of 29 (24.2%) of the error cases. The third highest type of errors was the error at the second digit level of the code covering 8 (6.7%) of the error cases. The numbers of cases due to the error at the fourth digit level of the code and due to the incorrect sequence of primary procedure code were consistent with 4 (6.7%) error cases per each type of coding errors. Lastly, the numbers of error cases due to the error at the third digit level of the code and due to up-coding were also consistent, with 2 (1.7%) error cases per each type of coding errors. Table 4.67 shows the distributions of the type of coding errors which occurred in the assignment of the primary procedure codes among O&G type of cases.

Table 4.67 Distributions of the Type of Coding Errors of Primary Procedure Codes in O&G Case-Type

Type of Error	No. of Error Cases	%
Under-coding	39	32.5
Wrong Selection of Primary Procedure Code	29	24.2
Error at Second Digit Level	8	6.7
Error at Fourth Digit Level	4	3.3
Principal Procedure Incorrectly Sequenced	4	3.3
Error at Third Digit Level	2	1.7
Up-coding	2	1.7

ii. Comparisons of Top Primary Procedure Code Assigned in O&G Case-Type Before and After the Re-Coding Process

Table 4.68 shows the comparisons of the distributions of the top 10 primary procedure codes assigned before and after the re-coding process within O&G type of cases. From the distributions of the top 10 primary procedure codes assigned before and after the re-coding process, it is noticeable that, there were four common codes that were frequently used by both of the coders. The four codes are 74.1 (Low cervical caesarean section), 75.69 (Repair of other current obstetric laceration), 72.79 (Other vacuum extraction) and 73.4 (Medical induction of labour). The four common codes listed before and after the re-coding process implies that the level of agreement between the in-house coder and the Independent Senior Coder in the assignment of primary procedure code in

O&G case type is fair. This is proven by the Cohen Kappa output of k = 0.023.

Among cases that were grouped under O&G type of case before the re-coding process, code 74.1 was identified as the code with the highest frequency for its primary procedure. As apparent in Table 4.68, before the re-coding processthis code was assigned to 48 (42.5%) cases. However, after the re-coding process, 26 (54.2%) of the cases which were assigned to code 74.1 before the re-coding process were re-assigned to other primary procedure code. Majority of these 26 cases were re-assigned to code 88.38 (Other computerized axial tomography) and 75.69 (Repair of other current obstetric laceration), whereby 8 (16.7%) of the cases were re-assigned to code 88.38 and 7 (14.6%) of the cases were re-assigned to code 75.69 after the re-coding process. A more detailed comparison of the changes which occurred due to coding errors within cases that were assigned to the top 10 primary procedure codes assigned before the re-coding process is illustrated in Table 4.69.

It is apparent from Table 4.68 that the frequency of cases assigned to code 74.1 was still the highest even after the re-coding process. After the re-coding process, the total number of cases that were assigned to code 74.1 has reached 53 (45.3%) cases, showing an increment of 2.8%. However, even though code 74.1 remained as the highest frequency for primary procedure codes after the re-coding process from the 53 cases, only 22 (41.5%) of the cases were assigned to the similar primary procedure codes as before the re-coding process. This indicates that more than 50.0% of the cases assigned to the highest frequency primary procedure code after the re-coding process were originally assigned to the wrong primary procedure code. Evidently, it implies a poor agreement between the in-house coders and the Independent Senior Coder in the assignment of primary procedure code among O&G cases.

Table 4.68 Comparisons of Top 10 Primary Procedure Code Assigned Before and After the Re-Coding Process within O&G Case-Type

		Before Re-Coding Process				After Re-Coding Process		
		n = 113	n =*			n = 117	n =**	
No.	Codes	Description	Frequency (%)*	No. of Error Cases (%)	Codes	Description	Frequency (%)**	No. of Cases Without Coding Errors (%)
1.	74.1	Low cervical caesarean section	48 (42.5)	26 (54.2)	74.1	Low cervical caesarean section	53 (45.3)	22 (41.5)
2.	75.69	Repair of other current obstetric laceration	21 (18.6)	18 (85.7)	88.38	Other computerized axial tomography	27 (23.1)	0 (0.0)
3.	73.6	Episiotomy	20 (17.7)	19 (95.0)	75.69	Repair of other current obstetric laceration	17 (14.5)	3 (17.6)
4.	72.71	Vacuum extraction with episiotomy	6 (5.3)	6 (100.0)	72.7	Vacuum Extraction	8 (6.8)	0 (0.0)
5.	72.79	Other vacuum extraction	5 (4.4)	5 (100.0)	72.79	Other vacuum extraction	2 (1.7)	0 (0.0)
6.	73.4	Medical induction of labour	4 (3.5)	4 (100.0)	73.59	Other manually assisted delivery	2 (1.7)	1 (50.0)
7.	75.34	Other fetal monitoring	4 (3.5)	4 (100.0)	88.78	Diagnostic ultrasound of gravid uterus	2 (1.7)	0 (0.0)
8.	73.3	Failed forceps	2 (1.8)	2 (100.0)	57.94	Insertion of indwelling urinary catheter	1 (0.9)	0 (0.0)
9.	74.99	Other caesarean section of unspecified type	1 (0.9)	1 (100.0)	72.1	Low forceps operation with episiotomy	1 (0.9)	0 (0.0)
10.	75.4	Manual removal of retained placenta	1 (0.9)	1 (100.0)	73.4	Medical induction of labour	1 (0.9)	0 (0.0)

Kappa value = 0.023 p <0.001

Table 4.69 Changes Among the Top 10 Primary Procedure Code Among O&G Case-Type due to Coding Errors

	Before Re-Coding Process n = 116			After Re-Coding Process n =*		
No.	Original Primary Procedure Code	No. of Cases* (%)	No. of Cases with Similar Primary Procedure Code (%)	Cases With New Primary Diagnosis Code due to Coding Error		
				New Primary Procedure Code	Description	No. Cases (%)
1.	74.1 (Low cervical caesarean section)	48 (42.5)	22 (45.8)	88.38	Other computerized axial tomography	8 (16.7)
				75.69	Repair of other current obstetric laceration	7 (14.6)
				72.7	Vacuum extraction	2 (4.2)
				72.79	Other vacuum extraction	2 (4.2)
				88.78	Diagnostic ultrasound of gravid uterus	2 (4.2)
				73.4	Medical induction of labor	1 (2.1)
				73.59	Other manually assisted delivery	1 (2.1)
				74.9	Caesarean section of unspecified type	1 (2.1)
				74.4	Caesarean section of other specified type	1 (2.1)
				None	None	1 (2.1)
2.	75.69 (Repair of other current obstetric laceration)	21 (18.6)	3 (14.3)	74.1	Low cervical caesarean section	9 (42.9)
				88.38	Other computerized axial tomography	5 (23.8)
				72.7	Vacuum extraction	2 (9.5)
				72.1	Low forceps operation with episiotomy	1 (4.8)

#	Procedure code	n (%)	n (%)	Code	Associated procedure	n (%)
3.	73.6 (Episiotomy)	20 (17.7)	1 (5.0)	88.78	Diagnostic ultrasound of gravid uterus	1 (4.8)
				74.1	Low cervical caesarean section	8 (40.0)
				88.38	Other computerized axial tomography	7 (35.0)
				75.69	Repair of other current obstetric laceration	3 (15.0)
				72.7	Vacuum extraction	1 (5.0)
				73.59	Other manually assisted delivery	1 (5.0)
4.	72.71 (Vacuum extraction with episiotomy)	6 (5.3)	0 (0.0)	74.1	Low cervical caesarean section	3 (50.0)
				75.69	Repair of other current obstetric laceration	2 (33.3)
				88.38	Other computerized axial tomography	1 (16.7)
5.	72.79 (Other vacuum extraction)	5 (4.4)	0 (0.0)	74.1	Low cervical caesarean section	2 (40.0)
				88.38	Other computerized axial tomography	2 (40.0)
				72.7	Vacuum extraction	1 (20.0)
6.	73.4 (Medical induction of labor)	4 (3.5)	0 (0.0)	74.1	Low cervical caesarean section	2 (50.0)
				88.38	Other computerized axial tomography	1 (25.0)
				None		1 (25.0)
7.	75.34 (Other fetal monitoring)	4 (3.5)	0 (0.0)	74.1	Low cervical caesarean section	2 (50.0)
				75.69	Repair of other current obstetric laceration	1 (25.0)
				88.38	Other computerized axial tomography	1 (25.0)
8.	73.3 (Failed forceps)	2 (1.8)	0 (0.0)	72.7	Vacuum extraction	1 (50.0)
				88.38	Other computerized axial tomography	1 (50.0)
9.	74.99 (Other cesarean section of unspecified type)	1 (0.9)	0 (0.0)	72.7	Vacuum extraction	1 (100.0)
10.	75.4 (Manual removal of retained placenta)	1 (0.9)	0 (0.0)	88.38	Other computerized axial tomography	1 (100.0)

d. Coding Errors of Secondary Procedure Code of O&G Case-Type

In the assignment of secondary procedure code within O&G type of cases, the coding errors rate was higher at the first level of coding error calculation than at the second level. At the first level of coding error calculation of secondary procedure codes in O&G type of cases, coding errors occurred in 98 (84.5%) of the selected cases. On the other hand, at the second level of coding error calculation, from the 222 secondary procedure codes reviewed by the Independent Senior Coder, 212 (95.5%) of the codes were considered as error codes.

Before the re-coding process, the total number of secondary diagnosis codes assigned to the entire case was 117 codes and have increased up to 200 codes after the re-coding process by the Independent Senior Coder. The maximum number of secondary procedure codes assigned to the patient was 3, with the mean of 1.01 (SD 0.78). After the re-coding process by the Independent Senior Coder, the maximum number of secondary procedure code increased to 4 codes, with the mean of 1.68 (SD 1.37). The level of agreement between the in-house coder and the Independent Senior Coder in the number of secondary procedure code assigned per patient was poor with the kappa value of 0.052 (Table 4.70).

Table 4.70 Distributions of Total Number of Secondary Procedure Code Assigned to Patient Before and After the Re-Coding Process within O&G Case-Type

No. of Secondary Procedure Code	Before	After	Kappa value	p value
			0.052	<0.001
Total Nos of Code	117	200		
Max. Codes	3	4		
Mean (SD)	1.01 (0.78)	1.68 (1.37)		

i. Comparison of Number of Secondary Procedure Code Before and After the Re-Coding Process in O&G Case-Type

From the 116 cases selected under O&G case-type, 30 (25.9%) of the cases were unassigned to any secondary procedure code before the re-coding process. From these 30 cases, 19 (63.3%) of the cases were identified as coding error cases. Table 4.71 shows the distributions of coding error cases by the number of secondary procedure code among cases assigned to O&G case type. As apparent in the table, the highest coding errors rate was among cases that were assigned to 3 and above secondary procedure code (100.0%). A chi-square test was conducted to determine the association between the number of secondary procedure code and coding errors. The result was proven to be statistically insignificant with the X^2 value of 1.319, p > 0.05 (Table 4.71).

Table 4.71 Distributions of Coding Error Cases by Number of Secondary Procedure Code within O&G Case-Type

No. of Secondary Procedure Code	No. of Case without Coding Error	%	No of Case with Coding Error/s	%	Total	%
0	2	6.7	28	93.3	30	100.0
1	2	3.4	57	96.6	59	100.0
2	2	8.7	21	91.3	23	100.0
3 and above	0	0.0	4	100.0	4	100.0

X^2 = 1.319, df =3, p =0.725

Table 4.72 shows the distributions of the number of secondary procedure code assigned to a patient before and after the re-coding process. Before the re-coding process, the maximum number of secondary procedure code assigned to the patient in O&G case type was three covering 4 (3.4%) of the cases. However, after the re-coding process, the number of case that was assigned to 4 secondary procedure codes has decreased to 1 (25.0%) case and the remaining cases were re-assigned to 3 types of secondary procedure codes.

On the other hand, after the re-coding process in total there were 37 (31.1%) cases that were assigned to 3 secondary procedure codes. Apparently, from these 37 cases, only 1 (2.7%) case was assigned to the same number of secondary procedure code after the re-coding process. The maximum number of secondary procedure code assigned to the patient in O&G case type increased to 4 codes after the re-coding process was performed by the Independent Senior Coder covering up to 9 (7.6%) cases. Data analysis showed that, out of these 9 cases, 6 (66.7%) of the cases were originally assigned to 1 secondary procedure code before the re-coding process. The increment of the number of cases that were assigned to 3 and more secondary procedure codes showed that the tendency of the O&G cases to be under-coded was high. This finding was aligned with the output of the commonest type of error of secondary procedure code in O&G case type namely, under-coding.

Table 4.72 Comparison of Number of Secondary Procedure Code Assigned per Patient Before and After the Re-Coding Process Within O&G Case-Type

No.	Before Re-Coding Process					After Re-Coding Process				
	n =116					n =119				
	No. of Secondary Procedure Code	No. of Cases (%) *	No. of Cases With Similar number of Secondary Diagnosis Code After Re-Coding Process (%)	n = *		No. of Secondary Procedure Code	No. of Cases (%)**	No. of Cases With Similar number of Secondary Diagnosis Code as Before Re-Coding Process (%)	n = **	
				No. of Errors Cases with Lower No of Secondary Procedure Code After Re-Coding Process (%)	No. of Errors Cases with Higher No of Secondary Procedure Code After Re-coding process (%)				No. of Errors Cases with Lower No of Secondary Procedure Code Before Re-Coding Process (%)	No. of Errors Cases with Higher No of Secondary Procedure Code Before Re-Coding Process (%)
1.	0	30 (25.9)	11 (36.7)	0 (0.0)	19 (63.3)	0	33 (27.7)	11 (33.3)	0 (0.0)	22 (66.7)
2.	1	59 (51.0)	15 (25.4)	16 (27.1)	28 (47.4)	1	27 (22.7)	15 (55.6)	2 (7.4)	10 (37.0)
3.	2	23 (19.8)	3 (13.0)	12 (52.2)	8 (34.8)	2	13 (10.9)	3 (23.1)	8 (61.5)	2 (15.4)
4.	3	4 (3.4)	1 (25.0)	3 (75.0)	0 (0.0)	3	37 (31.1)	1 (2.7)	36 (97.3)	0 (0.0)
5.	4	N/A	N/A	N/A	N/A	4	9 (7.6)	0 (0.0)	9 (100.0)	0 (0.0)

ii. Type of Coding Errors of Secondary Procedure Code within O&G Case-Type

Data analysis in this study shows that the most common type of error in the assignment of secondary procedure code within cases grouped under O&G case-type was under-coding. From the 222 secondary procedure codes reviewed by the Independent Senior Coder, 109 (49.1%) of the codes were undercoded by the in-house coder. The second highest type of errors found within the secondary procedure codes was the wrong selection of secondary procedure code covering up to 64 (28.8%) of the error cases. Up-coding was the third highest type of error in which 25 (11.3%) of error cases were due to this type error. The fourth highest type of error in the assignment of secondary procedure within O&G type of cases were the error at the third digit level, in which 9 (4.1%) of the error cases were identified with this type of error. In the assignment of secondary procedure code within O&G type of cases, the least common type of errors was the error at the second digit level of the code. There were only 5 (2.3%) cases reported which contained this type of error in their assignment of secondary procedure code. The distributions of the type of coding errors in the assignment of secondary procedure code are illustrated in Table 4.73.

Table 4.73 Distributions of Type of Coding Errors of Secondary Procedure Code within O&G Case-Type

Type of Error	No. of Error Cases	%
Under-coding	109	49.1
Wrong Selection of Secondary Procedure Code	64	28.8
Up-coding	25	11.3
Error at Third Digit Level	9	4.1
Error at Second Digit Level	5	2.3

iii. **Comparisons of Top 10 Secondary Procedure Code Assigned Before and After the Re-Coding Process within O&G Case-Type**

Before the re-coding process, there were only ten types of secondary procedure codes assigned to the O&G type of cases. Among these ten codes, the highest frequency code assigned as the secondary procedure was code 75.34 (Other fetal monitoring), in which the number of cases assigned to this code has reached 75 (64.1%) cases. Out of these 75 cases, 68 (90.7%) of the cases were coded with at least one wrong secondary procedure code by the in-house coder. After the re-coding process by the Independent Senior Coder, the number of cases assigned to code 75.34 as its secondary procedure code has declined to 4 (2.0%) cases and all these 4 cases were originally codified with the same secondary procedure as after the re-coding process by the Independent Senior Coder.

After the re-coding process by the Independent Senior Coder, in total there were 14 types of secondary procedure codes assigned to O&G cases. The code with the highest frequency was code 88.38 (Other computerized axial tomography) in which it was assigned to 72 (36.0%) of the cases. However, as seen in Table 4.74, none of the cases that were assigned to code 88.38 after the re-coding process was originally assigned accurately for its secondary procedure code before the re-coding process. From Table 4.74, it is also notable that only cases that were assigned to codes 75.34 and 73.4 after the re-coding process was assigned accurately to its secondary procedure codes before the re-coding process by the Independent Senior Coder.

To sum it up, as apparent in Table 4.74, there were 5 secondary procedure codes that were frequently assigned by both coders. This showed a moderate agreement regarding the type of codes that were commonly used by both coders. However, the coding errors rate of secondary procedure code in cases that were grouped under O&G case type was exceptionally high in comparison to the coding errors rate in Medical and Surgical case type, specifically at the second level of coding error calculation. Similar to the assignment of the secondary diagnosis code, in O&G type of cases, the high similarity of the disease treated in this case type could possibly be related to the difficulties among the in-house coder to determine the accurate secondary procedure code to the patient.

Table 4.74 Comparisons of Top Secondary Procedure Code Assigned within O&G Case-Type

		Before Re-Coding Process				After Re-Coding Process		
			n = 117	n = *			n = 200	n = **
No.	Codes	Description	Frequency (%) *	No. of Error Cases (%)	Codes	Description	Frequency (%) **	No. of Cases Without Coding Errors (%)
1.	75.34	Other fetal monitoring	75 (64.1)	68 (90.7)	88.38	Other computerized axial tomography	72 (36.0)	0 (0.0)
2.	73.4	Medical induction of labour	17 (14.5)	14 (82.4)	57.94	Insertion of indwelling urinary catheter	50 (25.0)	0 (0.0)
3.	73.3	Failed forceps	8 (6.8)	8 (100.0)	97.64	Removal of other urinary drainage device	50 (25.0)	0 (0.0)
4.	99.04	Transfusion of packed cells	4 (3.4)	4 (100.0)	75.69	Repair of other current obstetric laceration	9 (4.5)	0 (0.0)
5.	74.1	Low cervical caesarean section	3 (2.6)	3 (100.0)	75.34	Other fetal monitoring	4 (2.0)	4 (100.0)
6.	75.69	Repair of other current obstetric laceration	3 (2.6)	3 (100.0)	99.04	Transfusion of packed cells	4 (2.0)	0 (0.0)
7.	89.26	Gynaecological examination	3 (2.6)	3 (100.0)	88.78	Diagnostic ultrasound of gravid uterus	3 (1.5)	0 (0.0)
8.	88.78	Diagnostic ultrasound of gravid uterus	2 (1.7)	2 (100.0)	66.39	Other bilateral destruction or occlusion of fallopian tubes	2 (0.5)	0 (0.0)
9.	75.4	Manual removal of retained placenta	1 (0.9)	1 (100.0)	72.52	Other partial breech extraction	2 (0.5)	0 (0.0)
10.	74.3	Other Intrauterine Operations On Foetus and Amnion	1 (0.0)	1 (100.0)	73.4	Medical induction of labour	2 (0.5)	2 (100.0)

4.4.4 Coding Errors of Paediatric Case-Type

Coding error cases detected within cases that were grouped under paediatric case type was the third highest among the four case types, in which the number of error cases was 102 (87.9%) cases. Among the paediatric type of cases, the coding errors were mostly high in the assignment of its secondary diagnosis code covering up to 84 (72.4%) cases. Fewer errors were found in the assignment of the secondary procedure code where the numbers of error cases were only 29 (25.0%) cases. Table 4.75 summarised the distributions of coding error cases in paediatric case type by the coding item.

Table 4.75 Distributions of Coding Errors Cases by Coding Item in Paediatric Case-Type

Coding Items	Total Case Reviewed	No. of Case without Coding Error (%)	No. of Case with Coding Error/s (%)	Kappa Value	p value
Primary Diagnosis	116	58 (50.0)	58 (50.0)	0.460	<0.001
Secondary Diagnosis	116	32 (27.6)	84 (72.4)	0.261	<0.001
Primary Procedure	116	55 (47.4)	61 (52.6)	0.013	<0.001
Secondary Procedure	116	87 (75.0)	29 (25.0)	0.202	<0.001

Cohen's Kappa Test was conducted to determine the level of agreement between the in-house coder and the Independent Senior Coder in the assignment of codes among the paediatric type of cases. In this case type, the output of the kappa test showed that among the paediatric cases, the level of agreement in the assignment of primary diagnosis code is higher than primary procedure code (kappa value of 0.460 vs. 0.013, respectively). On the other hand, with regards to the number of secondary diagnosis code and the number of the secondary procedure code assigned per patient, the kappa agreement is higher in the assignment of secondary diagnosis code than secondary procedure code (kappa value 0.261 vs. 0.202, respectively).

a. **Coding Errors of Primary Diagnosis Code within Paediatric Case-Type**

In paediatric case type, at the first level of coding error calculation within primary diagnosis codes, coding errors occurred in 58 (56.0%) of the selected cases. The second level of coding error calculation within primary diagnosis codes also showed the same percentage of errors; 56.0% in respect to the similar number of the denominator in both level of calculations; n=116.

i. **Type of Coding Errors in Primary Diagnosis Within Paediatric Case-Type**

In the assignment of the primary diagnosis code for the paediatric type of cases, the highest type of errors was the error at the fourth digit level of the code, comprising of 29 (25.0%) of the error cases. The second highest type of errors was the error at the third digit level covering 10 (8.6%) of the error cases. The third highest type of coding errors was the error at the second digit level of the code covering 9 (7.8%) of the error cases. Following this, the Independent Senior Coder has identified 7 (6.0%) cases where the primary diagnosis code was incorrectly sequenced. The least common type of error identified in the assignment of primary diagnosis code within the paediatric type of cases was the wrong selection of primary diagnosis code with 3 (2.6%) number of error cases. Table 4.76 shows the distributions of the types of coding errors in the assignment of the primary diagnosis code among the paediatric type of cases.

Table 4.76 Distribution of Type of Coding Errors of Primary Diagnosis Code in Paediatric Case-Type

Type of Error	No. of Error Cases	%
Error at Fourth Digit Level	29	25.0
Error at Third Digit Level	10	8.6

Error at Second Digit Level	9	7.8
Primary Diagnosis Incorrectly Sequenced	7	6.0
Wrong Selection of Primary Diagnosis Code	3	2.6

ii. Top 10 Highest Frequency Primary Diagnosis Codes Before and After The Re-Coding Process within Paediatric Case-Type

Table 4.78 shows the comparisons of the top 10 primary diagnosis codes assigned to patients before and after the re-coding process in the paediatric case type. As seen in the table, from the ten listed codes, there were six common codes that were frequently chosen by both coders in the assignment of the primary diagnosis code. The codes were P59.9 (Neonatal jaundice, unspecified), P22.1 (Transient tachypnoea of newborn), P36.9 (Bacterial sepsis of newborn, unspecified), P23.9 (Congenital pneumonia, unspecified), P55.1 (ABO isoimmunization of fetus and newborn) and P22.0 (Respiratory distress syndrome of newborn). The similarity of the distributions of the high-frequency primary diagnosis codes among the paediatric type of cases indicating a moderate agreement between the in-house coder and the Independent Senior Coder in the assignment of primary diagnosis code. This is supported by the output of the bivariate analysis using Cohen's Kappa Test with the kappa value of 0.460.

It is apparent as it is shown in Table 4.78 that the highest frequency for primary diagnosis code before and after the re-coding process was associated with neonatal jaundice. Before the re-coding process the highest frequency for primary diagnosis code was P59.9 covering 47 (40.5%) cases. However, after the re-coding process the highest frequency for the primary diagnosis code was P59.8 (Neonatal jaundice from other specified causes) covering 27 (25.0%). Interestingly code P59.8 was not among the highest frequency primary diagnosis code before the re-coding process. To compare the both highest frequency primary diagnosis code before and after the re-coding process the highest frequency code assigned after the re-coding process shows a more detailed description of the cause of jaundice when compared to the highest frequency primary diagnosis code before the re-coding process. This indicates a broader knowledge of the Independent Senior Coder than the in-house coder.

From Table 4.78 it is notable that in total there were 81 cases that were assigned to the top 10 primary diagnosis codes before the re-coding process by the Independent Senior Coder. From these 81 cases, 47 (58.0%) of the cases were codified with a wrong primary diagnosis code by the in-house coder. The highest errors rate was involved cases that were assigned to code P07.3 (Other preterm infants) before the re-coding process. As apparent in the table, all cases that were assigned to code P07.3 as its primary diagnosis code before the re-coding process were assigned to the wrong primary diagnosis code.

On the other hand, after the re-coding process was performed by the Independent Senior Coder, there were 82 cases assigned to the top 10 primary diagnosis codes assigned after the re-coding process. From these 82 cases, 40 (48.8%) of the cases involved coding error cases. As visible in Table 4.97, the highest coding errors rate involved cases that were assigned to code P59.8 (Neonatal jaundice from other specific causes), P12.2 (Epicardial subaponeurotic haemorrhage due to birth injury) and P20.9 (Intrauterine hypoxia, unspecified).

Table 4.77 Top 10 Primary Diagnosis Code Assigned Before and After Re-Coding Process within Paediatric Case-Type

		Before Re-Coding Process				After Re-Coding Process		
		n = 116	n = *			n = 108	n = **	
No.	Codes	Description	Frequency (%) *	No. of Error Cases (%)	Codes	Description	Frequency (%) **	No. of Cases With Unchanged Primary Diagnosis Code (%)
1.	P59.9	Neonatal jaundice, unspecified	47 (40.5)	30 (63.8)	P59.8	Neonatal jaundice from other specified causes	27 (25.0)	0 (0.0)
2.	P22.1	Transient tachypnoea of newborn	13 (11.2)	1 (7.7)	P59.9	Neonatal jaundice, unspecified	15 (13.9)	14 (93.3)
3.	P36.9	Bacterial sepsis of newborn, unspecified	8 (6.9)	4 (50.0)	P22.1	Transient tachypnoea of newborn	14 (13.0)	12 (85.7)
4.	P23.9	Congenital pneumonia, unspecified	7 (6.0)	1 (14.3)	P23.9	Congenital pneumonia, unspecified	6 (5.6)	6 (100.0)
5.	P07.3	Other preterm infants	4 (3.4)	4 (100.0)	P36.9	Bacterial sepsis of newborn, unspecified	4 (3.7)	4 (100.0)
6.	P55.1	ABO isoimmunization of fetus and newborn	4 (3.4)	3 (75.0)	P55.1	ABO isoimmunization of fetus and newborn	4 (3.7)	2 (50.0)
7.	P22.0	Respiratory distress syndrome of newborn	3 (2.6)	1 (33.3)	P70.4	Other neonatal hypoglycaemia	4 (3.7)	2 (50.0)
8.	P24.0	Neonatal aspiration of meconium	3 (2.6)	1 (33.3)	P12.2	Epicardial subaponeurotic haemorrhage due to birth injury	3 (2.8)	0 (0.0)
9.	J38.0	Paralysis of vocal cords and larynx	2 (1.7)	1 (50.0)	P22.0	Respiratory distress syndrome of newborn	3 (2.8)	2 (66.7)
10.	P07.1	Other low birth weight new born	2 (1.7)	1 (50.0)	P20.9	Intrauterine hypoxia, unspecified	2 (1.9)	0 (0.0)

Kappa Value = 0.460, p <0.001

Table 4.79 shows the changes which occurred due to coding errors among the top 10 primary diagnosis codes assigned before the re-coding process within paediatric case type. As seen in the table, code P59.9 was the highest frequency for primary diagnosis code which was assigned to paediatric cases, which comprised of 47 (40.5%) of the cases. From these 47 cases, only 17 (36.1%) of the cases were assigned to similar primary diagnosis code after the re-coding process by the Independent Senior Coder. Mostly, cases that were assigned to code P59.9 before the re-coding process was re-assigned to code P59.8 after the re-coding process by the Independent Senior Coder (8 cases; 38.3%).

From Table 4.79, it is also notable that none of the cases that were assigned to code P07.3 before the re-coding process were assigned to the similar primary diagnosis code after the re-coding process by the Independent Senior Coder. In total, there were 4 cases that were assigned to code P07.3 as its primary diagnosis code before the re-coding process by the Independent Senior Coder. After the re-coding process, 2 (50.0%) of the cases were re-assigned to code P59.8. The remaining 2 (50.0%) cases were re-assigned to code P12.2 and P20.9 with 1 case for each code.

To sum it up, coding errors of primary diagnosis code in paediatric case type was moderate. The errors rate reported in this case type (58.0%) was the second lowest after surgical case type. The level of agreement between the in-house coder and the Independent Senior Coder was moderate with the kappa value of 0.460. This indicates a moderate knowledge of the in-house coders on the diagnosis codes associated with paediatric cases. It is also worth to note that, the highest frequency of primary diagnosis code before and after the re-coding process was associated with neonatal jaundice. However, the code that was frequently assigned by the Independent Senior Coder shows a more detailed condition of the patient. This implies that even though the knowledge of the in-house coders in the assignment of primary diagnosis code was moderate, the in-house coders still need to enhance their coding skill to be able to assign a more detailed and accurate code during the coding process.

Table 4.78 Changes in the Top 10 Primary Diagnosis Code Assigned Before the Re-Coding Process in Paediatric Case-Type due to Coding Errors

No.	Before Re-Coding Process n = 116			After Re-Coding Process n = *		
	Original Primary Diagnosis Code	No. of Cases* (%)	No. of Cases with Similar Primary Diagnosis Code (%)	Cases With New Primary Diagnosis Code due to Coding Error		
				New Primary Diagnosis Code	Description	No. Cases (%)
1.	P59.9 (Neonatal jaundice, unspecified)	47 (40.5)	17 (36.1)	P59.8	Neonatal jaundice from other specified causes	18 (38.3)
				P55.1	ABO isoimmunization of fetus and newborn	2 (4.3)
				P58.4	Neonatal jaundice due to drugs or toxins transmitted from mother or given to newborn	1 (2.1)
				J38.0	Paralysis of vocal cords and larynx	1 (2.1)
				M25.1	Fistula of joint	1 (2.1)
				P24.0	Neonatal aspiration of meconium	1 (2.1)
				P58.2	Neonatal jaundice due to infection	1 (2.1)
				P58.8	Neonatal jaundice due to other specified excessive haemolysis	1 (2.1)
				P59.3	Neonatal jaundice from breast milk inhibitor	1 (2.1)
				P70.4	Other neonatal hypoglycaemia	1 (2.1)
				P92.0	Vomiting in newborn	1 (2.1)

HOW MUCH IS THE COST OF CODING ERRORS?

2.	P22.1 (Transient tachypnoea of newborn)	13 (11.2)	12 (92.3)	P22.0	Respiratory distress syndrome of newborn	1 (7.7)
3.	P36.9 (Bacterial sepsis of newborn, unspecified)	8 (6.9)	4 (50.0)	P12.2	Cephalhematoma due to birth injury	1 (12.5)
				P59.8	Neonatal jaundice from other specified causes	1 (12.5)
				P70.4	Other neonatal hypoglycaemia	1 (12.5)
				P81.8	Other specified disturbances of temperature regulation of newborn	1 (12.5)
4.	P23.9 (Congenital pneumonia, unspecified)	7 (6.0)	6 (85.7)	P55.1	ABO isoimmunization of fetus and newborn	1 (14.3)
5.	P07.3 (Other preterm infants)	4 (3.4)	0 (0.0)	P59.8	Neonatal jaundice from other specified causes	2 (50.0)
				P12.2	Epicranial subaponeurotic haemorrhage due to birth injury	1 (25.0)
				P20.9	Intrauterine hypoxia, unspecified	1 (25.0)
6.	P55.1 (ABO isoimmunization of fetus and newborn)	4 (3.4)	1 (25.0)	P22.1	Transient tachypnoea of newborn	1 (25.0)
				P59.8	Neonatal jaundice from other specified causes	1 (25.0)
				P59.9	Neonatal jaundice, unspecified	1 (25.0)
7.	P22.0 (Respiratory distress syndrome of newborn)	3 (2.6)	2 (66.7)	P23.9	Congenital pneumonia, unspecified	1 (33.3)
8.	P24.0 (Neonatal aspiration of meconium)	3 (2.6)	2 (66.7)	P28.0	Primary atelectasis of newborn	1 (33.3)
9.	J38.0 (Paralysis of vocal cords and larynx)	2 (1.7)	1 (50.0)	P28.8	Other specified respiratory conditions of newborn	1 (50.0)
10.	P07.1 (Other low birth weight new born)	2 (1.7)	1 (50.0)	P59.0	Neonatal jaundice associated with preterm delivery	1 (50.0)

b. Coding Errors of Secondary Diagnosis Code within Paediatric Case-Type

The coding error rates among paediatric case types are higher at the second level of coding error calculation than at the first level of coding, error calculation. At the first level of the calculation the coding errors occurred in 84 (72.4%) of the selected cases. On the other hand, at the second level of the calculation, from the 246 secondary diagnosis codes reviewed by the Independent Senior Coder during the re-coding process within paediatric cases, 193 (78.5%) of the codes were considered as error codes.

Among the paediatric cases, after the re-coding process the number of cases that were assigned to at least one secondary diagnosis code after the re-coding process has increased by 36.8%. Before the re-coding process there were 62 cases that were assigned to at least one secondary diagnosis code. After the re-coding process however, at least 1 secondary diagnosis code was assigned to 87 cases that were grouped under paediatric case type. Before the re-coding process the total numbers of codes assigned as secondary diagnosis code across the cases that were assigned to paediatric case type were 127 codes and have grossly been increased to 208 codes after the re-coding process. Before the re-coding process the maximum number of codes assigned per patient was 6 codes, with the mean of 1.11 (SD: 1.41). On the other hand, the maximum number of codes assigned per patient has increased to 12 codes, with the mean of 1.91 (SD: 1.85) after the re-coding process. The level of agreement between the Independent Senior Coder and in-house coder on the number of secondary diagnosis code assigned per patient was tested using Cohen's Kappa test and the result showed a fair agreement with the kappa value of 0.261 (Table 4.79).

Table 4.79 Distributions of the Number of Secondary Diagnosis Codes Assigned Before and After the Re-Coding Process within Paediatric Case-Type

No. of Secondary Diagnosis Code	Before	After	Kappa value	p value
			0.261	<0.001
Total No. of Code	127	208		
Max. Codes	6	12		
Mean (SD)	1.11 (1.41)	1.91 (1.85)		

i. **Comparisons of Number of Secondary Diagnosis Code Assigned per Patient Before and After the Re-Coding Process in Paediatric Case-Type**

Table 4.80 shows the comparisons of the number of secondary diagnosis codes that were assigned per patient before and after the re-coding process among cases that were assigned to paediatric case-type. The level of agreement between the in-house coder and the Independent Senior Coder in the assignment of the number of secondary diagnosis code in cases that were assigned to paediatric case-type was fair, with the kappa value of 0.261.

As seen in Table 4.80, in total there were 56 (48.3%) cases that were unassigned to any secondary diagnosis code before the re-coding process. From these 56 cases, only 19 (33.9%) cases remained unassigned to any secondary diagnosis code after the re-coding process was performed by the Independent Senior Coder. The 37 (66.1%) remaining cases were assigned to at least 1 secondary diagnosis code after the re-coding process. Before the re-coding process, the maximum number of secondary diagnosis codes assigned to the patient in paediatric case type was 6 codes with the number of the case was 1 (0.9%). However, after the re-coding process, this case was assigned to 2 number of secondary diagnosis code.

After the re-coding process, in total there were 2 (1.8%) cases that were assigned to more than 6 secondary diagnosis codes. The highest number of secondary diagnosis codes assigned to the patient in paediatric case type after the re-coding process was 12 codes. Data analysis shows that there was 1 (0.9%) case that was assigned with 12 secondary diagnosis codes and this case was originally assigned to only 1 secondary diagnosis code before the re-coding process was performed by the Independent Senior Coder.

Table 4.80 Comparisons of Number of Secondary Diagnosis Code Assigned per Patient Before and After the Re-Coding Process in Paediatric Case-Type

	Before Re-Coding Process						After Re-Coding Process			
	n =116		n = *			n = 108		n = **		
No.	No. of Secondary Diagnosis Code	No. of Cases (%)*	No. of Cases with Similar No of Secondary Diagnosis Code After Re-Coding Process (%)	No. of Cases With Lower No of Secondary Diagnosis Code After Re-Coding Process (%)	No. of Cases With Higher No of Secondary Diagnosis Code After Re-Coding Process (%)	No. of Secondary Diagnosis Code	No. of Cases (%)**	No. of Cases with Similar No of Secondary Diagnosis Code After Re-Coding Process (%)	No. of Cases With Lower No of Secondary Diagnosis Code Before Re-Coding Process (%)	No. of Cases With Higher No of Secondary Diagnosis Code Before Re-Coding Process (%)
1.	0	56 (48.3)	19 (33.9)	0 (0.0)	37 (66.1)	0	21 (19.4)	17 (81.0)	0 (0.0)	4 (19.0)
2.	1	26 (22.4)	12 (46.2)	3 (11.5)	11 (42.3)	1	32 (29.6)	13 (40.6)	13 (40.6)	6 (18.8)
3.	2	15 (12.9)	5 (33.3)	1 (6.7)	9 (60.0)	2	26 (24.1)	4 (15.4)	18 (69.2)	4 (15.4)
4.	3	10 (8.6)	1 (10.0)	6 (60.0)	4 (40.0)	3	14 (13.0)	1 (7.1)	12 (85.7)	1 (7.1)
5.	4	5 (4.3)	2 (25.0)	3 (75.0)	0 (0.0)	4	10 (9.3)	2 (20.0)	7 (70.0)	1 (10.0)
6.	5	3 (2.6)	0 (0.0)	3 (0.0)	0 (0.0)	5	2 (1.9)	0 (0.0)	2 (100.0)	0 (0.0)
7.	6	1 (0.9)	0 (0.0)	1 (100.0)	0 (0.0)	6	1 (0.9)	0 (0.0)	1 (100.0)	0 (0.0)
8.	N/A	N/A	N/A	N/A	N/A	10	1 (0.9)	0 (0.0)	1 (100.0)	0 (0.0)
9.	N/A	N/A	N/A	N/A	N/A	12	1 (0.9)	0 (0.0)	1 (100.0)	0 (0.0)

k= 0.261, p < 0.001

Table 4.81 shows the distribution of coding error cases by the number of its secondary diagnosis codes. It is notable in the table that the highest coding error rates (100.0%) involved cases that were assigned to 4 and above secondary diagnosis code. This implies that the in-house coder has difficulties to codify cases with a higher number of secondary diagnosis code. A chi-square test was ran to determine the association between the number of secondary diagnosis code and coding errors. The result was statistically insignificant with chi-square value of 3.369, p>0.05.

Table 4.81 Distributions of Coding Errors Cases by Number of Secondary Diagnosis Codes in Paediatric Case-Type

No. of Secondary Diagnosis Code	No. of Case without Coding Error	%	No. of Case with Coding Error/s	%	Total	%
0	11	19.6	45	80.4	56	100.0
1	2	7.7	24	92.3	26	100.0
2	2	13.3	13	86.7	15	100.0
3	1	10.0	9	90.0	10	100.0
4 and above	0	0.0	9	100.0	9	100.0

X^2 = 3.369 df =4, p =0.498

ii. Type of Coding Errors of Secondary Diagnosis Code within Paediatric Case-Type

Data analysis of this study shows that the commonest type of error in the assignment of secondary diagnosis code across cases that were assigned to paediatric case type was under-coding. From the 246 secondary diagnosis codes reviewed by the Independent Senior Coder, 114 (46.3%) of the codes were being under-coded by the in-house coder. The second highest type of errors found within the secondary diagnosis codes was the error at the second digit level with the number of error case of 30 (12.2%) cases. The error at the assignment of the fourth digit level of the code was the third highest type of error in the paediatric type of cases in which 24 (9.8%) of error codes were reported due to this type of error. The fourth highest type of error in the assignment of secondary diagnosis code within the paediatric type of cases was up-coding, in which 17 (6.9%) cases were reported with this type of error. Lastly, the least common type of errors was the error at the fourth digit level of the code in which there were 8 (3.3%) cases that were reported with this type of errors. The details of the type of coding errors in the assignment of secondary diagnosis code among the surgical type of cases are illustrated in Table 4.82.

Table 4.82 Distributions of Type of Coding Errors in Secondary Diagnosis Code within Paediatric Case-Type

Type of Error	No. of Error Cases	%
Under-coding	114	46.3
Error at Second Digit Level	30	12.2
Error at Fourth Digit Level	24	9.8
Up-coding	17	6.9
Error at Third Digit Level	8	3.3

iii. **Comparisons of Top 10 Secondary Diagnosis Code Assigned Before and After the Re-Coding Process within Paediatric Case-Type**

Table 4.83 below shows the comparison of the top 10 secondary diagnosis codes assigned before and after the re-coding process in paediatric case type. It is notable that in Table 4.83, codes that were associated with neonatal jaundice and feeding are among the most frequently used codes by both of the coders, before and after the re-coding process. Also as seen in the table, from the 10 listed codes, there were 5 codes that were commonly used by both of the coders during the assignment of secondary diagnosis coder. The codes were P59.9 (Neonatal jaundice, unspecified), P70.4 (Other neonatal hypoglycaemia), P36.9 (Bacterial sepsis of newborn, unspecified), P05.1 (Small gestational age), and P12.0 (Cephalhematoma due to birth injury).

Before the re-coding process, code P59.9 was the code with the highest frequency assigned as secondary diagnosis code in paediatric case type covering 22 (17.3%) of the cases. From these 22 cases assigned to code P59.9 as its secondary diagnosis code before the re-coding process, 19 (86.4%) of the cases contained at least one error for its secondary diagnosis code in it. On the other hand, after the re-coding process, code P59.9 was still listed as the top 10 secondary diagnosis code with the number of cases assigned to this code reduced to 20 (9.6%) cases. The highest frequency for secondary diagnosis code after the re-coding process was for the code P92.3, which covers 22 (10.6%) of the cases. From these 22 cases, only 1 (4.5%) of the case was assigned to code P92.3 with accurate secondary diagnosis codes.

From the 78 cases that contain at least one of the top 10 highest secondary diagnosis code assigned before the re-coding process 67 (85.9%) of the cases were the coding error cases. The highest coding error rates (100.0%) involved cases that were assigned to the code P07.3 (Other preterm infants) and P22.0 (Respiratory distress syndrome of newborn) as its secondary diagnosis code. On the other hand, after the re-coding process from the 103 cases which contained at least one of the top 10 highest secondary diagnosis code after the re-coding process, 96 (93.2%) of the cases contained at least one error secondary diagnosis code in it. It is also notable in Table 4.83 that all of the cases assigned to codes P70.0 (Syndrome of infant of mother with gestational diabetes), P07.1 (Other low birth weight), P05.1 and P70.4 as its secondary diagnosis code, contained at least one error secondary diagnosis code in it.

To sum it up, in paediatric case type, even though the total number of cases assigned to this case type has decreased after the re-coding process, the total number of secondary diagnosis code has increased from 127 codes before the re-coding process to 208 codes after the re-coding process. The number of cases listed in the top 10 secondary diagnosis codes has also increased from 78 cases before the re-coding process to 103 cases after the re-coding process. The increasing pattern of the number of secondary diagnosis codes assigned to cases in paediatric cases after the re-coding process is parallel with the most common type of errors identified within this case type namely undercoding.

Table 4.83 Comparisons of Top 10 Secondary Diagnosis Code Assigned within Paediatric Case-Type

| | | Before Re-Coding Process | | | After Re-Coding Process | | | |
| | | n =127 | n =* | | | n = 208 | n =** |
No.	Codes	Description	Frequency (%)*	No. of Error Cases (%)	Codes	Description	Frequency (%)**	No. of Cases Without Coding Errors (%)
1.	P59.9	Neonatal jaundice, unspecified	22 (17.3)	19 (86.4)	P92.3	Underfeeding of newborn	22 (10.6)	1 (4.5)
2.	P92.9	Feeding problem of newborn, unspecified	16 (12.6)	15 (93.8)	P59.9	Neonatal jaundice, unspecified	20 (9.6)	2 (10.0)
3.	P70.4	Other neonatal hypoglycaemia	7 (5.5)	6 (85.7)	P70.0	Syndrome of infant of mother with gestational diabetes	14 (6.7)	0 (0.0)
4.	P36.9	Bacterial sepsis of newborn, unspecified	6 (4.7)	4 (66.7)	P07.1	Other low birth weight	10 (4.8)	0 (0.0)
5.	P70.1	Syndrome of infant of a diabetic mother	6 (4.7)	5 (83.3)	P36.9	Bacterial sepsis of newborn, unspecified	8 (3.8)	1 (12.5)
6.	P22.1	Transient tachypnoea of newborn	5 (3.9)	4 (80.0)	P05.1	Small for gestational age	6 (2.9)	0 (0.0)
7.	P05.1	Small for gestational age	4 (3.1)	3 (75.0)	P12.0	Cephalhematoma due to birth injury	6 (2.9)	1 (16.7)
8.	P07.3	Other preterm infants	4 (3.1)	4 (100.0)	P70.4	Other neonatal hypoglycaemia	6 (2.9)	0 (0.0)
9.	P12.0	Cephalhematoma due to birth injury	4 (3.1)	3 (75.0)	P92.8	Other feeding problems of newborn	6 (2.9)	1 (16.7)
10.	P22.0	Respiratory distress syndrome of newborn	4 (3.1)	4 (100.0)	P59.0	Neonatal jaundice associated with preterm delivery	5 (2.4)	1 (20.0)

c. Coding Errors of Primary Procedure Code within Paediatric Case-Type

Among the paediatric type of cases, the number of cases assigned as paediatric case-type in MY-DRG® grouper has decreased from 116 cases to 108 cases. However, in comparisons to the number of cases, the percentage of cases assigned to primary procedure code was higher after the re-coding process. Prior to the re-coding process, from the 116 cases assigned to paediatric case type, 93 (80.2%) of the cases were codified with primary procedure code. After the re-coding process, from the 108 cases assigned to paediatric case type, 95 (88.0%) of the cases were codified with primary procedure code.

In this case-type, the coding error rates were higher at the second level of coding error calculation when compared to the calculation at the first level. At the first level of calculation, the coding errors rate was 52.6% covering 61 of error cases. On the contrary, at the second level of calculation, from the 105 primary procedure codes reviewed by the Independent Senior Coder 61 (58.1%) of the codes were considered as error codes.

i. Type of Coding Errors of Primary Procedure Code In Paediatric Case-Type

In the assignment of the primary procedure code within paediatric cases, most of the codes were being under-coded, in which 30 (28.6%) of error cases were reported due to this type of error. The second highest type of errors was up-coding where the number of error cases has reached 15 (14.3%) cases. The third highest type of errors was the error at the second digit level of the code covering 6 (5.7%) of the error cases. The fourth highest type of errors was due to the wrong selection of the primary procedure code in which the number of error cases was reported as 5 (4.8%) cases. The errors due to primary procedure code being incorrectly sequenced were the fifth highest, with the number of error cases of 3 (2.9%). The least common type of errors in the assignment of primary procedure codes in paediatric cases were due to the error at the third and fourth digit level with 1 (1.0%) error case per each type of error. Table 4.84 shows the distributions of the type of coding errors which occurred within the assignment of the primary procedure codes in paediatric cases.

Table 4.84 Distributions of the Type of Coding Errors of Primary Procedure Codes in Paediatric Case-Type

Type of Error	No. of Error Cases	%
Under-coding	30	28.6
Up-coding	15	14.3
Error at Second Digit Level	6	5.7
Wrong Selection of Primary Procedure Code	5	4.8
Principal Procedure Incorrectly Sequenced	3	2.9
Error at Third Digit Level	1	1.0
Error at Fourth Digit Level	1	1.0

ii. Comparisons of Top 10 Primary Procedure Code Assigned in Paediatric Case-Type Before and After the Re-Coding Process

Table 4.85 shows the comparisons of the top 10 primary procedure codes assigned before and after the re-coding process within paediatric cases. As shown in the table, from the ten listed codes, seven of the codes were commonly assigned by both of the coders in the assignment of the primary procedure code among paediatric cases. The codes are 99.83 (Other phototherapy), 87.44 (Routine chest x-ray, so described), 88.72 (Diagnostic ultrasound of heart), 34.04 (Insertion of intercostal catheter for drainage), 88.71 (Diagnostic ultrasound of head and neck), 18.11 (Otoscopy) and 99.04 (Transfusion of packed cells). Even though the distributions of the frequently used codes by both of the coders are more similar in paediatric cases than for other cases, the kappa agreement between both of the coders in the assignment of primary procedure code was poor with the kappa value of 0.013. This implies that the frequently used codes by both coders have a high possibility to be assigned to different cases before and after the audit.

Table 4.85 Comparisons of Top 10 Primary Procedure Code Assigned Before and After the Re-Coding Process within Paediatric Case-Type

	Before Re-Coding Process				After Re-Coding Process			
			n = 93	n = *			n = 95	n = **
No.	Codes	Description	Frequency (%)*	No. of Error Cases (%)	Codes	Description	Frequency (%)**	No. of Cases Without Coding Errors (%)
1.	99.83	Other phototherapy	32 (34.4)	15 (46.9)	99.83	Other phototherapy	65 (68.4)	16 (24.6)
2.	87.44	Routine chest x-ray, so described	18 (19.4)	17 (94.4)	87.44	Routine chest x-ray, so described	7 (7.4)	1 (14.3)
3.	93.9	Non-invasive mechanical ventilation	11 (11.8)	11 (100.0)	88.72	Diagnostic ultrasound of heart	5 (5.3)	0 (0.0)
4.	88.72	Diagnostic ultrasound of heart	3 (3.2)	3 (100.0)	88.71	Diagnostic ultrasound of head and neck	3 (3.2)	0 (0.0)
5.	34.04	Insertion of intercostal catheter for drainage	2 (2.2)	2 (100.0)	18.11	Otoscopy	1 (1.1)	0 (0.0)
6.	87.17	Other x-ray of skull	2 (2.2)	2 (100.0)	31.42	Laryngoscopy and other tracheoscopy	1 (1.1)	0 (0.0)
7.	88.71	Diagnostic ultrasound of head and neck	2 (2.2)	2 (100.0)	34.04	Insertion of intercostal catheter for drainage	1 (1.1)	0 (0.0)
8.	18.11	Otoscopy	1 (1.1)	1 (100.0)	89.52	Electrocardiogram	1 (1.1)	0 (0.0)
9.	88.19	Other x-ray of abdomen	1 (1.1)	1 (100.0)	96.33	Gastric lavage	1 (1.1)	0 (0.0)
10.	99.04	Transfusion of packed cells	1 (1.1)	1 (100.0)	99.04	Transfusion of packed cells	1 (1.1)	0 (0.0)

Kappa value = 0.013 p <0.001

In paediatric case-type, the highest frequency of code assigned as a primary procedure code was mutual for before and after the re-coding process, namely for the code 99.83. However, data after the re-coding process showed a higher number of cases assigned to this code. Before the re-coding process, there were 32 (34.4%) of the cases that were assigned to code 99.83 as its primary procedure code. However, after the re-coding process, the number of cases assigned to this code has increased to 65 (68/4%) cases. Interestingly, from the 65 cases assigned to code 99.83 after the re-coding process 20 (30.8%) of the cases were unassigned to any primary procedure code before the re-coding process by the in-house coder. This indicates a significant number of under-coding cases in the assignment of the primary procedure code in the paediatric case-type.

Table 4.86 below shows the changes which occurred due to coding errors among the top 10 primary procedure codes assigned before the re-coding process. As seen in the table, before the re-coding process, there were 32 (34.4%) cases assigned to code 99.83 as its primary procedure code. After the re-coding process, from these 32 cases, 15 (46.9%) of the cases were identified as error cases. From these 15 error cases, 7 (41.2%) of the cases were unassigned to any primary procedure code after the re-coding process by the Independent Senior Coder. On the other hand, 3 (17.6%) of the error cases were re-assigned to code 87.44 as its primary procedure code. From Table 4.86 it is also notable that, either than cases that were assigned to code 99.83 and 87.44, all the cases that were assigned to the top 10 primary procedure codes assigned before the re-coding process were assigned to inaccurate primary procedure codes. Majority of the cases were re-assigned to code 99.83, which has the highest frequency to be assigned as primary procedure code, both before and after the audit.

To sum it up, at the first level of the coding error calculation, the coding errors rate (52.6%) identified in the paediatric case type was the second highest among all the case types. Even though the selection of the common code to be assigned to the primary procedure of the patient was almost similar by both of the coders, the output from the kappa test indicates a poor agreement between both of the coders. This indicates a poor knowledge of the procedure carried out across cases assigned to paediatric cases among the in-house coder.

Table 4.86 Changes Among the Top 10 Primary Procedure Code Assigned Among Paediatric Case-Type due to Coding Errors

No.	Before Re-Coding Process n = 93			After Re-Coding Process n = *		
	Original Primary Procedure Code	No. of Cases * (%)	No. of Cases with Similar Primary Procedure Code (%)	Cases With New Primary Procedure Code due to Coding Error		
				New Primary Procedure Code	Description	No. Cases (%)
1.	99.83 (Other phototherapy)	32 (34.4)	17 (54.1)	None	None	7 (41.2)
				87.44	Routine chest x-ray, so described	3 (17.6)
				18.11	Otoscopy	1 (5.9)
				39.95	Haemodialysis	1 (5.9)
				88.71	Diagnostic ultrasound of head and neck	1 (5.9)
				88.72	Diagnostic ultrasound of heart	1 (5.9)
				99.04	Transfusion of packed cells	1 (5.9)
2.	87.44 (Routine chest x-ray, so described)	18 (19.4)	1 (55.6)	99.83	Other phototherapy	8 (44.4)
				None	None	5 (27.8)
				88.72	Diagnostic ultrasound of heart	2 (11.1)
				34.04	Insertion of intercostal catheter for drainage	1 (5.6)

3.	93.9 (Non-invasive mechanical ventilation)	11 (11.8)	0 (0.0)	96.33	Gastric lavage	1 (5.6)
				None	None	4 (36.4)
				99.83	Other phototherapy	3 (27.3)
				31.42	Laryngoscopy and other tracheoscopy	1 (9.1)
				87.17	Other x-ray of skull	1 (9.1)
				87.44	Routine chest x-ray, so described	1 (9.1)
				88.71	Diagnostic ultrasound of head and neck	1 (9.1)
4.	88.72 (Diagnostic ultrasound of heart)	3 (3.2)	0 (0.0)	87.44	Routine chest x-ray, so described	1 (33.3)
				99.83	Other phototherapy	1 (33.3)
				None	None	1 (33.3)
5.	34.04 (Insertion of intercostal catheter for drainage)	2 (2.2)	0 (0.0)	89.52	Electrocardiogram	1 (50.0)
				99.83	Other phototherapy	1 (50.0)
6.	87.17 (Other x-ray of skull)	2 (2.2)	0 (0.0)	87.44	Routine chest x-ray, so described	1 (50.0)
				99.83	Other phototherapy	1 (50.0)
7.	88.71 (Diagnostic ultrasound of head and neck)	2 (2.2)	0 (0.0)	99.83	Other phototherapy	2 (100.0)
8.	18.11 (Otoscopy)	1 (1.1)	0 (0.0)	99.83	Other phototherapy	1 (100.0)
9.	88.19 (Other x-ray of abdomen)	1 (1.1)	0 (0.0)	99.83	Other phototherapy	1 (100.0)
10.	99.04 (Transfusion of packed cells)	1 (1.1)	0 (0.0)	None	None	1 (100.0)

d. Coding Errors of Secondary Procedure Code in Paediatric Case-Type

The coding errors rate of secondary procedure code in cases assigned to paediatric cases was higher at the second level of coding error calculation than the first level of calculation. At the first level of coding error calculation, the coding errors rate was 25.0%, covering 29 (25.0%) of the cases. At the second level of coding error calculation, from the 55 secondary procedure codes reviewed by the Independent Senior Coder, 47 (85.5%) of the codes were considered as error codes.

In paediatric case type, before and after the re-coding process, the total number of secondary diagnosis codes assigned to the entire case was 30 codes. Before the re-coding process, the maximum number of secondary procedure codes assigned to the patient was 3, with the mean of 0.26 (SD 0.56). After the re-coding process, the maximum number of secondary procedure code increased to 8 codes, with the mean of 0.28 (0.94). The level of agreement between the in-house coder and the Independent Senior Coder in the number of secondary procedure code assigned per patient was poor with the kappa value of 0.202 (Table 4.87).

Table 4.87 Distributions of Total Number of Secondary Procedure Code Assigned to Patient Before and After the Re-Coding Process within Paediatric Case-Type

No. of Secondary Procedure Code	Before	After	Kappa value	p value
			0.202	<0.001
Total No of Code	30	30		
Max. Codes	3	8		
Mean (SD)	0.26 (0.56)	0.28 (0.94)		

i. Comparison of Number of Secondary Procedure Code Before and After the Re-coding process in Paediatric Case-Type

Before the re-coding process, from the 116 cases assigned to paediatric cases, 91 (78.4%) of the cases were unassigned to any secondary procedure code. From these 91 cases, 10 (11.0%) of the cases were identified as coding error cases. Table 4.88 shows the distributions of error cases by the number of secondary procedures codes assigned to the patient in paediatric case type. As seen in the table, before the re-coding process, the coding errors rate (100.0%) was the highest among cases that were assigned to 2 and above secondary procedure code. A Chi-Square test was conducted to determine the association between the number of secondary procedure code and coding errors. The result was proven to be statistically insignificant with the X^2 value of 0.980, p >0.05 (Table 4.88).

Table 4.88 Distributions of Coding Errors Cases by Number of Secondary Procedure Code within Paediatric Case-Type

No. of Secondary Procedure Code	No. of Case without Coding Error	%	No. of Case with Coding Error/s	%	Total	%
0	13	14.2	78	84.8	92	100.0
1	3	15.0	17	85.0	20	100.0
2	0	0.0	4	100.0	4	100.0
3 and above	0	0.0	1	100.0	1	100.0

X^2 = 0.980, df =3, p =0.806

Table 4.89 shows the distributions of the number of secondary procedure code assigned to the patient before and after the re-coding process. As seen in the table, the number of cases that were unassigned to any secondary procedure code was consistent before and after the re-coding process(91 cases). However, as seen in the table, even though the number of cases without secondary procedure code was similar before and after the re-coding process, the cases without secondary procedure code after the re-coding process was unnecessarily the similar case as before the re-coding process. Apparently, from the 91 cases without secondary procedure code before the re-coding process 10 (11.0%) of the cases were assigned to at least one secondary procedure code after the re-coding process

It is also notable from Table 4.89 that, before the re-coding process by the Independent Senior Coder, the maximum number of secondary procedure code assigned to the patient assigned to paediatric case-type was 3 covering 1 (0.9%) case. However, after the re-coding process, this case has been re-assigned with only one secondary procedure code by the Independent Senior Coder. On the other hand, after the re-coding process, in total there were 2 (1.9%) cases that were assigned to more than 3 secondary procedure codes. On the other hand, the maximum number of secondary procedure code assigned to paediatric cases after the re-coding process was eight codes covering 1 (0.9%) case. Interestingly, this case was originally unassigned to any secondary procedure code before the re-coding process by the Independent Senior Coder. This implies poor skills of the in-house coder in assigning not only the accurate secondary procedure code but also the accurate number of secondary procedure code among paediatric cases.

Table 4.89 Comparison of Number of Secondary Procedure Code Assigned per Patient Before and After the Re-Coding Process within Paediatric Case-Type

No		Before Re-Coding Process					After Re-Coding Process				
		n =116					n =108				
	No. of Secondary Procedure Code	No. of Cases (%) *	No. of Cases With Similar number of Secondary Diagnosis Code After Re-Coding Process (%)	n =*			No. of Secondary Procedure Code	No. Of Cases (%)**	No. Of Cases With Similar Number Of Secondary Diagnosis Code As Before Re-Coding Process (%)	n =**	
				No. of Errors Cases with Lower No of Secondary Procedure Code After Re-Coding Process (%)	No. of Errors Cases with Higher No of Secondary Procedure Code After Re-Coding Process (%)					No. of Errors Cases with Lower No of Secondary Procedure Code Before Re-Coding Process (%)	No. of Errors Cases with Higher No of Secondary Procedure Code Before Re-Coding Process (%)
1.	0	91 (78.4)	81 (89.0)	0 (0.0)	10 (11.0)		0	91 (84.3)	75 (82.4)	0 (0.0)	16 (17.6)
2.	1	20 (17.2)	6 (30.0)	13 (65.0)	1 (5.0)		1	12 (11.1)	5 (41.7)	5 (41.7)	2 (16.7)
3.	2	4 (3.4)	1 (25.0)	1 (25.0)	2 (50.0)		2	3 (2.8)	0 (0.0)	3 (100.0)	0 (0.0)
4.	3	1 (0.9)	0 (0.0)	1 (100.0)	0 (0.0)		4	1 (0.9)	0 (0.0)	1 (100.0)	0 (0.0)
5.	4	N/A	N/A	N/A	N/A		8	1 (0.9)	0 (0.0)	1 (100.0)	0 (0.0)

ii. Type of Coding Errors of Secondary Procedure Code in Paediatric Case-Type

Data analysis in this study shows that there were only four types of coding errors that were identified in the assignment of secondary procedure code across cases assigned to the paediatric type of cases. The commonest type of error in the assignment of secondary procedure code within paediatric cases was under-coding covering 25 (45.5%) of the error cases. The second highest type of errors of secondary procedure codes in paediatric case type was up-coding covering 19 (34.5%) of the error cases. The wrong selection of the secondary procedure code was the third highest type of error consisting of 2 (3.6%) of error cases were due to these type errors. The least type of error in the assignment of secondary procedure code in the paediatric type of cases was the error at the third digit level of the code covering 1 (1.8%) error case. The distributions of the type of coding errors in the assignment of secondary procedure code within paediatric case type are illustrated in Table 4.90.

Table 4.90 Distributions of Type of Coding Errors of Secondary Procedure Code within Paediatric Case-Type

Type of Error	No. of Error Cases	%
Under-coding	25	45.5
Up-coding	19	34.5
Wrong Selection of Secondary Procedure Code	2	3.6
Error at Third Digit Level	1	1.8

iii. Comparisons of Top 10 Secondary Procedure Code Assigned Before and After the Re-coding process within Paediatric Case-Type

Table 4.91 shows a comparison of the secondary procedure codes that were assigned with the highest frequency in the paediatric case type before and after the re-coding process. As seen in the table, before the re-coding process, there were only seven types of codes were used by the in-house coders to codify the secondary procedure codes to the cases assigned to paediatric case type. On the other hand, after the re-coding process, there were more than ten types of secondary procedure codes assigned by the Independent Senior Coder to the paediatric cases. The more diversified codes used by the Independent Senior Coder indicates his broader knowledge of the coding process compared to the in-house coders. As also notable in the table, from the seven listed codes before the re-coding process, 5 of the codes were commonly used by the Independent Senior Coder and the in-house coders during the assignment of secondary procedure codes of the paediatric type of cases.

Before the re-coding process, code 87.44 (Routine chest x-ray, so described) was the highest assigned secondary procedure code with the number of cases assigned to this code was 12 (40.0%). From these 12 cases, 9 (75.0%) of the cases were assigned to at least one error secondary procedure code. After the re-coding process, code 87.44 was listed as the second highest assigned secondary procedure code in paediatric case type with 4 (13.3%) number of cases.

After the re-coding process. code 88.72 (Diagnostic ultrasound of heart) was the highest assigned secondary procedure code assigned in paediatric case type with 5 (16.7%) number of cases. From these 5 cases, only 1 (20.0%) of the case was originally assigned to the same secondary procedure code. Before the re-coding process, the number of cases assigned to code 88.72 was 2 (6.7%) cases and from these 2 cases, only 1 (50.0%) case was codified with accurate secondary procedure code. As also seen in Table 4.91, besides codes 88.72, 87.44, 99.83 (Other phototherapy) and 93.9 (Respiratory therapy), all the cases that were assigned to the top 10 highest secondary procedure codes after the re-coding process were originally assigned to at least one wrong secondary procedure code.

To sum it up, the number of secondary procedure code assigned to paediatric cases was the lowest compared to the other case types. Also, the type of secondary procedure code assigned to paediatric cases was fewer than other case types. However, at the second level of coding error calculation, the coding errors rate of secondary procedure code in Paediatric case type was the second highest (85.5%) compared to another case type. This shows that even though the types of secondary procedure code that were commonly assigned to paediatric cases were fewer than other case types, the in-house coders still having difficulties to assign the accurate secondary procedure code to the patient. This has given a poor reflection of the in-house coder's skills in assigning the secondary procedure code.

Table 4.91 Comparisons of Top 10 Secondary Procedure Code Assigned within Paediatric Case-Type

		Before Re-Coding Process				After Re-Coding Process			
			n = 30	n = *				n = 30	n = **
No.	Codes	Description	Frequency (%) *	No. of Error Cases (%)		Codes	Description	Frequency (%) **	No. of Cases Without Coding Errors (%)
1.	87.44	Routine chest x-ray, so described	12 (40.0)	9 (75.0)		88.72	Diagnostic ultrasound of heart	5 (16.7)	1 (20.0)
2.	93.9	Respiratory therapy	6 (20.0)	5 (83.3)		87.44	Routine chest x-ray, so described	4 (13.3)	3 (75.0)
3.	99.83	Other phototherapy	5 (16.7)	4 (80.0)		96.6	Enteral infusion of concentrated nutritional substances	3 (10.0)	0 (0.0)
4.	88.72	Diagnostic ultrasound of heart	2 (6.7)	1 (50.0)		99.83	Other phototherapy	3 (10.0)	1 (33.3)
5.	89.52	Electrocardiogram	2 (6.7)	2 (100.0)		88.19	Other x-ray of abdomen	2 (6.7)	0 (0.0)
6.	96.6	Enteral infusion of concentrated nutritional substances	2 (6.7)	0 (0.0)		93.9	Respiratory therapy	2 (6.7)	1 (50.0)
7.	96.04	Insertion of endotracheal tube	2 (6.7)	2 (100.0)		34.04	Insertion of intercostal catheter for drainage	1 (3.3)	0 (0.0)
8.	NIL	NIL	NIL	NIL		38.9	Puncture of vessel	1 (3.3)	0 (0.0)
9.	NIL	NIL	NIL	NIL		38.92	Umbilical vein catheterization	1 (3.3)	0 (0.0)
10.	NIL	NIL	NIL	NIL		38.93	Venous catheterization, not elsewhere classified	1 (3.3)	0 (0.0)

4.5 Coding Errors by Severity Level

From the descriptive analysis, this study pointed that majority of the selected cases were assigned to severity level I with the number of cases was 297 (64.0) cases followed by severity level II with 124 (26.7%) cases. The cases were least assigned to severity level III with the number of cases was 43 (9.3%), respectively.

From Table 4.92, it was notable that the coding errors rate was the highest (95.3%) among the cases that were originally assigned to severity level III. The second highest errors rate (92.7%) was among the cases with severity level II. A chi-square test was run to determine the relationship between the severity level and coding error and the result was statistically significant with $X^2(2) = 17.66$, $p < 0.001$ (Table 4.117).

Table 4.92 Distributions of Error Cases by Severity Level

Type of Severity Level	No. of Case without Coding Error (%)	No. of Case with Coding Error/s (%)	Total (%)
I	38 (12.8)	259 (87.2)	297 (100.0)
II	9 (7.3)	115 (92.7)	124 (100.0)
III	2 (4.7)	41 (95.3)	43 (100.0)

$X^2 = 17.66$, df =2, p <0.001

Table 4.92 below shows the distributions of the severity level after the re-coding process. As seen in the table, the number of severity level I cases has decreased from 297 cases to 211 (45.5%) cases. There is an increment of severity III cases from 43 cases to 61 (52.6%) cases and also increment in severity II cases from 124 cases to 184 (39.7%). From the table, it is also notable there are 6 (1.3%) cases that were unassigned to any group of severity level as these cases were identified as ungroupable cases. A Cohen Kappa test was conducted to identify the level of agreement in the assignment of severity level before and after the re-coding process. The results showed a fair agreement in the assignment of severity level before and after the re-coding process with the kappa value of k = 0.284.

Table 4.93 Distributions of Severity Level After the Re-coding Process

		New Severity				
		X	I	II	III	Total
Original Severity Level	I	3	173	103	18	297
	II	1	31	71	21	124
	III	4	7	10	22	43
	Total	8	211	184	61	464

k = 0.284, p <0.001

4.6 Coding Errors by Type of CMG

This study demonstrates that, from the 415 coding error cases, 69 (16.7) of the error cases show changes in the assignment of its CMG group after the re-coding process. Table 4.94 below shows the comparisons of the distributions of coding error cases by the top 10 highest volume CMG groups before the re-coding process. From the table, before the re-coding process in comparisons to the total number of cases assigned to the CMG group, cases that were assigned to CMG group B (Hepatobiliary and pancreatic system) shows the highest coding errors rate (100.0%). On the other hand, among the top 10 CMG groups before the re-coding process the lowest coding errors rate (82.4%) was among cases that were assigned to CMG group H (Eye and Adnexa).

Before the re-coding process from the 32 types of CMG groups in the MY-DRG Casemix system used by this tertiary hospital, 21 types of CMG groups were used to group the selected cases. After the re-coding process by the Independent Senior Coder, there were 22 types of CMG groups that were used to group the selected cases in this study. The new CMG group that was reported after the re-coding process was CMG group X (Error CMG). There were 6 cases that were re-grouped under this group. All of the cases were from paediatric case-type where there was no information on birth weight re-corded in the patients' medical record.

From Table 4.94, it is notable that before the re-coding process the highest volume was for deliveries (CMG group O) and newborn and neonatal groups (CMG group P) with the number of cases 116 cases per group (25.0%). It is worth to note from the table that, the incidence of coding errors has impacted the assignment of CMG group of one error case that was assigned to CMG group O before the re-coding process. This error case was re-assigned to CMG W (Female reproductive system) after the re-coding process. On the other hand, the incidence of coding errors has caused changes in the assignment of CMG group of eight error cases that were assigned to CMG P before the re-coding process. Interestingly, data analysis showed that from the eight error cases, six of the cases were re-assigned to CMG group X (Error CMG) after the audit.

The coding errors have impacted the distributions of the highest volume CMG groups after the re-coding process. The CMG group O remained as the highest volume CMG group after the re-coding process whereas CMG group P was the second highest volume CMG group. Due to the coding errors, after the re-coding process the number of cases assigned to CMG group O has increased to 119 (25.6%) cases. From these 119 cases, 115 of the cases were the similar cases as before the re-coding process and the additional 4 cases were originally assigned to CMG group W before the re-coding process.

In comparisons of the distributions of the top 10 highest volume CMG groups before and after the re-coding process, both lists showed a similar top 10 CMG groups but with a different number of the case. The bivariate analysis resulted in an almost perfect agreement of kappa value in determining the level of agreement of CMG group before and after the re-coding process ($k=0.829$, $p<0.001$). This implies that the coding errors detected in this study were less likely impacted the assignment of CMG groups of the error cases.

Table 4.94 Top 10 Highest Frequency CMG Before and After the Re-Coding Process

		Before Re-Coding Process					After Re-Coding Process	
		n =464	n =*	n =**				n =464
No.	CMG Code	Description	Frequency (%)*	No. of Case with Coding Error/s (%)**	Error Cases with Changes in CMG	CMG Code	Description	Frequency (%)***
1.	O	Deliveries	116 (25.0)	110 (94.8)	1 (25.0)	O	Deliveries	119 (25.6)
2.	P	Newborns & Neonates	116 (25.0)	100 (86.2)	8 (8.0)	P	Newborns & Neonates	108 (23.3)
3.	K	Digestive system	40 (8.6)	33 (82.5)	8 (24.2)	K	Digestive system	43 (9.3)
4.	W	Female reproductive system	32 (6.9)	27 (90.0)	11 (40.7)	W	Female reproductive system	28 (6.0)
5.	M	Musculosketal system & connective tissue	20 (4.3)	17 (85.0)	3 (17.6)	M	Musculosketal system & connective tissue	24 (5.2)
6.	I	Cardiovascular system	19 (4.1)	18 (94.7)	6 (33.3)	N	Nephro-urinary system	19 (4.1)
7.	N	Nephro-urinary system	18 (3.9)	18 (88.9)	5 (31.3)	I	Cardiovascular system	17 (3.7)
8.	H	Eye and Adnexa	17 (3.7)	14 (82.4)	4 (28.6)	H	Eye and Adnexa	14 (3.0)
9.	L	Skin, subcutaneous tissue & breast	13 (2.8)	12 (92.3)	3 (25.0)	L	Skin, subcutaneous tissue & breast	13 (2.8)
10.	B	Hepatobiliary & pancreatic system	12 (2.6)	12 (100)	3 (25.0)	B	Hepatobiliary & pancreatic system	12 (2.6)

$k=0.829, p<0.001$

4.7 Coding Errors by MY-DRG® Groups

The coding error cases identified in this study have led changes in the assignment of MY-DRG® code among the 307 (74.0%) of the error cases. Before the re-coding process, there were 164 types of MY-DRG® groups assigned to the selected cases. However, after the re-coding process, the number of MY-DRG® groups assigned to the selected cases has grossly increased to 194 groups. Table 4.95 below shows the comparisons of the top 10 highest volume MY-DRG® groups assigned to the selected cases before and after the audit.

From Table 4.95, it could be derived that the highest coding errors rate (100.0%) was involving cases that were assigned to MY-DRG® group O-6-12-II (Vaginal delivery with other procedure excluding sterilization and/or dilation & curettage-moderate) and P-8-08-I (Neonate, birth-weight >2499 grams with respiratory distress syndrome & congenital pneumonia-minor). It is also notable from the table that among 15 error cases that were assigned to MY-DRG® group O-6-12-II before the re-coding process 12 (80.0%) of the cases were re-assigned to other MY-DRG® groups after the re-coding process. On the other hand, from the 11 error cases that were assigned to MY-DRG® group P-8-08-I before the re-coding process, 7 (63.6%) of the cases were re-assigned to other MY-DRG® groups after the re-coding process. Another worth to note information from Table 4.95 was, error cases that were assigned to code H-1-30-I (Intraocular & lens operations-minor) shows the highest percentage (100.0%) of error cases with changes in the assignment of its MY-DRG® groups.

As seen in Table 4.95, before the re-coding process, the highest assigned MY-DRG® code was P-8-17–I (Neonate, birth-weight >2499 grams without complex operation-mild) with the number of cases assigned to this code was 47 (10.1%) cases. Data analysis revealed that from these 47 cases, 39 (83.0%) of the cases were the coding error cases. Another striking finding during the data analysis is, from the 39 (83.0%) error cases, 35 (89.7%) of the error cases were re-assigned to other MY-DRG® group after the re-coding process. A more in-depth descriptive analysis shows that, from these 35 cases, 13 (37.1%) of the cases were re-assigned to MY-DRG® P-8-17-II (Neonate, birth-weight >2499 grams without complex operation-moderate) after the audit.

Data analysis showed that, after the re-coding process by the Independent Senior Coder, code P-8-17-II (Neonate, Birth-Weight >2499 Grams Without Complex Operation-Moderate) was the highest MY-DRG® code. After the re-coding process, in total there were 22 (4.7%) cases that were assigned to this code. This showed an increment of 46.7% from the total number of case before the re-coding process by the Independent Senior Coder. Interestingly, from the 22 cases assigned to MY-DRG® P-8-17-II after the re-coding process, 12 (54.5%) of the cases were originally assigned to MY-DRG® P-8-17-I. This shows that although the DRG group of the cases were similar, after the re-coding process, these cases were re-assigned to a higher level of severity. This also implies that majority of the paediatric cases were being under-coded before the re-coding process leading to a high volume of severity level I cases before the re-coding process.

To sum it up, as apparent in the Table 4.95, the total number of cases assigned to the top 10 highest MY-DRG® group is higher before the re-coding process compared to after the re-coding process. This indicates that after the re-coding process, without the coding errors, the selected cases were re-assigned to a more varieties type of MY-DRG® group. A kappa test was conducted to identify the level of agreement in the assignment of MY-DRG® group before and after the re-coding process. The test shows a fair agreement with a kappa value of 0.211 ($p<0.001$).

Table 4.95 Top 10 Highest MY-DRG® Code Before and After The Re-Coding Process

No.	Before Re-Coding Process					After Re-Coding Process		
	DRG Code	Description	n =464 Frequency (%) *	n =* No. of Error Cases (%) **	n =** Error Cases with Changes in DRG code	DRG Code	Description	n =464 Frequency (%) ***
1.	P-8-17-I	Neonate, birth-weight >2499 grams without complex operation-mild	47 (10.1)	39 (83.0)	35 (89.7)	P-8-17-II	Neonate, birth-weight >2499 grams without complex operation-moderate	22 (4.7)
2.	O-6-13-I	Vaginal delivery-mild	27 (5.8)	26 (96.3)	20 (76.9)	O-6-13-I	Vaginal delivery-mild	22 (4.7)
3.	O-6-10-I	Caesarean Section-minor	25 (5.4)	22 (88.0)	15 (68.2)	O-6-12-I	Vaginal delivery with other procedure excluding sterilization &/or dilation & curettage-minor	22 (4.7)
4.	O-6-12-I	Vaginal delivery with other procedure excluding sterilization &/or dilation & curettage-minor	25 (5.4)	24 (96.0)	20 (83.3)	O-6-13-II	Vaginal delivery-moderate	21 (4.5)
5.	O-6-12-II	Vaginal delivery with other procedure excluding sterilization &/or dilation & curettage-moderate	15 (3.2)	15 (100.0)	12 (80.0)	O-6-12-II	Vaginal delivery with other procedure excluding sterilization &/or dilation & curettage-moderate	20 (4.3)
6.	P-8-17-II	Neonate, birth-weight >2499 grams without complex operation-moderate	15 (3.2)	13 (86.7)	10 (76.9)	P-8-17-I	Neonate, birth-weight >2499 grams without complex operation-mild	17 (3.7)
7.	O-6-13-II	Vaginal delivery-moderate	12 (2.6)	11 (91.7)	8 (72.7)	O-6-10-I	Caesarean section-minor	16 (3.4)
8.	P-8-08-I	Neonate, birth-weight >2499 grams with respiratory distress syndrome & congenital pneumonia-minor	11 (2.4)	11 (100.0)	7 (63.6)	O-6-10-II	Caesarean section-moderate	15 (3.2)
9.	H-1-30-I	Intraocular & lens operations-minor	10 (2.2)	7 (70.0)	7 (100.0)	P-8-13-I	Neonate, birth-weight 2000-2499 grams without complex operation-mild	12 (2.6)
10.	P-8-08-II	Neonate, birth-weight >2499 grams with respiratory distress syndrome & congenital pneumonia-moderate	10 (2.2)	9 (90.0)	7 (77.8)	P-8-08-I	Neonate, birth-weight >2499 grams with respiratory distress syndrome & congenital pneumonia-minor	9 (1.9)

$k = 0.211, p < 000.1$

4.8 Coding Errors by Completeness of Admission Form

During the data analysis, the completeness of admission form for each case was also being accessed to determine its impact towards the accuracy of coding. Findings from this study indicate that, in total, there were only 30 cases were filled up with complete information in their admission form whereas 433 of the cases were filled with incomplete admission form. Table 4.96 below shows the distributions of coding error cases by the completeness of admission form.

It is apparent in the table that majority of the cases were filled up with incomplete admission form. The coding errors rate (90.5%) was the highest among cases with incomplete admission form. In the data analysis, a chi-square test was conducted to access the relations between coding errors and completeness of admission form. The result was statistically significant with $X^2(1) = 204.25$, p<0.001.

Table 4.96 Distributions of Error Cases by Completeness of Admission Form

Type of Admission Form	No. of Cases without Coding Errors	%	No. of Cases with Coding Errors	%	Total	%
Complete	8 (26.7)	26.7	22 (73.3)	73.3	30	100.0
Not Complete	41 (9.5)	9.5	393 (90.5)	90.5	434	100.0

$X^2 = 204.25$, df= 1 p<0.001

4.9 Coding Errors by Completeness of Discharge Summary

In this study, the completeness of discharge summary was also examined to access its relations with coding errors. Findings from this study indicate that, in total, there were only 27 cases were filled up with complete information in their discharge summary whereas 437 of the cases were filled with incomplete discharge summary. Table 4.97 below shows the distributions of coding error cases by the type of discharge summary.

Table 4.97 Distributions of Coding Error Cases by Completeness of Discharge Summary

Type of Discharge Summary	No. of Case without Coding Error	%	No. of Case with Coding Error/s	%	Total	%
Complete	25	92.6	2	7.4	27	100.0
Not Complete	24	5.5	413	94.5	437	100.0

$X^2 = 213.67$, df= 1, p< 0.001

As apparent in the Table 4.97, the coding errors rate (94.5%) was the highest among cases with incomplete discharge summary. A bivariate analysis using chi-square test was conducted to determine the association between completeness of discharge summary and coding errors. The result was proven to be statistically significant with $X^2(1) = 213.67$, p<0.001.

The output of the descriptive analysis revealed that in the discharge summary, the information of the secondary procedure and the secondary diagnosis was most likely to be incomplete compared to the information of primary diagnosis and primary procedure. Among the 464 selected cases, 374 (80.6%) of the selected cases were filled with incomplete information on their secondary procedure phrases. Also, 298 (64.2%) of the discharge summaries were with incomplete information of their secondary diagnosis phrases. On the other hand, there were 55 (11.9%) cases with incomplete information of their primary diagnosis phrase in the discharge summary and 160 (34.5%) of the cases with incomplete information of their primary procedure phrase in the discharge summary. This implies that the doctors are most likely to unrecognised the importance of secondary procedure and secondary diagnosis in the implementation of Casemix system as the provider payment tool.

4.10 Coding Erros by Coder's Characteristic

In this study, to identify factors influencing coding errors, the coder's characteristic has been examined. In the year 2013, there were 8 clinical coders serving under the Clinical Coding Unit in this tertiary hospital. They were aged between 28 years old to 39 years old with none of them are from the clinical background. From the 8 coders, 2 (37.5%) of the coders have been working under this unit for more than 5 years. All the coders who have been working for more than 5 years have received 15 types of in-house training related to coding. However, there were none of the coders have received any coding training outside the hospital.

Table 4.98 shows the distributions of coding error cases by coder's characteristic. As seen in the table, from the 464 selected cases, 96 (20.7%) of the cases were codified by the coders with a length of service more and equal than ten years. On the other hand, among the 368 (79.3%) cases it was codified by the coders with a length of service less than ten years. It is notable from the table that the highest coding errors rate (91.7%) was involving cases that were codified by coders more and equal than ten years.

Table 4.98 Distributions of Coding Errors by Coder's Characteristic

Variables	No. of Case without Coding Errors (%)	No. of Case with Coding Errors (%)	X^2 value	df	p value
Length of Service			0.636	1	0.425
More and equal than 10 years	8 (8.3)	88 (91.7)			
Less than 10 years	41 (11.1)	327 (88.9)			
Educational Level			0.636	1	0.425
Non-Degree Holder	8 (8.3)	88 (91.7)			

Degree Holder	41 (11.1)	327 (88.9)			
Number of Training Attended			2.489	1	0.081
Less than 5	30 (9.1)	299 (90.9)			
More and equal than 5	19 (14.1)	116 (85.9)			

Data analysis from this study also showed that there were 96 (20.7%) cases that were codified by the non-degree holder coder. In contrast, there were a total of 368 (79.3%) of cases that were codified by a -degree holder coder. It is notable from the table that the highest coding error rate (91.7%) was for cases that were codified by the non-degree coders.

As apparent in the Table 4.98, in total there were 329 (70.9%) cases that were codified by the coders that have attended less than five in-house coding training. On the other hand, there were a total of 125 (26.9%) cases that were codified by a coder that has more and equal than five in-house training. It is notable from the table that the highest coding errors rate (90.9%) was involving cases that were codified by the coders with less than five in-house training.

A bivariate analysis using chi-square test was conducted to access the relations between coder's characteristic and coding errors involving coder's length of service, coder's educational level and the number of training attended by the coders. As can be seen in Table 4.98, none of these variables shows up as statistically significant.

4.11 Coding Errors by Doctor's Characteristic

During the data analysis, this study also examined the doctor's characteristic to determine its association with coding errors. The data on doctor's characteristic was retrieved from the Human Resource Department, UKMMC. The variables that were examined were the doctor's length of service and educational background. In total, this study managed to retrieve doctor's information for only 376 (81.0%) cases. These doctors were responsible in writing the discharge summary of the selected cases.

Table 4.99 below shows the distributions of coding error cases by doctor's characteristic. As can be seen in the table, most of the discharge summary was written by doctors with 2 years working experience with the total number of 170 (36.7%) cases. On the other hand, there were only 4 (0.9%) discharge summary that was written by the doctor's with more and equal to 3 years working experience. From the table, it could be understood that the highest coding errors rate (97.2%) was involving discharge summary written by a doctor with less than one-year working experience.

Table 4.99 Distributions of Coding Errors by Doctor's Characteristic

Variables	No. of Cases without Coding Errors (%)	No. of Cases with Coding Errors (%)	X^2 value	df	p value
Length of Service			4.122	3	0.127
Less than 1 year	1 (2.8)	35 (97.2)			
1 year	13 (7.8)	153 (92.2)			
2 years	24 (14.1)	146 (85.9)			
More and equal to 3 years	1 (25.0)	3 (75.0)			
Educational Level			0.014	1	0.905
Degree Holder	38 (10.4)	327 (89.6)			
Master Holder	1 (9.1)	10 (90.9)			

As written in Table 4.99, in this study there were two level of educations among the doctors namely degree holder and master holder. In total there were 365 (78.7%) of the discharge summaries was written by the degree holder's doctor. Interestingly, the highest coding errors rate (90.9%) was involving discharge summary that was written by the master holder's doctor. The higher percentage could be contributed by the smaller number of denominator among master holder's doctor than degree holder's doctor.

A bivariate analysis using chi-square test was conducted to access the relations between doctor's characteristic and coding errors involving doctor's length of service and educational level. As can be seen in Table 4.99, none of these variables show up as statistically significant.

4.12 Multiple Logistic Regression on Factors Influencing Coding Errors

In this study, a multivariate analysis using the logistic regression was applied to control the confounding effect of many other variables that potentially could influence the coding errors. The dependent variable was coding error cases and Table 4.100 showed the independent variables used in the model.

The output from the logistic regression indicates that there were no significant relations between coding errors and coder's also doctor's characteristic. As apparent in Table 4.101, discipline, incomplete admission form and incomplete discharge summary could influence the coding errors.

The completeness of the admission form and the completeness of the discharge summary were the most important factors that influenced the coding errors. The re-coding process by the Independent Senior Coder identified that the regular coding process that was conducted in this hospital was performed according to the discharge summary alone. It is apparent from Table 4.101 that the incidence of coding errors is almost 216 times more likely to occur among cases with incomplete admission form (OR = 215.014, 95% Confidence limits = 48.096 – 962.022). Also, from the table, it is understood that the incidence of coding errors is almost 150 times more likely to occurred among cases with incomplete discharge summary (OR = 143.056, 95% Confidence limits = 40.323 – 507.521).

During the descriptive analysis, it was revealed that the lowest coding errors rate (82.8%) was among the surgical cases whereas the highest coding errors rate (94.8%) was among the O&G cases. The findings from the multivariate analysis showed that the O&G cases are almost quadruple times more likely to be coded wrongly than surgical cases (OR = 3.819, 95% Confidence limits = 1.473 – 9.901). On the other hand, medical cases are almost triple time more likely to be coded wrongly than surgical cases (OR = 2.839, 95% Confidence limits = 1.196 – 6.739). It is also understood from the table that, the possibilities of the paediatric cases to be coded wrongly than surgical discipline could not be determined statistically ($p > 0.005$).

Table 4.100 Description of Variables used in Multiple Logistic Regression

Variables	Values	
A. Dependent		
Coding Error Case	Dummy :	Non Error Case = 0
		Error Case = 1
B. Independent		
i) Case-type	Dummy :	Surgical : 0 (Reference Group)
		Medical : 1
		O&G : 2
		Paediatric : 3
ii) Admission Form	Dummy :	Complete Admission Form = 0 (Reference Group)
		Incomplete Admission Form = 1
iii) Discharge Summary	Dummy:	Complete Discharge Summary = 0 (Reference Group)
		Incomplete Discharge Summary = 1
iv) Severity Level	Dummy :	Severity Level I = 0 (Reference Group)
		Severity Level II = 1
		Severity Level III = 2
v) Coder's Length of Service	Dummy :	Less than 10 years = 0 (Reference Group)
		More and equals to 10 years = 1

vi) Coder's Educational Level	Dummy :	Degree Holder = 0 (Reference Group) Non-Degree Holder = 1
vii) Coder's Coding Training	Dummy :	More and equals to 5 = 0 (Reference Group) Less than 5 = 1
viii) Doctor's Length of Service	Dummy :	More and equal to 3 year = 0 (Reference Group) Less than 1 year =1 1 year = 2 2 years = 3
ix) Doctor's Educational Background	Dummy :	Degree Holder = 0 (Reference Group) Master Holder = 1

Table 4.101 Multiple Logistic Regression of Factors Influencing Coding Errors

Variables	B	S.E	Wald	p value	OR	95% Confidence Limits
Disciplines						
Medical	1.043	0.441	5.594	0.018	2.839	1.196 - 6.739
O&G	1.340	0.486	7.604	0.006	3.819	1.473 - 9.901
Paediatric	0.329	0.370	0.787	0.375	1.389	0.672 - 2.870
Incomplete Admission Form	5.371	0.764	49.391	<0.001	215.014	48.096 – 962.022
Incomplete Discharge Summary	5.369	0.764	49.346	<0.001	143.056	40.323 – 507.521
Severity Levels						
II	0.628	0.387	2.633	0.105	1.875	0.878 - 4.005
III	1.101	0.745	2.187	0.139	3.008	0.699 - 12.946
Coders' with 10 years or more Lengths of Service	-0.322	0.405	0.631	0.427	0.725	0.328 - 1.603

Coders with less than 5 Coding Trainings Sessions	0.490	0.313	2.453	0.117	1.632	0.884 - 3.015
Non-Degree Holder's Coders	-0.322	0.405	0.631	0.427	0.725	0.328 - 1.603
Doctors' Lengths of Service						
Less than 1 year	2.457	1.537	2.555	0.110	11.667	0.574 - 237.200
1 year	1.367	1.190	1.319	0.251	3.923	0.381 - 40.439
2 year	0.956	1.203	0.631	0.427	2.600	0.246 - 27.453
Master Holder's Doctor	0.170	1.060	0.026	0.873	1.185	0.148 - 9.461

4.13 UKMMC's Potential Hospital Revenue

UKMMC's potential hospital revenue shows a massive increment after the re-coding process. In total, the potential hospital revenue has escalated by 39.1% from RM1,672,922.13 to RM2,327,226.00. Table 4.102 below shows the comparisons of the UKMMC's potential hospital revenue before and after the re-coding process.

Before the re-coding process by the Independent Senior Coder, the mean of the potential hospital revenue in UKMMC was RM3,508.45 (SD: RM3,276.35). As also apparent in the table, with the coding error cases, the minimum potential hospital revenue that could be potentially gained per patient was RM1,020.24. Also, with the coding error cases, the maximum potential hospital revenue that could be potentially gained per patient was RM39,993.00.

On the other after the re-coding process by the Independent Senior Coder, the mean of the potential hospital revenue in UKMMC was RM5,015.57 (SD: RM12,101.59). After the re-coding process, due to the ungroupable cases, the minimum potential hospital revenue that could be potentially gained per patient was RM0.00 whereas the maximum potential hospital revenue that could be potentially gained per patient has increased to RM233,318.94.

Table 4.102 Comparisons of Total Potential Hospital Revenue Before and After the Re-Coding Process

	Total Potential Hospital Revenue	Mean (SD)/ Patient	Minimum Potential Hospital Revenue / Patient	Maximum Potential Hospital Revenue / Patient	t value	p value
					-2.648	0.008
Before	1,672,922.13	3,508.45 (3,276.35)	1,020.24	39,993.00		
After	2,327,226.07	5,015.57(12,101.59)	00.00	233,318.94		

*All amount are shown in Ringgit Malaysia (RM)

A bivariate analysis using paired sample t-test was conducted to access the statistical significant of the difference between the total potential hospital revenue before and after the re-coding process. From Table 4.102 it can be concluded that, the difference was proven to be statistically significant with t (463) = -2.648, p = 0.008.

4.13.1 Total Potential Hospital Revenue by Case-Type

This sub topic presents the difference of the total potential hospital revenue before and after the re-coding process according to the four case-type selected by this study namely, medical, surgical, O&G and paediatric. Table 4.103 below shows the distributions of total potential hospital revenue before and after the re-coding process according to the case-type.

The highest difference of hospital potential revenue before and after the re-coding process was involving cases assigned to the paediatric case-type with a total difference of RM 589,031.32. On the other hand, the lowest difference of hospital potential revenue before and after the re-coding process was involving cases assigned to O&G case-type with a total difference of RM 18,237.61. Next sub-topic illustrates a more detailed explanation on the total potential hospital revenue before and after the re-coding process according to the case-type.

Table 4.103 Comparisons of Total Potential Hospital Revenue Before and After the Re-Coding Process by Case-Type

Case-Type	Total Potential Hospital Revenue	Mean (SD) / Patient	Minimum Potential Hospital Revenue / Patient	Maximum Potential Hospital Revenue / Patient	t value	p value
Medical					-3.044	0.003
Before	351,450.99	3,003.85 (1,964.02)	1,020.24	15,836.25		
After	437,255.91	3,363.51 (3,224.79)	1,160.00	24,547.17		
Surgical					0.753	0.453
Before	619,472.01	5,340.28 (5,617.46)	1,530.00	39,993.00		
After	625,701.30	6,257.01 (5,317.15)	1,524.42	30,723.31		
O&G					-0.768	0.444
Before	395,988.45	3,413.69 (1,300.82)	2,614.74	14,767.32		
After	414,226.06	3,480.89 (1,331.68)	2,614.74	14,767.32		
Paediatric					-2.398	0.018
Before	261,010.68	2,269.66 (948.37)	1,412.00	6,098.51		
After	850,042.00	7,798.56 (23,896.31)	1,343.35	233,318.94		

*All amount are shown in Ringgit Malaysia (RM)

a. Total Potential Hospital Revenue Before and After the Re-Coding Process in Medical Case-Type

Before the re-coding process, the total potential hospital revenue under medical case type was RM351,450.99 with the mean of potential hospital revenue of RM3,003.85 (SD: RM1,964.02). In this case type, the minimum potential hospital revenue that could be potentially gained per patient before the re-coding process was RM1,020.24 and the maximum potential hospital revenue that could be potentially gained per patient was RM15,836.25.

After the re-coding process, the total potential hospital revenue has increased to RM437,255.91 with the mean of potential hospital revenue of RM3,363.51 (RM1,160.00). The minimum potential hospital revenue that could be potentially gained per patient shows an increasing pattern of the amount of RM 1,160.00 after the re-coding process. In addition, the maximum potential hospital revenue that could be potentially gained per patient also increased to RM24,547.17 after the re-coding process.

A bivariate analysis using paired sample t-test was conducted to access the statistical significance of the difference between the total potential hospital revenue before and after the audit in the medical case-type. From Table 4.103 above, it can be concluded that the difference was proven to be statistically significant with t (115) = -3.044, p = 0.003.

b. Total Potential Hospital Revenue Before and After the Re-Coding Process in Surgical Case-type

Before the re-coding process, the total potential hospital revenue under surgical case type was RM619,472.01 with the mean of the potential hospital revenue of RM5,340.28 (SD: RM5,617.46). In this case type, the minimum potential hospital revenue that could be potentially gained per patient before the re-coding process was RM 1,530.00 and the maximum potential hospital revenue that could be potentially gained per patient was RM39,993.00.

On the other hand, after the re-coding process, the total potential hospital revenue has increased to RM625,701.30 with the mean of the potential hospital revenue of RM6,257.01 (RM5,317.15). However, the minimum potential hospital revenue that could be potentially gained per patient shows a decreasing pattern with the amount of RM1,524.42 after the re-coding process. In addition, the maximum potential hospital revenue that could be potentially gained per patient also decreased to RM30,723.31 after the re-coding process.

A bivariate analysis using paired sample t-test was conducted to access the statistical significance of the difference between the total potential hospital revenue before and after the re-coding process in the surgical case type. From Table 4.103 above, it can be concluded that, even though there was a slight improvement in the total income after the re-coding process, the difference was proven to be statistically insignificant with t (115) = 0.753, p = 0.453.

c. Total Potential Hospital Revenue Before and After the Re-Coding Process in O&G Case-Type

Before the re-coding process, the total potential hospital revenue under O&G case type was RM395,988.45 with the mean of the potential hospital revenue of RM3,413.69 (SD: RM1,300.82). In this case type, the minimum potential hospital revenue that could be potentially gained per patient before the re-coding process was RM2,614.74 and the maximum potential hospital revenue that could be potentially gained per patient was RM14,767.32.

After the re-coding process, the total potential hospital revenue has increased to RM414,226.06 with the mean of the potential hospital revenue of RM3,480.89 (RM1,331.68). Interestingly, in this case-type, after the re-coding process the minimum and maximum potential hospital revenue that could be potentially gained per patient shows no changes with before the re-coding process.

A bivariate analysis using paired sample t-test was conducted to access the statistical significance of the difference between the total potential hospital revenue before and after the re-coding process in the O&G case type. From Table 4.103 above, it can be concluded that, even though there was a slight improvement in the total income after the re-coding process, the difference was proven to be statistically insignificant with t (115) = -0.768, p = 0.444.

d. Total Potential Hospital Revenue Before and After the Re-Coding Process in Paediatric Case-Type

Before the re-coding process, the total potential hospital revenue under paediatric case type was RM261,010.68 with the mean of the potential hospital revenue of RM2,269.66 (SD: RM948.37). Among cases that were assigned to paediatric case-type, the minimum potential hospital revenue that could be potentially gained per patient before the re-coding process was RM1,412.00 and the maximum potential hospital revenue that could be potentially gained per patient was RM6,098.51.

After the re-coding process, the total potential hospital revenue has grossly increased to RM850,042.00 with the mean of the potential hospital revenue of RM7,798.56 (RM23,896.31). In this case type, after the re-coding process, the minimum potential hospital revenue that could be potentially gained per patient has decreased to RM1,343,00. However, the maximum potential hospital revenue that could be potentially gained per patient has dramatically increased to RM233,318.94 after the re-coding process.

A bivariate analysis using paired sample t-test was conducted to access the statistical significance of the difference between the total potential hospital revenue before and after the re-coding process in the paediatric case type. From Table 4.103 above, it can be concluded that the difference was proven to be statistically insignificant with t (115) = -2.398, p = 0.018.

4.13.2 Total Potential Hospital Revenue by Severity Level

This sub topic presents the difference between the total potential hospital revenue before and after the re-coding process according to the severity level. Table 4.104 below shows the distributions of total potential hospital revenue before and after the re-coding process according to severity level. The highest difference of hospital potential revenue before and after the re-coding process was involving cases assigned to the severity level II with a total difference of RM 638,889.10.

Table 4.104 Comparisons of Total Potential Hospital Revenue Before and After the Re-Coding According to Severity Level

Severity Level	Total Potential Hospital Revenue	Mean (SD) /Patient	Minimum Potential Hospital Revenue / Patient	Maximum Potential Hospital Revenue / Patient	t value	p value
Level I					-4.133	<0.001
Before	835, 178.64	2,812.05 (1,263.50)	1,020.24	6,564.00		
After	602, 892.47	2,857.31 (1,382.66)	1,160.19	11,535.05		
Level II					-2.477	0.015
Before	516,977.43	4,169.17 (3,279.93)	1,371.75	28,796.41		
After	1,155,866.52	6,281.88 (17,916.02)	1,459.39	233,318.94		
Level III					-0.804	0.026
Before	275, 766.06	6,413.16 (7,888.08)	2,371.83	39,993.00		
After	568, 467.08	9,023.29 (10,018.87)	1,852.02	40,183.69		

a. **Total Potential Hospital Revenue Among Severity Level I Cases**

Before the re-coding process, there were 297 cases of severity level I. The total potential hospital revenue that could be gained by this hospital from these 297 severity level I cases was RM835,178.64 with the mean of the potential hospital revenue of RM2,812.05 (RM1,263.50). Before the re-coding process, the minimum potential hospital revenue that could be gained per patient assigned to severity level I was RM1,020.24. On the other hand, the maximum potential hospital revenue that could be gained per patient before the re-coding process was RM6,564.00.

After the re-coding process, the number of severity level I cases have decreased to 211 cases. Subsequently, the total potential hospital revenue that could be gained from these 211 cases was RM602, 892.47 with the mean of the potential hospital revenue RM2,857.31 (RM1,382.66). Without the coding error cases, the minimum potential hospital revenue that could be gained per patient among severity level I cases was RM1,160.19. Meanwhile, the maximum potential hospital revenue per patient among severity level I case has increased to RM11,535.05 after the re-coding process.

A paired sample t-test was conducted to determine the statistical significance of the difference between the total potential hospital revenue before and after the re-coding process of the severity level I cases. From Table 4.104 it can be concluded that the difference was proven to be statistically insignificant with $t(296) = -4.133$, $p < 0.001$.

b. Total Potential Hospital Revenue Among Severity Level II Cases

Before the re-coding process, there were 124 severity level II cases. The total potential for the hospital revenue that could be gained by this hospital from these 124 severity level II cases is RM516,977.43 with the mean of the potential hospital revenue of RM4,169.17 (RM3,279.93). Before the re-coding process by the Independent Senior Coder, the minimum potential hospital revenue that could be gained per patient among the severity level II patient was RM1,371.75. On the other hand, the maximum potential hospital tariff that could be charged to severity level II patient before the re-coding process was RM28,796.41.

After the re-coding process, the number of severity level II cases has increased to 184 cases. The total potential hospital revenue that could be gained from these 184 cases was RM1,155,866.52 with the mean of potential hospital tariff of RM6,281.88 (RM17,916.02). Without the coding error cases, the minimum potential hospital revenue that could be gained per patient among these severity level II cases was RM1,459.39. Meanwhile, the maximum potential hospital revenue that could be gained among severity level II cases has dramatically increased to RM233,318.94 after the re-coding process.

A paired sample t-test was conducted to determine the statistical significance of the difference between the total potential hospital revenue before and after the re-coding process among the severity level II cases. From Table 4.104 it can be concluded that the difference was proven to be statistically insignificant with t (123) = -2.447, p = 0.015.

c. **Total Potential Hospital Revenue Among Severity Level III Cases**

Before the re-coding process, there were 42 severity level III cases. The total potential hospital revenue that could be gained by this hospital from these 42 severity level III cases is RM275,766.06 with the mean of potential hospital revenue of RM6,413.16 (RM7,888.08). Before the re-coding process, the minimum potential hospital revenue per patient that could be gained among severity level III cases was RM2,371.83. On the other hand, the maximum potential hospital revenue per patient that could be gained among severity level III cases before the re-coding process was RM39,993.00.

After the re-coding process the number of severity level III cases has increased to 61 cases. The total potential hospital revenue that could be gained from these 61 cases was RM568,467.08 with the mean income of RM9,023.29 (10,018.87). Without the coding error cases, the minimum potential hospital revenue per patient among cases assigned to severity level III was RM 1,852.02. Meanwhile, the maximum potential hospital revenue per patient that could be gained among cases assigned to severity level III was RM40,183.69 after the audit.

A paired sample t-test was conducted to determine the statistical significance of the difference between the total potential hospital revenue before and after the re-coding process among the severity level III cases. From Table 4.104 it can be concluded that the difference was proven to be statistically insignificant with t (41) = -0.804, p = 0.026.

4.13.3 Top 10 MY-DRG® with Highest Total Potential Hospital Revenue

Table 4.105 below shows the comparison of the top 10 MY-DRG® groups with highest total potential hospital revenue before and after the re-coding process. As apparent in the table, before the re-coding process the total potential hospital revenue of the cases assigned to the top 10 highest potential hospital revenue MY-DRG® group was RM575, 175.46. The highest volume of potential hospital revenue was from MY-DRG® group O-6-10-I (Caesarean section – mild) with the total potential hospital revenue amounting to RM97, 925.75. The hospital tariff assigned to cases under MY-DRG® group O-6-10-I was RM3,917.03. In total there were 25 cases that were assigned to MY-DRG® group O-6-10-I before the audit.

After the re-coding process, the potential hospital revenue of the cases assigned to the top 10 highest potential hospital revenue MY-DRG® group has reached RM919,709.97. This shows an increment of 59.9% of the potential hospital revenue of the cases assigned to the top 10 MY-DRG® groups with the highest potential revenue before the re-coding process. Data analysis from this study also highlighted that the MY-DRG® group P-8-02-II (Neonate birth weight <1000 grams with complex operation – Mild) was the MY-DRG® group with the highest potential hospital revenue after the re-coding process. The hospital tariff that was assigned to MY-DRG® group P-8-02-II was RM233,318.94. Interestingly, before the re-coding process, the MY-DRG® group P-8-02-II was not assigned to any of the selected cases.

Table 4.106 below shows the distributions of top 10 cases with highest potential loss of hospital revenue. From the table, it is notable that majority of the top 10 cases with highest potential loss of hospital revenue were among the paediatric cases. All the cases with a potential loss amounting to more than RM30,000.00 were assigned to a wrong birth weight before the re-coding process reflecting a poor quality of documentation, which could affect the accuracy of clinical coding in this hospital. As also apparent in the table, the highest potential loss was involving a case that was initially assigned to MY-DRG® group P-8-17-III (Neonate, birthweight >2499 grams without complex operation – Severe) before the re-coding process with the hospital tariff amounting to RM3,292.00. However, after the re-coding process this case was re-assigned to MY-DRG® group P-8-02-II (Neonate, birthweight <1000 Grams With Complex Operation – Moderate) with the hospital tariff amounting to RM233,318.94. A total potential loss of hospital revenue for this one case has reached RM230,026.94.

Table 4.105 Comparisons of the Top 10 MY-DRG® Group With Highest Potential Hospital Revenue Before and After the Re-Coding Process

	Before			After		
No.	MY-DRG® Code	Description	Total Potential Hospital Revenue	MY-DRG® Code	Description	Total Potential Hospital Revenue
1.	O-6-10-I	Caesarean section - Mild	97,925.75	P-8-02-II	Neonate, birth weight <1000 grams with complex operation - Mild	233,318.94
2.	O-6-13-I	Vaginal delivery - Mild	71,361.26	P-8-12-III	Neonate, birth weight 1500 - 1999 grams without complex operation - Severe	120,551.07
3.	O-6-12-I	Vaginal delivery with fallopian tube destruction &/or dilation & curettage - Mild	70,514.00	P-8-03-II	Neonate, birth weight <1000 grams without complex operation - Mild	106,124.60
4.	P-8-17-I	Neonate, birthweightt >2499 grams without complex operation - Mild	66,364.96	O-6-10-II	Caesarean section - Moderate	78,912.90
5.	H-1-30-I	Intraocular & lens operations - Mild	52,495.65	O-6-12-II	Vaginal delivery with fallopian tube destruction &/or dilation & curettage - Moderate	65,587.20
6.	O-6-12-II	Vaginal delivery with fallopian tube destruction &/or dilation & curettage - Moderate	49,715.10	P-8-13-III	Neonate, birth weight 2000 - 2499 grams without complex operation - Severe	65,316.09
7.	O-6-10-II	Caesarean section - Moderate	47,347.74	O-6-13-II	Vaginal delivery - Moderate	63,088.83
8.	P-8-17-II	Neonate, birthweight >2499 grams without complex operation - Moderate	42,800.00	O-6-10-I	Caesarean section - Mild	62,672.48
9.	H-1-20-III	Orbital & extraocular operation – Severe	39,993.00	P-8-17-II	Neonate, birth weight >2499 grams without complex operation - Moderate	62,085.54
10.	M-1-50-III	Operation of soft tissues – Severe	36,658.00	O-6-12-I	Vaginal delivery with fallopian tube destruction &/or dilation & curettage - Mild	62,052.32

*All amount are shown in Ringgit Malaysia (RM)

Table 4.106 Top 10 Cases with Highest Potential Loss of Revenue

No.	Hospital Tariff Before	Hospital Tariff After	Potential Loss Due to Coding Errors	MY-DRG* Group Before	Description	New MY-DRG* Code After	Description
1.	3,292.00	233,318.94	230,026.94	P-8-17-III	Neonate, birthweight >2499 grams without complex operation - Severe	P-8-02-II	Neonate, birthweight <1000 Grams With Complex Operation - Moderate
2.	2,149.00	53,062.30	50,913.30	P-8-14-I	Neonate, birthweight >2499 Grams With Complex Congenital Abnormalities - Mild	P-8-03-II	Neonate, birthweight <1000 Grams Without Complex Operation - Moderate
3.	2,521.00	53,062.30	50,541.30	P-8-15-II	Neonate, birthweight >2499 Grams With Aspiration Syndrome - Moderate	P-8-03-II	Neonate, birthweight <1000 Grams Without Complex Operation - Moderate
4.	2,933.00	40,183.69	37,250.69	P-8-08-II	Neonate, birthweight >2499 Grams With Respiratory Distress Syndrome & Congenital Pneumonia	P-8-12-III	Neonate, birthweight 1500 - 1999 Grams Without Complex Operation - Severe
5.	3,292.00	40,183.69	36,891.69	P-8-17-II	Neonate, birthweight >2499 grams without complex operation - Moderate	P-8-12-III	Neonate, birthweight 1500 - 1999 Grams Without Complex Operation - Severe
6.	2,298.57	26,549.22	24,250.65	B-4-14-II	Laparoscopic Cholecystectomy	B-1-10-III	Pancreas & Liver Operations - Severe
7.	1,412.00	21,772.03	20,360.03	P-8-17-I	Neonate, birthweight >2499 grams without complex operation - Mild	P-8-13-III	Neonate, birthweight 2000 - 2499 Grams Without Complex Operation - Severe
8.	4,362.00	24,547.17	20,185.17	M-1-50-I	Operation of soft tissues - Mild	M-4-21-III	Other Musculoskeletal System & Connective Tissue Disorders - Severe
9.	6,099.09	24,547.17	18,448.08	J-4-21-II	Respiratory System Signs, Symptoms & Other Disorders - Moderate	M-4-21-III	Other Musculoskeletal System & Connective Tissue Disorders - Severe
10.	2,822.00	20,747.07	17,925.07	P-8-17-II	Neonate, Birthweight >2499 Grams Without Complex Operation - Moderate	P-8-12-II	Neonate, birthweight 1500 - 1999 Grams Without Complex Operation - Moderate

*All amount are shown in Ringgit Malaysia (RM)

4.13.4 Top 10 CMGs With Highest Total Potential Hospital Revenue

Table 4.107 shows the comparisons of the top 10 CMGs with highest total potential hospital revenue before and after the re-coding process. As apparent in the table, before the re-coding process, the total potential of the hospital revenue was among the top 10 CMGs with the highest total potential hospital revenue amounting to RM1,390,806.09. The potential hospital revenue for CMGs O (Deliveries) was the highest reaching RM395,988.66. The minimum potential hospital revenue among cases assigned to CMGs O before the re-coding process was RM2,614.74. Meanwhile the maximum potential hospital revenue among cases that were assigned to CMGs O after the re-coding process, was RM14, 767.32.

After the re-coding process, the total potential hospital revenue that could be gained from the top 10 CMGs with highest potential hospital revenue has escalated to RM2,085,379.12. This shows an increment of 49.9% of the total potential hospital revenue among top 10 CMGs with highest total potential hospital revenue before the re-coding process. As can be seen in Table 4.112, after the re-coding process, CMGs P (Newborn & Neonates) was the CMGs with highest potential hospital revenue. The total potential hospital revenue after the re-coding process from CMGs P was RM849,948.37. The minimum potential hospital revenue from this CMGs after the re-coding process was RM1,343.35 whereas the maximum potential hospital tariff was RM233,318.94.

From the output of the total potential hospital revenue among top 10 CMGs with the highest potential hospital revenue, it can be concluded that, without the coding errors cases, this hospital could generate almost twice from the total potential hospital revenue with coding errors cases. The cases assigned to CMGs P especially showed a huge increment from RM261,010.68 before the re-coding process to RM847,948.37 after the audit by the Independent Senior Coder.

Table 4.107 Comparisons of the Top 10 CMGs With Highest Potential Hospital Revenue Before and After the Re-Coding Process

No	CMG Group	Descriptions	Before					CMG Group	Descriptions	After			
			Total Potential Hospital Revenue	Mean Potential hospital revenue (SD)	Min Potential Hospital Revenue / Patient	Max Potential Hospital Revenue / Patient				Total Potential hospital revenue	Mean Potential hospital revenue (SD)	Min Potential Hospital Revenue / Patient	Max Potential Hospital Revenue / Patient
1.	O	Deliveries	395,988.55	3,413.69 (1,300.81)	2,614.74	14,767.32	P	Newborns & Neonates	847,948.37	7,851.37 (24,001.32)	1,343.35	233,318.94
2.	P	Newborns & Neonates	261,010.68	2,269.65 (948.37)	1,412.00	6,098.51	O	Deliveries	414,226.06	3480.89 (1,331.68)	2,614.74	14,767.32
3.	M	Musculoskeletal system & connective tissue	151,524.24	7,576.21 (7,761.94)	3,579.78	36,658.00	M	Musculoskeletal system & connective tissue	212,699.99	8,862.49 (7,949.21)	2,094.43	30,723.31
4.	H	Eye and Adnexa	127,184.33	7,481.43 (8,409.73)	2,834.00	39,993.00	K	Digestive system	151,582.87	3,525.18 (2,327.64)	1,160.19	11,372.56
5.	W	Female reproductive system	121,461.19	3,795.66 (1,585.16)	2,308.00	8,586.00	W	Female reproductive system	101,083.52	3,610.12 (1,300.63)	2,238.89	6,825.63
6.	K	Digestive system	115,522.52	2,888.06 (1,799.47)	1,160.19	8,958.00	H	Eye and Adnexa	86,456.32	6,175.45 (1,129.60)	5,293.78	9,823.78
7.	N	Nephro-urinary system	57,790.25	3,210.56 (1,582.32)	1,359.41	5,778.00	N	Nephro-urinary system	84,739.26	4,459.96 (3,873.20)	1,359.41	16,624.04
8.	U	Ear, nose, mouth & throat	57,713.66	9,618.94 (9,504.14)	4,792.33	28,796.41	U	Ear, nose, mouth & throat	76,143.77	9,517.97 (8,294.91)	4,792.33	28,796.41
9.	G	Central nervous system	51,899.20	4,718.10 (5,654.06)	1,275.02	20,901.00	B	Hepatobiliary & pancreatic system	64,493.34	5,374.44 (7,290.80)	1,473.00	26,549.22
10.	I	Cardiovascular system	50,711.47	2,669.02 (1,001.21)	1,371.75	4,600.00	L	Skin, subcutaneous tissue & breast	46,005.62	3,538.89 (2,585.02)	1,370.07	11,278.66

* All amount are shown in Ringgit Malaysia (RM)

4.14 Bivariate Analyses on Factors Influencing Loss of Potential Hospital Revenue in Casemix System

This section presents the output on the factors influencing loss of hospital revenue in Casemix System. Table 4.108 below shows the distributions of variable that was measured by this study to identify factors influencing loss of potential hospital revenue in using Casemix system as the provider payment tools.

Table 4.108 Distributions of Factors Influencing Loss of Potential Hospital Revenue is Casemix System

Variable	No. of Cases without Error in the Assignment of HT (%)	No. of Cases with Error in the Assignment of HT (%)	Total (%)	X^2	df	p-value
Type of Primary Diagnosis Code				16.084	1	<0.001
Accurate	101 (43.3)	132 (56.7)	233 (100.0)			
Error	58 (25.8)	173 (74.2)	231 (100.0)			
Type of Secondary Diagnosis Code				49.901	1	<0.001
Accurate	58 (66.7)	29 (33.3)	87 (100.0)			
Error	101 (26.8)	276 (73.2)	377 (100.0)			
Type of Primary Procedure Code				0.323	1	0.570
Accurate	58 (25.4)	170 (74.6)	228 (100.0)			
Error	101 (42.8)	135 (57.2)	236 (100.0)			
Type of Secondary Procedure Code				8.293	1	0.004
Accurate	81 (41.8)	113 (58.2)	194 (100.0)			
Error	78 (28.9)	192 (71.1)	270 (100.0)			
Type of Severity Level				155.64	1	<0.001
Accurate	158 (59.0)	109 (41.0)	268 (100.0)			
Error	0 (0.0)	196 (100.0)	196 (100.0)			
Type of Case-Type				26.523	1	<0.001
Accurate	159 (40.1)	236 (59.7)	395 (100.0)			
Error	0 (0.0)	69 (100.0)	69 (100.0)			

Type of Admission Form				24.095	1	<0.001
Complete	21 (70.0)	9 (30.0)	30 (100.0)			
Incomplete	138 (31.8)	296 (68.2)	434 (100.0)			
Type of Discharge Summary				24.539	1	<0.001
Complete	21 (77.8)	6 (22.2)	27 (100.0)			
Incomplete	138 (31.6)	299 (68.4)	437 (100.0)			

From the bivariate analysis using Chi-Square test, the factors that were believed to cause loss of hospital revenue in casemix System were cases with coding errors at any of the coding items; primary diagnosis code, secondary diagnosis code, primary procedure code and secondary procedure code, cases with errors at the assignment of severity level, cases with errors at the assignment of case type, cases with incomplete admission form as well as incomplete discharge summary. Further explanation on these factors are being explained in the next section.

4.14.1 Association between Coding Errors of Primary Diagnosis Code and Potential Loss of Hospital Revenue

In using Casemix system as the provider payment tools, the wrong assignment of primary diagnosis code could highly relate to the potential loss of hospital revenue. It was identified that from the 231 (49.7%) error cases of the primary diagnosis code, 173 (74.2%) of the cases were identified with errors in the assignment of its potential hospital tariff. Before the re-coding process, the total amount of the potential hospital revenue of these 231 cases was RM845,355.94 and has escalated to RM1,444,127.99 after the re-coding process. This implies that the coding errors of primary diagnosis code occurred in this study could cause a potential loss of hospital revenue.

From Table 4.108 above, it is notable that the highest percentage (74.2%) of cases with changes in the assignment of hospital tariff was in cases with an error in the assignment of primary diagnosis code. A chi-square test was conducted to access the association between coding errors at primary diagnosis code and assignment of hospital tariff. As apparent in Table 4.108, it was statistically proven that cases with errors in the assignment of the primary diagnosis code would face changes in the assignment of their hospital tariff with the chi-square value of X^2 (1) = 16.084, p <0.001.

4.14.2 Association between Coding Errors of Secondary Diagnosis Code Potential Loss of Hospital Revenue

In the casemix system, the coding errors in the assignment of secondary diagnosis code could affect the accuracy of the severity of illness of the case. The wrong assignment of severity level subsequently would affect the potential hospital revenue of the case. In this study, after the re-coding process, from the 377 (81.3%) error cases of secondary diagnosis codes, 276 (73.2%) of the cases were assigned to a wrong hospital tariff. Before the re-coding process, the total amount of the potential hospital revenue of these 276 cases was RM845,355.94 and has escalated to RM1,444,127.99 after the re-coding process. Similarly to error cases of the primary diagnosis code, the increasing patterns of the total potential hospital revenue after the re-coding process implies that the coding errors of secondary diagnosis code occurred in this study could cause a potential loss of hospital revenue.

From Table 4.108 above, it is notable that the highest percentage (73.2%) of cases with changes in the assignment of its hospital tariff was in cases with an error in the assignment of secondary diagnosis code. A chi-square test was conducted to access the association between coding errors at primary diagnosis code and the assignment of hospital tariff. As apparent in Table 4.108, it was statistically proven that cases with errors in the assignment of secondary diagnosis codes could relate to the changes in the hospital tariff with the chi-square value of X^2 (1) = 49.901, p <0.001.

4.14.3 Association between Coding Errors of Primary Procedure Code and Potential Loss of Hospital Revenue

According to the MY-DRG® grouper used in the casemix system, the coding errors in the assignment of primary procedure code could affect the accuracy of the case-type of the patient. The wrong assignment of case-type could also possibly affect the potential hospital revenue of the case. In this study, from the 236 (50.9%) error cases of primary procedure code, 135 (57.2%) of the cases were assigned to a wrong hospital tariff. Before the re-coding process the total amount of the potential hospital revenue of these 236 cases was RM1,436,687.06 and has escalated to RM1,835,493.64 after the re-coding process. Even though after the re-coding process there was an increment in the total potential hospital revenue among error cases of primary procedure code, the increment was not drastic in comparisons to the increment among cases with errors of the primary diagnosis code, and errors of secondary diagnosis code.

From Table 4.108 above, it is notable that the highest percentage (74.6%) of cases with changes in the assignment of hospital tariff was among cases without an error in the assignment of primary procedure code. This implies that, in UKMMC, the majority of the coding errors occurred in the assignment of primary procedure code does not reflect the assignment of the case-type of the case. A chi-square test was conducted to access the association between coding errors of primary procedure code and assignment of hospital tariff. As apparent in Table 4.108, the association between cases with errors in the assignment of primary procedure code and assignment of hospital tariff was statistically insignificant with the chi-square value of $X^2 (1) = 0.323$, $p > 0.05$.

4.14.4 Association between Coding Errors of Secondary Procedure Code and Potential Loss of Hospital Revenue

In the assignment of MY-DRG® code, a wrong assignment of secondary procedure code could affect the assignment of the case-type of the patient. This subsequently could impact the assignment of the hospital tariff of the case. From the 270 (58.2%) error cases of secondary procedure code, 192 (71.1%) of the cases were assigned to a wrong hospital tariff. Before the re-coding process the total amount of the potential hospital revenue of these 270 cases was RM1,027,730.14 and has increased to RM1,267,594.87 after the re-coding process. This indicates that in UKMMC, the coding errors of secondary procedure code could relate to the potential loss of hospital revenue.

From Table 4.108 above, it is notable that the highest percentage (71.1%) of cases with changes in the assignment of its hospital tariff was in cases with an error in the assignment of secondary procedure code. A chi-square test was conducted to access the association between coding errors of secondary procedure code and assignment of hospital tariff. As apparent in Table 4.108 the association between cases with errors in the assignment of secondary procedure code and assignment of hospital tariff was statistically significant with the chi-square value of X^2 (1) = 8.293, p = 0.004.

4.14.5 Association between Coding Error Cases with Errors of Severity Level and Potential Loss of Hospital Revenue

Due to the coding errors, from 464 selected cases, 196 (42.2%) of the cases showed changes in the assignment of their severity level after the re-coding process. Data analysis from this study indicates all 196 cases with errors of severity level were assigned to a wrong potential hospital tariff before the re-coding process. The total potential hospital revenue for this 196 cases before the re-coding processwas RM711,228.95 and has dramatically increased to RM1,318,295.55 after the re-coding process. This shows that coding errors that caused a wrong assignment of severity level would also lead to a potential loss of hospital revenue.

From Table Table 4.108 above, it is notable that the highest percentage (100.0%) of cases with changes in the assigment of its hospital tariff was in coding error cases with an error in the assignment of severity level. A chi-square test was conducted to access the association between errors in the assignment of severity level and assignment of hospital tariff. As apparent in Table Table 4.108 it was statistically proven that coding error cases with errors in the assignment of severity level would highly relate to changes in the assignment of hospital tariff with the chi-square value of $X^2 (1) = 155.64$, $p< 0.001$.

4.14.6 Association between Coding Error Cases with Errors of Case-Type and Potential Loss of Hospital Revenue

From the 464 selected cases, the coding errors incidence in UKMMC has causes changes in the assignment of case-type of 69 (14.8%) error cases. It was also identified that all these 69 cases have changes in the assignment of its hospital tariff. The total potential hospital revenue for these 196 cases before the re-coding process was RM268,169.34 and has increased to RM308,675.30 after the re-coding process. This shows that coding errors that caused a wrong assignment of case-type would lead to a potential loss of hospital revenue.

From Table 4.108 above, it is notable that the highest percentage (100.0%) of cases with changes in the assignment of its hospital tariff was in coding error cases with an error in the assignment of case-type. A chi-square test was conducted to access the association between cases with errors in the assignment of case-type and assignment of hospital tariff. As apparent in Table 4.108, it was statistically proven that coding error cases with errors in the assignment of case-type would highly relate to changes in the assignment of hospital tariff with the chi-square value of X^2 (1) = 26.523, p< 0.001.

4.14.7 Association between Cases with Incomplete Admission Form Potential Loss of Hospital Revenue

Among the 464 cases selected in this study, there were 434 (93.5%) cases with incomplete patient's information in their admission form. From these 434 cases, 296 (68.2%) of the cases were assigned to a wrong potential hospital tariff before the re-coding process. The total potential hospital revenue for these 296 cases before the re-coding process was RM1, 512,469.12 and has increased to RM2,218,712.49 after the re-coding process. This shows that coding error cases with incomplete admission form would lead to a potential loss of hospital revenue.

From Table 4.108 above, it is notable that the highest percentage (68.2%) of cases with changes in the assignment of its hospital tariff was in cases with incomplete admission form. A chi-square test was conducted to access the association between incomplete admission form and assignment of hospital tariff. As apparent in Table 4.108, it was statistically proven that cases with incomplete admission form would relate to errors in the assignment of hospital tariff with the chi-square value of X^2 (1) = 24.095, p< 0.001.

4.14.8 Association between Cases with Discharge Summary and Potential Loss of Hospital Revenue

Among the 464 selected cases, there were 436 (94.0%) cases with incomplete discharge summary. From these 436 cases with incomplete discharge summary, 299 (68.3 %) of the cases were assigned to a wrong potential hospital tariff before the re-coding process was performed. The total potential hospital revenue for this 299 cases before the re-coding process was RM1,510,364.84 and has increased to RM2,215,988.74 after the re-coding process.

This shows that coding error cases with incomplete discharge summary would lead to a potential loss of hospital revenue.

From Table 4.108 above, it is notable that the highest percentage (68.4%) of cases with changes in the assignment of its hospital tariff occurred in cases with an incomplete discharge summary. A chi-square test was conducted to access the association between incomplete discharge summary and assignment of the hospital tariff. As apparent in Table 4.108, it was statistically proven that cases with incomplete discharge summary would relate to errors in the assignment of hospital tariff with the chi-square value of $X^2 (1) = 24.539$, p< 0.001.

4.15 Multiple Logistic Regression on Factors Influencing Accuracy of Assignment of Potential Hospital Tariff

In this study, a multivariate analysis using the logistic regression was applied to control the confounding effect of many other variables that potentially could influence the accuracy of the assignment of hospital tariff. The dependent variable was error cases with changes in the assignment of hospital tariff and Table 4.109 shows the independent variables used in the model.

The output from the multivariate analysis indicates that there were no significant relations between errors in the assignment of the hospital tariff and cases with errors in their primary procedure code. As apparent in Table 4.110, coding errors in the primary diagnosis code, secondary diagnosis code, secondary procedure code, cases with errors in the assignment of its severity level and case type as well as cases with incomplete admission forms and discharge summary will affect the accuracy of the assignment of the hospital tariff.

Error cases that led to the wrong assignment of severity level were the most important factor that influenced the assignment of hospital tariff. An error case with the error at the assignment of its severity level was 65.416 times higher (OR = 65.416, 95% Confidence limits = 23.601 – 181.314) to be assigned with an incorrect potential hospital tariff than cases with an accurate assignment of its severity level. A case with an error in the assignment of its secondary diagnosis code is 5.465 times more likely (OR = 5.465, 95% Confidence limits = 3.319 – 9.017) to be assigned with incorrect hospital tariff than cases with accurate primary diagnosis code. From Table 4.110, it could also be concluded that cases that were assigned with incorrect hospital tariff were likely to be among cases with errors in the assignment of the primary diagnosis code, errors in the assignment of the secondary procedure codes, error cases with errors in the assignment of the case type, cases with incomplete admission form and cases with incomplete discharge summary than cases with accurate assignment of its potential hospital tariff.

Table 4.109 Description of Variables used in Multiple Logistic Regression

Variables		Values
A. Dependent		
• Error Cases with Changes in the Assignment of Hospital Tariff	• Dummy:	• No Change = 0 • With Changes = 1
B. Independent		
i) Coding Error Case of Primary Diagnosis Code	Dummy :	Error Case = 0 (Reference Group) Non Error Case =1
ii) Coding Error Case of Secondary Diagnosis Code	Dummy :	Error Case = 0 (Reference Group) Non Error Case =1
iii) Coding Error Case of Primary Procedure Code	Dummy:	Error Case = 0 (Reference Group) Non Error Case =1
iv) Coding Error Case of Secondary Procedure Code	Dummy :	Error Case = 0 (Reference Group) Non Error Case =1

v) Coding Error Case with Error in Severity Level	Dummy :	Error Case = 0 (Reference Group) Non Error Case =1
vi) Coding Error Case with Error in Case-Type	Dummy :	Error Case = 0 (Reference Group) Non Error Case =1
vii) Coding Error Case with Incomplete Admission Form	Dummy :	Error Case = 0 (Reference Group) Non Error Case =1
viii) Coding Error Case with Incomplete Discharge Summary	Dummy :	Error Case = 0 (Reference Group) Non Error Case =1

Table 4.110 Results of the Analysis Using Multiple Logistic Regressions on Factors Influencing the Hospital Tariff

Variables	B	S.E	Wald	p value	OR*	95% Confidence Limits
Coding Error Case of Primary Diagnosis Code	0.798	0.201	15.804	<0.001	2.221	1.499 - 3.292
Coding Error Case of Secondary Diagnosis Code	1.698	0.255	44.210	<0.001	5.465	3.313 - 9.017
Coding Error Case of Primary Procedure Code	0.156	0.274	0.322	0.570	1.168	0.683 - 1.999
Coding Error Case of Secondary Procedure Code	0.568	0.198	8.221	0.004	1.764	1.197 – 2.601
Coding Error Case with Error in the Assignment of Severity Level	4.181	0.520	64.604	<0.001	65.416	23.601 - 181.314
Error in Assignment of Case-type	2.271	0.526	18.620	<0.001	9.687	3.454 - 27.174
Incomplete Admission Form	2.026	0.474	18.252	<0.001	7.583	2.994 – 19.209
Incomplete Discharge Summary	1.868	0.448	17.362	<0.001	6.478	2.690 – 15.601

V DISCUSSION

5.1 Introduction

This chapter is presented in four sections. The first section discusses the quality of clinical coding in UKMMC. The second section discusses on the under-coding issue identified in this study. The third section discusses on the economic implications of the clinical coding errors. The final section discusses the limitations of the study.

5.2 Evaluation of Quality of Clinical Coding In UKMMC

This study was performed to analyse the economic impact of clinical coding errors in the implementation of the MY-DRG® Casemix System in UKMMC. In this study, a blinded audit methodology was employed to access the quality of clinical coding that is carried out in UKMMC. A comprehensive evaluation of clinical coding was carried out covering most of the aspects of clinical coding including the accuracy of the primary diagnosis code, secondary diagnosis code, primary procedure code and secondary diagnosis code.

Based on the outcome of the study, the quality of clinical coding in UKMMC can be concluded to be low. The low quality of clinical coding in UKMMC is translated through the higher percentage of coding errors rate in UKMMC in comparisons to coding errors rate reported by the other studies. The coding errors rate in UKMMC is far from reaching the average coding errors rate of preceding studies. The findings from this study highlights that, of the 464 selected cases, 415 (89.4%) of the cases were the coding errors cases. On the other hand, preceding studies elsewhere indicated that the average coding errors rate was 38.0% ranging from 28.0% to 59.4% (Bajaj et al. 2007; Campbell et al. 2001b; Curtis et al. 2002; Farhan et al. 2005; Haliasos et al. 2010; Mehrdad et al. 2010; Ping et al. 2009).

The higher coding errors rate reported in UKMMC is represented by the high percentage of cases with errors in the assignment of their secondary diagnosis code. It is worth to mention that 81.3% of the selected cases in this study contained at least one error secondary diagnosis code. The errors rate of secondary diagnosis code were found to be the highest among other coding items. This finding echoed the findings in preceding studies which indicated the challenges in assigning the code for secondary diagnosis phrase compared to other coding items (Bajaj et al. 2007; Hywel Dda University 2014).

The substantial amount of coding errors cases in UKMMC are also caused by the high number of error cases in the O&G speciality that was analysed. From the 116 cases selected from O&G speciality, 94.8% of the cases were detected with coding errors. There were only 6 cases that were codified accurately by the in-house coders for O&G case type. Subsequently, the O&G case type was the most case type containing coding error cases. Interestingly, this finding is contradicted with other studies in which, the coding errors rate among surgical cases are usually reported to be higher compared to O&G cases (Farhan et al. 2005; Weingart et al. 2002).

This study has identified the important factors that contribute to the poor quality of clinical coding in UKMMC. The first factor is the quality of the primary reference of clinical coding process which is the clinical documentation used during the clinical coding process. The second factor is due to the level of knowledge on the clinical coding among the coders. The third factor is due to the doctor's demographic information. Lastly, the final and important factor is due to the evaluation method employed by this study. The following subtopic will discuss these factors which relate to the poor quality of clinical coding in UKMMC.

5.2.1 Quality of the Discharge Summary

From the data analysis, this study has concluded that the main factor relating to the poor quality of clinical coding in UKMMC is due to the poor quality of the primary reference used during the clinical coding process. The documentation used as the primary reference of clinical coding process is the main source in determining the quality of clinical coding in an organisation. Accordingly, the absence of a good quality of primary reference of clinical coding process would affect the level of quality of clinical coding. It was highlighted in past study that the documentation used during the clinical coding process plays a vital role in ensuring the level of accuracy of the codes (Jameson & Reed 2007). Nevertheless, the questions on the quality and reliability of the documentation used during the clinical coding continue to rise (Hennessy et al. 2010).

In maintaining a good quality of coding, it is critical to use the most reliable, accurate and specific documentation as the primary reference of the clinical coding. However, it is debatable today on the kind of documents to be used as the primary references for the clinical coding process. The specific guidelines for selecting the best primary reference of clinical coding are still lacking. While some hospitals prefer to use the entire medical records, other might decide to use the discharge summaries alone (Ghaffari et al. 2010). It is worth to note that due to the voluminous patient's progress note in the patient medical records; this crucial material is not being used as the main reference during the clinical coding process in UKMMC. Instead, the clinical coding practice in this tertiary hospital is by using the discharge summary alone as the primary reference for the clinical coding process. Even though the usage of the discharge summary could reduce the time consumed by the coders during the clinical coding process, the information written by the doctors in the discharge summaries tend to be incomplete and lack important pieces of information that are vital for good clinical coding practice.

It is worth to note that the percentage of cases with complete information on discharge summary in UKMMC was only 5.4% (25/464). In comparisons to other studies, this figure is very low. For instance, a study conducted in Saudi Arabia reported 88.3% of cases with a complete discharge summary and another study by Bajaj et al. in 2007 indicates that in the United Kingdom the percentage of case with complete discharge summary was 69.0% (Bajaj et al. 2007; Farhan et al. 2005). Accordingly, the lower rate of cases with complete discharge summary in UKMMC compared to other studies indicates a poor quality of the primary reference of clinical coding process in UKMMC. This has subsequently resulted in the poor quality of clinical coding in UKMMC.

The quality of the discharge summary needs to be improved in order to increase the quality of clinical coding in UKMMC. Implementing a regular quality check for the discharge summary by the hospital managers is believed to potentially help improve the quality of the discharge summary in this hospital. However, more importantly, instead of the discharge summary, the use of medical records as the primary reference during the clinical coding process is more favourable as the medical record is considered as the complete reference that reflects the patient's condition (Van Walraven & Demers 2001). Past study also recommended that the best coding practice is by referring to the entire patient medical record (B. A. Reid et al. 2017b).

In comparisons to the completeness of the information written in the discharge summaries, the information written in the wordiness medical records is more reliable, specific and complete. The argument on the reliability of the discharge summaries due to the lack of information written is frequently raised (Kind et al. 2012; Kripalani et al. 2007). In addition, the information written in the discharge summaries has the tendency to be less specific than in the medical records. Evidently, in UKMMC, in regards to the top 10 most assigned primary diagnosis code to the selected cases, the most frequent code assigned by the Independent Senior Coder shows a higher specificity than the frequent code assigned by the in-house coder. Past study also has highlighted the misspecification of the diagnosis written by the doctor as the reason for the error in interpretation by coders in assigning clinical coding codes (Neuhaus et al. 2014). Even though as reported by past study that the discharge summaries are the essential communication tool during patient care transition, their role as a primary reference during clinical coding process needs to be re-evaluated as discharge summaries commonly do not reflect the specific condition of the patient (Kind et al. 2012). Accordingly, the findings from this study have proven that the information written in the medical records is to be more specific when compared to those written in the discharge summaries. Therefore, although by referring to the medical records the clinical coding process tend to be more time consuming, the practice of using the medical records as the primary reference of clinical coding could ensure a better quality of clinical coding in this hospital.

5.2.2 Coders' Knowledge on Coding Process

The quality of clinical coding in UKMMC is also influenced by the in-house coder's level of knowledge on coding rules and guidelines. Observation from the coders characteristic, it could be concluded that the in-house coder's level of knowledge on coding rules and guidelines is insufficient. This is reflected from the number of clinical coding training attended by the in-house coders. A formal clinical coding training before commencing the official clinical coding task is essential as clinical coding process is an error-prone process (O'Malley et al. 2005). Therefore, in achieving a good quality of clinical coding, the coders need to be equipped with a formal clinical coding training that would enhance and increase their skills in clinical coding. However, interestingly, from the eight coders serving the coding unit in the year of 2013, only three of the coders have received special coding training from the casemix expert during the early implementation of casemix system in UKMMC. On the other hand, the remaining five coders have only received in-house coding training from the senior coders. It is also worth to note that none of these coders has received any certified coding training outside of the hospital. Past study has stressed on the importance of receiving formal coding training which is conducted by the professionals to enhance the coder's coding skills (Bramley & Reid 2007). The lack of formal training on clinical coding might lead to a limited coding knowledge among the coders. Subsequently, this could result in a poor quality of coding in UKMMC. Thus proper training among coders especially among junior coders in UKMMC needs to be implemented to increase the quality of coding in UKMMC

Even though, the senior coders have received a special training on clinical coding, their participation in a regular coding training is still needed as the medical field is evolving in nature which causes the coding rules and guidelines to also evolve gradually (Heywood et al. 2016; O'Malley et al. 2005). It is worth to highlight that the senior coders do not receive any further professional coding training after attending the special coding training conducted by the casemix expert. Therefore, the knowledge transferred by the senior coders to junior coders need to be assessed since the senior coder's knowledge and skills may not be regularly updated. The on-the-job training given by the senior coders to the junior coders is an excellent practice as this practice could help junior coders to directly be exposed to ICD codes of the common disease treated in the hospital. Past study has highlighted on the effectiveness of the on-the-job training among coders, but it was stressed that the junior coders need to be trained by an experienced senior coder (Shepheard 2010). In continuing the on-the-job training practised by this hospital, it is imperative for the senior coders to receive a regular coding training by the professional and fully-trained coders. Past studies have highlighted that the coders need to receive a continuous coding training to ensure a high coding quality in the hospital (Bhangu et al. 2012; Hennessy et al. 2010). The continuous training would help to enhance and ensure the quality of the coding knowledge among senior coders that could contribute to a better quality of clinical coding in UKMMC.

The framework of the governance in the hospital could also contribute to the limited knowledge of the coding rules and guidelines among coders in UKMMC. Currently, the awareness of the importance of clinical coding is still limited among the hospital managers as evidenced by the lack of financial allocation to support the training of clinical coders. It was highlighted by the past study that the effort on improving the skills and knowledge of the coder depends on the funding allocation by the hospital managers on the coding-related programmes (Santos et al. 2008). Even though there is a strong will among the coders to improve their knowledge and skills in clinical coding, without adequate budget allocation given by the hospital, it is almost impossible for the coders to participate in those related clinical coding's training. The lack of attention by the hospital managers could retaliate the success of the knowledge improvement among coders. When clinical coding is not being one of the critical aspects of the framework of the governance in hospital, it also could demotivate coder's enthusiasm in the workplace resulting in poor quality of coding in UKMMC.

The limited knowledge on coding process relates to the poor quality of clinical coding could also be influenced by the voluminous workload of the in-house coders in UKMMC. The absence of clinical coding in the framework of the hospital's governance has caused unnecessary work allocation given by the hospital managers to the coders. It is worth noting that the number of coders employed by UKMMC is small in comparisons to the number of cases treated in this hospital. The limited number of coders and a high number of admissions have caused a high workload of coding task among the coders. Nevertheless, in UKMMC, despite the voluminous coding task, these coders are also required to perform other administrative tasks during their working hours. Past study has highlighted that the coder's heavy workload especially when it is unrelated to the coding process could cause distractions in the workplace and will affect the quality of the clinical coding (O'Malley et al. 2005).

As mastering coding rules and guidelines required a steep learning curve, the additional task unrelated to coding process could disrupt coders in mastering the skills required in the clinical coding process. Since in UKMMC the coders have not attended any certified clinical coding's training outside the hospital, it is crucial for them to have a full focus in performing the coding process as this could help the coders to familiarise themselves with coding's rules and guidelines. Therefore, in structuring the framework of the hospital's governance, it is crucial to eliminate or reduce unnecessary job task among the coders. This subsequently would help coders in expediting their development in acquiring knowledge on clinical coding. If the hospital managers could institute proper attention on the importance of improving coder's knowledge, it could help UKMMC in increasing the quality of clinical coding.

5.2.3 Implications of Doctors' Demographic towards Clinical Coding

The doctors' demographic could also potentially influence the poor quality of clinical coding identified in UKMMC. The past studies have stressed the significant effects of doctor's length of service towards the quality of coding (Farhan et al. 2005; Gibson & Bridgman 1998; Nouraei et al. 2016; Pongpirul, Walker, Winch, et al. 2011). It was argued that the awareness among junior doctors on the importance of the availability of the information written in the discharge summaries is low. Subsequently relates to the poor quality of clinical coding. The findings of this study echoed the finding on the effect of length of service of doctors towards the quality of clinical coding from the past studies.

The findings from this study revealed that the discharge summaries are usually written by junior doctors with one to three years of length of service. In regards to the number of length of service among junior doctors, it could be argued that the junior doctor's limited experience in the working field could highly relate to the impoverished awareness of the high quality of the discharge summaries that subsequently impacted the quality of coding in UKMMC. Good quality of coding depends on the good quality of primary reference of clinical coding written by the doctors. This is supported by past studies saying that the process of clinical coding is highly dependent on the written information provided by the doctors (Hennessy et al. 2010; Johnson et al. 2014). The insufficient experience among the junior doctors could relate to the low understanding of the importance of clinical coding that would link to a poor attitude in executing a good clinical coding output. Therefore, it could be argued that if the junior doctors write the discharge summary without extensive monitoring from the senior doctors, it is almost impossible for UKMMC to achieve a good quality of clinical documentation. Thus, good quality of clinical coding could be achieved if the senior doctors are supervising the documentation task completed by the junior doctors.

Besides, the understanding of the concept of casemix especially on the importance of documentation among doctors is highly required in ensuring a good quality of clinical coding in using casemix system as the provider payment tools. Past study has indicated that in employing casemix system as the provider's payment tool, it requires high cooperation by the hospital's staff especially doctors in documenting casemix's minimum data set primarily on the information of the patient's diagnosis and procedural phrases (Chin et al. 2013). It could be argued by this study that the exposure on the casemix system among the junior doctors might be limited as this system is not yet widely known in this country. Therefore this has led to the challenge among the hospital managers in constituting the enforcement in submitting well-written discharge summaries among the junior doctors that subsequently lead to the poor quality of clinical coding. This challenge is not new as past study which has highlighted the difficulties to embed the concept of casemix especially on the importance of documentation among the doctors (Dowling et al. 1995). Nevertheless, the effort to embed the concept of casemix among the junior doctors need to be taken actively by the hospital managers especially during the early period of the doctor's service. This would help the doctors to familiarise the crucial elements in the casemix system especially involving the documentation task.

As mentioned earlier, in achieving a good quality of clinical coding, good quality of the documentation is pivotal. However, as highlighted in past studies, documenting patient's clinical information is a challenging task in regards to the time required by the doctor to complete this responsibility (Callen et al. 2010; Ellen et al. 2006). It is widely known that the highest priority task of a doctor is to treat the patients. In the view of this, the doctors might ignore the importance of proper and complete documentation, especially among the junior doctors. This may due to the poor time management by the junior doctors. In the early year of their service, the junior doctors might focus on their core task namely treating the patient. Therefore, the documentation task might be neglected by most of the junior doctors as this task is a time-consuming task and does not carry an important weight as the doctor's core task. Notwithstanding, the poor documentation issues due to doctor's time constraint needs to be resolved by the hospital's managers in avoiding the coding quality in UKMMC to deteriorate further. Even though it is a time-consuming task, good quality of documentation, in the long run, could be beneficial to the hospital's governance as it could provide a good quality clinical coding data. The senior staff nurse, for example, could be assigned by the hospital's managers in helping doctors in ensuring a good quality of documentation used as the reference during the clinical coding process.

A good quality coded data subsequently would play a useful role in helping the hospital to increase their efficiency both in the administrative side and the financial side of the hospital. Therefore if the coding process conducted in this hospital continues to be conducted according to the discharge summary, the junior doctors need to be trained in filling up complete and accurate information in the document. The past studies also have emphasised that doctor needs to be exposed as early as possible with training in recording information which could help to decrease the coding error rates as well as to ease the coding process (Singh et al. 2015; Yao et al. 1999). The current quality of discharge summary written by the junior doctors in UKMMC is very poor indicating more than 90% of the summaries with incomplete patient's demographic or clinical information. Evidently, this has caused the great number of coding errors cases in UKMMC. Thus in UKMMC, the initiative to increase the awareness on the importance of the availability of data in the discharge summary needs to be embedded among the doctors specifically the junior doctors to improve the quality of clinical coding.

On the other hand, if the coding process in UKMMC is shifted from using the discharge summaries to the medical records, the effort to embed the awareness among junior doctors on the importance of clinical coding is still imperative. In constituting a good quality of clinical coding, the doctors need to be aware of the readability of the information written in the medical records. The usage of the abbreviation and also the uniqueness of the doctor's handwriting could cause an erroneous interpretation of the patient's condition during the coding process. Past studies have highlighted that one of the challenges to clinical coding practice was the illegible handwriting of the doctors (Adeleke et al. 2014; Heywood et al. 2016). Therefore, it is crucial for the doctors especially the junior doctors to understand the concept of well-written information neither in the discharge summary nor the medical record. The high quality of clinical coding lies in the written information of the patient's condition given by the doctors. Without these criteria, it could contribute to the difficulties in performing a good quality of clinical coding.

5.2.4 Evaluation Method

Another plausible cause relating to the result of poor quality of clinical coding in UKMMC is due to the strict methodology employed by this study. Firstly, according to the methodology employed by this study, the study was carried out by assessing the entire patient's medical records. This is due to the fact that the medical records may have a complete and essential information on the patient as well as the services provided to them (Pongpirul, Walker, Rahman, et al. 2011). As discussed before, in UKMMC, the written information in the discharge summaries may not reflect the whole information that is documented in the medical records. The coders only conducted the coding process according to the information given in the discharge summaries without doing any cross-checking with the medical records. As the possibility for the information written in the medical records to be varied from those written in discharge summaries is high, this could potentially contribute to a huge variation in the code assigned by Independent Senior Coder and the in-house coder leading to high coding error rates in UKMMC. If the evaluation was conducted by assessing the information written in discharge summaries alone, the coding error rate might not be as high as reported in this study. Nevertheless, without vetting through the entire medical records, there is a high tendency where this study could not access the actual quality of coding in UKMMC, as the reliability of the information written in discharge summaries is significantly low.

Secondly, according to the methodology of this study, the Independent Senior Coder that was appointed as the auditor was a highly trained coder. He has more than ten years of experience as clinical coders and has attended clinical coding course at national and international level. This auditor also has obtained professional training in coding leading to the high exposure on awareness of the importance of documentation. His broad knowledge in the coding field may contribute to the higher coding errors rate as the evaluation done by this Independent Senior Coder would be a thorough and stringent. In the coding process, the coder's judgement is considered more reliable than the doctor's judgement as the coder is the expert in assigning codes whereas doctors are the expert in diagnosing and treating the patients. Past study has reported a lower rate of clinical coding errors rate in the study that has assigned doctors as the auditor during clinical coding audit (Farhan et al. 2005; Haliasos et al. 2010). Doctor's limited time in performing coding task as well as lesser knowledge than the clinical coders in the coding rules and guidelines which could highly contribute to the lower coding errors rate reported by the previous study. Subsequently, the coding errors rate in UKMMC could be lower if the audit was performed by individual who is not a coding expert.

It is also highly believed that the methodology using blind coding audit conducted by this study has related to the high coding errors rate in UKMMC. There was a high potential that a lower coding errors rate could be reported if the auditor has access to the original code beforehand as was mentioned by Donoghue in his study in 1992 (Donoghue 1992). The accessibility of the original code could relate to a bias judgement during the evaluation resulting in a lower coding errors rate. In contrast, the clinical coding's evaluation using blind coding audit could contribute to a fairness in judgement during the evaluation, which implies the true quality of the coding in the hospital. This subsequently could relate to a higher coding errors rate as reported by this study.

Another potential reason for the high coding errors rate might also be due to the definition of the coding errors employed by this study. In this study, the errors at any digit level of the code were considered as a coding error where other studies may accept error at the fourth and fifth digit level (Campbell et al. 2001b; Yao et al. 1999). Commonly, the errors at the fourth and fifth digit level of the code does not reflect the assignment of MY-DRG code, and the percentage of cases with a wrong assignment of fourth and fifth digit level is significantly low when compared to the error at first, second and third digit level of the code (Zafirah et al. 2017). However for the epidemiological studies purposes, the accuracy of every level of the code is imperative as it reflects the specific condition of the patient. Therefore in the effort to assess the quality of clinical coding in UKMMC, a strict evaluation rule was adopted by this study. Subsequently, this stringent evaluation has significantly contributed to the high coding errors rate in UKMMC.

5.3 Issue of Under-Coding

Data analysis from this study has reported a high volume of under-coded cases in UKMMC. It has also not escaped the attention that among the 464 selected cases, 298 (64.2%) of the discharge summaries were with incomplete information of secondary diagnosis phrases. Subsequently, the under-coded secondary diagnosis code has affected the assignment of the severity level of the 42.7% (198/464) of the selected cases in this study. It is also important to note that from these cases with errors in the assignment of its severity level, 76.8% (152/198) of the cases were re-assigned to a higher level of severity after the audit by the Independent Senior Coder. The high volume of cases with the reassignment of severity level to a higher severity level after the audit indicating that the poor quality of clinical coding has caused a potential loss of revenue to UKMMC in which most of the cases were wrongly assigned to a lower potential hospital tariff than the actual hospital tariff. Accordingly, the under-coding issues that caused a substantial amount of potential loss reported by this study reflects a poor assignment of secondary diagnosis code in UKMMC.

In implementing casemix system as the provider payment tool, the accuracy of the assignment of secondary diagnosis code is very crucial. Before accessing the accuracy of the code assigned to the case, it is also important to access the accuracy of the number and types of secondary diagnosis code assigned to the case. According to the MY-DRG® grouper used by this tertiary hospital, the assignment of severity level depends on the number of secondary diagnosis codes assigned to the case. The importance of secondary diagnosis in casemix system is not a new finding as Averill et al. has reported in 1998 that the secondary diagnosis in casemix system, will determine patient's severity level of illness (Averill et al. 1998). However, despite the crucial role of secondary diagnosis in casemix system, the finding of this study indicated that the highest percentage of coding errors rate is among the secondary diagnosis codes. This indicates the negligence of the importance of secondary diagnosis code in the implementation of casemix system as the provider payment tools in UKMMC.

The under-coding cases have caused O&G cases to be listed as the highest case type which contains error cases. The coding errors rate of cases assigned to O&G case-type was substantially high covering 94.8% of the cases. The finding of this study contradicts the preceding studies as the coding errors rate among surgical cases is usually higher that O&G case (Farhan et al. 2005; Weingart et al. 2002). The primary factor contributing to the higher coding errors rate across cases that were assigned to the O&G case-type in UKMMC was the higher coding errors rate of secondary diagnosis code in which most of the cases were being under-coded by the original coders. The under-coding issue among O&G cases is not a new finding as past studies have reported a higher number of under-coded code than up-coded code across O&G cases (K.H. et al. 2006; Lydon-Rochelle et al. 2005; Romano et al. 2005). These two studies by K.H et al. (2006) and Romano et al. (2005) have highlighted the issue of under-reporting of diagnosis and procedure across O&G cases which relates to under-coding issue among O&G cases.

The underlying cause of higher coding errors rate of secondary diagnosis codes that relates to the wrong assignment of the severity level in this study is due to several factors. The first factor that could contribute to the poor reporting of secondary diagnosis code is due to the level of enforcement of casemix system in UKMMC in which this system is not being officially utilised in the hospital's governance yet. The second factor that could contribute to poor reporting of secondary diagnosis is due to the availability of rules and guidelines in documenting secondary diagnosis code in the framework of the governance of the hospital. The third factor that could contribute to the poor reporting of secondary diagnosis code is due to the structure of the discharge summary where not much information could be documented in the discharge summary. The last factor that could contribute to the higher errors rate of secondary diagnosis is due to the ambiguities of interpretation in reporting secondary diagnosis among healthcare givers. The following subtopic will discuss more in detail on these factors that contributed to the under-coding issue in UKMMC.

5.3.1 Poor Enforcement of Casemix System

The main factor contributing to the under-coding issue in UKMMC is due to the lack of awareness of the minimum data set that is required in casemix system as the provider payment tool. It is important to remember that currently in UKMMC, casemix system is only being used for research purposes and not to govern the hospital. The absence of the implementation of casemix system in the framework of the hospital's governance has influenced the lacking of the movement among hospital managers in creating awareness on the minimum data set of casemix system. This has caused the documentation process done by the doctors was carried out without having sufficient awareness of the minimum data set that is required in the casemix system. This has subsequently related to the high volume of cases with under-reported secondary diagnosis by the doctors.

In using casemix system as the provider payment tools, on top of the accuracy of the primary diagnosis code, the accuracy of secondary diagnosis code is also imperative as it reflects the patient's severity of illness during the hospital stay. The higher number of secondary diagnosis reported the higher possibility for the case to be assigned to a high severity level, which would contribute to a higher reimbursement rate. However, despite the importance of secondary diagnosis code in the implementation of casemix system as the provider payment tools, the importance of secondary diagnosis code is always being under-emphasised. This is not a new finding as it has been debated by the past studies that doctor has a higher tendency to under-evaluate the importance of secondary diagnosis (Callen et al. 2010; Dinescu et al. 2012; Farhan et al. 2005; Mahfouz et al. 2017; Yao et al. 1999). Nevertheless, the awareness on the crucial role of the secondary diagnosis code is imperative in ensuring the accuracy of the assignment of the severity level. The absence of the sufficient awareness generated by the hospital managers on the importance of secondary diagnosis code has been related to the under-reported secondary diagnosis code among the doctors, which subsequently relates to the under-coding issue. Therefore in resolving the under-coding issue in UKMMC, it is crucial to have casemix system in the framework of the hospital's governance in ensuring the movement on creating awareness on the minimum data set of casemix could be done aggressively.

The under-coding issue in UKMMC is also influenced by UKMMC's status as a teaching hospital and a non-profit hospital. As a teaching hospital that received funding by the government annually, adequate generation of hospital revenue is not yet an important subject which relates to the low existence of casemix system in the framework of the hospital's governance. Subsequently, the lacking of casemix system in the framework of the hospital's governance has caused the clinical coding process to not being given high priority in the financial management of the hospital. As mention before, currently this system is only being used for research purposes, where the impact of the poor quality of clinical coding does not truly impact the health financing of the hospital yet. It was debated by the past study that the under-coding issue among teaching hospital is substantially higher compared to the profit hospital because of the revenue of a teaching hospital is not influenced by the coded data (Elizabeth Goldman et al. 2011). Echoing the past study, in UKMMC since the problem of under-reported secondary diagnosis does not affect the financial management of UKMMC, the movement in improving the primary reference of clinical coding is lacking which is related to lower awareness in reporting secondary diagnosis in the discharge summaries.

As the adequate generation of hospital revenue is less important in the teaching hospital, the importance of secondary diagnosis code is not being emphasized by the hospital managers. In using casemix system as the provider payment tool, the missing secondary diagnosis could relate to the under-coding issue, which potentially relates to a revenue loss. Therefore in preparing UKMMC in managing its own health financing in future, it is imperative to improve the quality of secondary diagnosis coding to prevent any potential loss of revenue.

5.3.2 Unclear Rules and Guidelines

The under evaluation of the importance of the secondary diagnosis is due to the insufficient rules and guidelines set by the hospital managers in documenting the minimum data set that is required in using casemix system as the provider payment tools.

It is important to note that in casemix system, there are many secondary diagnosis used in compared to just a single principal diagnosis. Commonly, in calculating cost under casemix system, the complications occurred during the hospital stay carried more weight than the comorbidities presented on admission. However, it is worth mentioning that there is a huge ambiguity in determining if the secondary diagnosis was the complications or comorbidity (Chiu GA & Woodwards 2011; Elizabeth Goldman et al. 2011; Heywood et al. 2016; Johnson et al. 2014).

The under-coding issue could be influenced by the lack of clear rules and guidelines in documenting secondary diagnosis in the discharge summaries. The clear rules and guidelines of clinical coding is imperative to standardise the information reported by the doctors in the discharge summary or other clinical documentation (Heywood et al. 2016). In UKMMC, due to the governance factor, it is believed that there is an absence of the specific rules and guidelines in documenting the secondary diagnosis in the discharge summary, as this clinical coding process does not carry a heavy weight among the hospital managers. The absent of rules and guidelines on what is worth to be documented and coded especially involving the selection of complication and comorbidity which could relates to the under-coding issue. For instance, without the clear rules and guidelines on what is worth to be documented and coded according to the casemix system, doctors will have the tendency to document common disease such as hypertension, obesity or depression as the secondary diagnosis even though these diseases hardly attribute to the healthcare treatment or cost (Chen et al. 2009; Peng et al. 2016).

The unclear rules and guidelines in documenting the secondary diagnosis could also confuse doctors in reporting the secondary diagnosis, as the key person in documenting the discharge summaries is the junior doctors. Junior doctors limited experience in working field could cause difficulties and confusion in selecting the appropriate and relevant secondary diagnosis that is worth to be documented for coding purposes. Evidently, cases with more than 5 secondary diagnosis codes have a higher tendency to be under-reported by the doctors in UKMMC. Therefore, the constitution of the specific rules and guidelines in documenting secondary diagnosis code is crucial to help the doctors in documenting important complications in the discharge summaries. For instance, in current Canada coding's rules, the secondary diagnosis of hospitalisation such as hypertension, obesity, depression and diabetic are optional for coding as these diseases are commonly the patient's comorbidity (Peng et al. 2016). Another example is through a study by Chen et al., whereby it was discussed in his study that obesity and weight loss should not be coded as a secondary diagnosis as it could hardly attribute to healthcare treatment or cost (Chen et al. 2009). Therefore attention by the hospital managers to create clear rules and guidelines for documenting secondary diagnosis is imperative. This would help to increase consistency among doctors specifically the junior doctors in reporting secondary diagnosis, which subsequently eases the coders to codify accurate secondary diagnosis code.

5.3.3 Structural Limitations of Discharge Summary

The poor quality of clinical coding due to the high volume of under-coded cases in UKMMC is influenced by the structure of the primary reference of clinical coding process namely the discharge summaries. Even though the discharge summary is one of the crucial documents during the patient's discharged, the reliability of this document, as the primary reference for clinical coding is very low. It was highlighted by past study that the discharge summary is not a recommended source of document for clinical coding as in general information written in the discharge summary is less precise than in the patient's note (Pocklington & Al-Dhahir 2011). The discharge summaries work as a tool to comprehensively document the patient's condition during the hospital stay. Previous studies have stressed that the purpose of discharge summaries is to summarise important information during the patient's hospital stay and to accompany the patient during their discharge and for post-hospital continuity of care (Horwitz et al. 2013; Mahfouz et al. 2017). Therefore, due to its ultimate purpose as a tools to summarised patient's information, there are several design limitations in the discharge summaries mainly on the availability of enough columns in reporting the secondary diagnosis. The structural limitation of the discharge summaries has linked to the lack of specificity of the information written in it.

In UKMMC, due to the structural limitation of the discharge summaries, the practice of reporting precise and specific information of secondary diagnosis in the discharge summaries is a challenging task. Data analysis in this study has revealed that after the evaluation by the Independent Senior Coder the highest number of secondary diagnoses code assigned per patient was 18. Interestingly currently in UKMMC, there were only 15 spaces in the discharge summaries form to report the secondary diagnosis. This indicates that discharge summaries are not the best documents to be the primary reference during the coding process as the structural limitations of the discharge summaries could retaliate doctor in reporting the patient's condition in a detailed manner. Even though if doctors are aware of the importance of reporting precise information of secondary diagnosis, the lacking of adequate space in the discharge summaries would still relate to the under-coding issue. Therefore to resolve the under-coding issue, it is the best for the coders to conduct the coding process according to the medical records until the hospital managers launched the enforcement of documenting adequate information of secondary diagnosis in the discharge summaries. This may include the restructuring of the design of the discharge summaries to allow doctors in reporting patient's secondary diagnosis in a more precise and more specific manner.

5.3.4 Ambiguities in Interpretation

As casemix system is not yet included formally in the current governance in UKMMC, the interpretation among doctors on the patient's clinical condition in the discharge summaries is varies. The variation of interpretation on patient's clinical condition is linked to the absent of the rules and guidelines in documenting the discharge summaries. This subsequently has contributed to the high volume of under-coding cases in UKMMC especially among O&G cases. In general, cases that are being assigned to O&G case type is usually a complex case as there is a higher tendency for the treatment of the patient may involves treatment in the emergency department as well as operation theatre. For this reason, O&G patients are commonly attended by various types of caregivers such as doctors, nurses and midwives.

It is worth to note that, the higher number of caregivers intervened for one patient, the higher the possibility for the case to be coded wrongly. This is due to the accuracy of the information transferred by each caregiver. Moreover, among O&G cases, there is an inconsistency among doctors in describing the condition of the patient (Romano et al. 2005). For instance, in ICD 10, there are four codes that refer to pre-eclampsia (O14.0 O14.1, O14.2, O14.9) where each code indicates a different level of severity of the pre-eclampsia. Without specific and accurate information written by doctors or any other caregivers on the severity of the patients, it would relate to under-coding issue. A consistency in reporting patient's condition during the treatment is imperative as without the consistency, the responsible doctors in documenting the discharge summary could underestimate a patient's condition leading to the under-reported information in the discharge summaries.

In resolving undercoding issue in UKMMC, the constitution of clear rules and guidelines for reporting patient's condition is crucial. With clear rules and guidelines, it could help to increase the consistency among doctors in reporting the severity level of the patients. The absence of clear rules and guidelines for reporting the patient's condition, each doctor might describe the severity level of the patient with different keywords. Lydon-Rochelle et al. (2005) has also highlighted in their study that there are ambiguities among doctors, nurses and also midwives in documenting the labour status of a patient especially involving caesarean deliveries. The ambiguities, especially in the use of the word to describe patient's level of severity in the discharge summaries, would cause erroneous assumptions among coders during the coding process (Johnson et al. 2014). Therefore in the effort to improve the quality of coding among O&G cases, it is important to conduct a discussion among doctors, coders and hospital managers in summarising important keywords to indicate the complexity of the cases treated across O&G cases. It is imperative for the doctors to use a standardised term and keyword in documenting patient's condition and coders need to be exposed to the meaning of each term and keywords to avoid any error during the coding process.

5.4 Economic Implication

The poor quality of clinical coding has caused the substantial amount of loss towards the potential hospital revenue in UKMMC. It is worth mentioning that, the output of this study shows that without the clinical coding errors, UKMMC's potential revenue has increased by 39.1% and showed a huge increment in the maximum potential hospital tariff chargeable to a patient. Data analysis revealed that most of the cases with potential loss of revenue were assigned to a lower severity level than the actual severity level before the audit, which reflects the poor quality of secondary diagnosis coding in UKMMC. In overall, the clinical coding errors in UKMMC have caused an average loss of RM1,410.14 per patient. The average loss of hospital revenue per patient in UKMMC deemed higher than average loss of revenue reported in past studies. Past studies have indicated that the average loss of revenue per patient due to clinical coding was

RM869.50 (USD264.97), ranging from RM504.42 (USD153.72) to RM1,312.64 (USD400.01) (Haliasos et al. 2010; Nouraei et al. 2009; Razik et al. 2013). This implies that the current quality of clinical coding in UKMMC could give a ramification impact towards the hospital's health financing if casemix system is being employed as the provider payment tools in the near future.

If the casemix system is being included in the structure of the hospital governance, the current quality of clinical coding is far from being beneficial to the hospital's financing. Although through DRG based payment by casemix system there is a high chance for a case to be up-coded for the financial benefits of the hospital and the attended doctors, the culture of up-coding cases for profit gain is still impossible in UKMMC (Marini & Street 2007; Soonman 2003). The combinations of current hospital governance, doctors' level of awareness of clinical coding as well as coder's level of knowledge in the coding field shows a higher tendency for a case to be undercoded than to be upcoded which relates to the adverse economic impact of clinical coding towards hospital's financing. The negative economic implication detected in this study echoed past studies that stress on the adverse effect of coding errors toward hospital financing. For instance, Burns et al. in a study on a systematic review on clinical coding conducted in 2012 reported a revenue loss of EUR443,371 (RM200,838.11) due to the coding errors in the year of 2009. Ping et al. (2009) also reported in his study on consequences of clinical coding errors in a teaching hospital at Australia that coding errors leads to a loss of revenue of AU 575,300 (RM1,685,564.19). Besides that, in the year of 2009, a loss of revenue of EUR30,000 (RM135,790.12) which is equivalent to 10% of the loss to the department which was reported by Beckley et al. (2009) in a study on coding errors at the Department of Urology in The United Kingdom. Another study by Curtis et al. (2002) also reported a revenue loss due to coding errors amounting to USD39,000 (RM127,978.50) for trauma patients at a tertiary centre in Australia.

Data analysis from this study has revealed the most influential factor that could contribute to the loss of revenue is the wrong assignment of the severity level of the case. It is worth mentioning again that the wrong assignment of severity level is due to the wrong assignment of secondary diagnosis code. Past study by Beckley et al. (2009) has also reported that cases with errors in the assignment of secondary diagnosis resulted in losing money for the hospital. This loss of revenue due to the wrong assignment of severity level is related to the low awareness of the importance of clinical coding in UKMMC. This emphasises the importance of clinical coding is translated from the poor enforcement by the hospital managers in monitoring the quality of documentation used as the primary reference during the coding process, namely the discharge summaries. This has subsequently caused a massive undercoding issue, which relates to the substantial number of cases with the wrong assignment of severity level relating to a massive potential loss of revenue to the hospital. Clearly, data analysis from this study has revealed a potential loss of revenue amounting to RM607,066.66 among cases with an error in the assignment of its severity level. This shows that 91.1% of the total amount of potential loss of revenue in UKMMC is contributed by the cases with errors in the assignment of severity level.

The poor quality of primary reference of clinical coding process has related to other far-reaching consequences towards the assignment of hospital tariff. Besides the lack of availability of data on secondary diagnosis, the current quality of discharge summaries shows poor quality of information of the birth weight for the neonatal patient. In assigning the DRG code for neonatal cases, the availability of the birth weight is crucial which without the birth weight the case would be assigned to the ungroupable case. In using Casemix system as the provider payment tools, the assignment of hospital tariff is impossible for the ungroupable cases. To ensure a neonate case is assigned to the accurate DRG group, the accuracy of birth weight is also important. This failure in documenting the accurate birth weight could relate to the huge loss of potential hospital revenue. Evidently, this study has shown that the biggest loss of revenue involves neonatal case with errors in the assignment of primary diagnosis code as well as inaccurate information of birth weight reported in the discharge summary. The next subtopic will discuss on the factor influencing to the ungroupable case and the importance of birth weight in the assignment of hospital tariff.

5.4.1 Ungroupable Case

One of the crucial findings from this study is the decreasing pattern of the minimum hospital tariff assigned to a patient after the evaluation of the quality of clinical coding conducted by this study. This decreasing pattern in the minimum potential tariff chargeable to a patient after the audit is due to the ungroupable case. After the audit, due to the missing information on birth weight, there were eight ungroupable cases identified in this study, and interestingly, all these eight cases were assigned to paediatric discipline before the audit. In total there were 8 cases detected by this study with a poor quality of documentation specifically on the birthweight that has caused the ungroupable issue. It is worth to note that the birthweight information of these 8 cases was unwritten, both in the discharge summaries or in the medical records. Form these eight ungroupable cases; UKMMC could potentially lose an amount of RM20,773.00 with an average potential loss of RM2,596.62 per patient.

The birthweight of neonates is one of the vital data that is required during the grouping process (Paranjothy et al. 2005). Past studies rarely report the missing of the ungroupable issue due to invalid birthweight. Commonly, the major factor contributing to the ungroupable cases is due to the invalid primary diagnosis code (Ghaffari et al. 2010; B. Reid & Sutch 2008). This indicates that the level of awareness among doctors on the minimum data set that is required in implementing casemix system as the provider payment tools is significantly low. The poor monitoring by hospital managers on the availability of minimum data set of casemix could highly affect the revenue of the hospital if the hospital is using casemix is their provider payment tools (Kind et al. 2012). The lack of movement in educating the hospital's staff especially among the doctors on the minimum data set of casemix could influence the level of awareness on these crucial data. Subsequently, the literacy of casemix's minimum data set is imperative and needs to be embedded among doctors at the early years of their service to make the reporting of these data would become a usual practice in the hospital.

5.4.2 Importance of Birthweight

The audit of this study revealed that the highest potential lost was among the cases that were assigned to paediatric case-type. Besides the coding errors, the poor documentation of newborn's birthweight also has affected the assignment of hospital tariff, which caused a huge loss to the hospital. As mentioned before, according to the DRG grouper used by UKMMC, the information of the neonate's birth weight is crucial during the grouping process, and failure in submitting the accurate birth weight of neonate, it would relate to the wrong assignment of DRG group. Hendrik and Juliane (2013) also emphasised in their study in German in the year of 2013 on the importance of reporting accurate information of neonate's birth weight to ensure the accurate DRG group of the case. Significantly, according to casemix system used in UKMMC, a very small difference in the birth weight's gram could result in a different assignment of DRGs group, as well as a wrong assignment of hospital tariff with the difference up to RM100,000.00.

For instance in UKMMC, the highest potential loss of income detected within the paediatric cases was amounting more than RM200,000.00. In this case, on top of the errors in the assignment of the primary diagnosis code, the birthweight of the neonate also was wrongly reported. Accordingly, the assignment of this case has shifted from P-8-17-III (Neonate, Birth-weight > 2499 g Without Complex Operation-Mild) to P-8-02-III (Neonate, Birth-weight < 1000 g With Complex Operation – Major) with the increment of hospital tariff from RM3,292.00 to RM233,319.00. It is also worth to note that there were more than five paediatric cases with potential losses of revenue amounting to more than RM20,000.00.

During the evaluation of the quality of clinical coding, it was identified that all the neonatal cases with normal birth weight were recorded with 2850 gram as their birth weight in the discharge summaries. The crosschecked of medical record revealed that there is a huge disparity of the information on birth weight written in the medical record and the discharge summary. This incidence relates to the lack of awareness among doctors in reporting accurate patient's information in the discharge summaries. Therefore, if casemix system in being included in the framework of the hospital's governance as their provider payment tools, it is essential to ensure high accuracy of documentation to avoid the ungroupable issue. The ungroupable patient could not be imposed to any amount of tariff during their discharge relates to potential loss of revenue to the hospital. The inaccurate documentation of birth weight also could relate to the wrong assignment of DRG group that accordingly will result in a potential loss of income to UKMMC.

5.5 Study Limitations

There are few limitations in conducting this study. In total, there are two major limitations of this study. The first limitation is the selection of the cases. The second limitation is the measurement of the coder's knowledge and ability. The final limitation is the accuracy of the diagnosis assigned by doctors. This section will discuss the limitations that were encountered by this study.

Firstly, it is important to note that the ethical approval for this study was submitted on April 2014 and was granted in June 2014. Therefore, during the ethical approval submission, this study has requested to audit the coded cases of the year of 2013. Accordingly, the quality of the clinical coding might be increased, as year to year, the coders are more exposed to the clinical coding process and have gained much experience in conducting the coding process. Subsequently, the coding error rates reported by this study might do not reflect the current clinical coding quality in UKMMC.

Secondly, the output of this study might not reflect the true abilities of the coders. In this study, the suggested level of knowledge of the coders is according to the comparisons of the clinical coding errors cases with the number of training attended by the coders during their service period. This might not reflect the true abilities of the coders as this study's methodology does not access the coder's ability according to their regular coding's practice in a specific manner. This is due to the main focus of this study in finding the best coding practice that could be conducted in UKMMC. Accordingly, this relates to the comparisons of the clinical coding output according to the patient's medical records with the output according to the discharge summaries. The underlying cause of the clinical coding errors in UKMMC could be caused by other the non-coder errors and not due to the coder's lack of ability.

Lastly, this study focused on the coder errors according to the information documented by the doctors. There is no assessment conducted on the accuracy of the diagnosis assigned by the doctors. Therefore doctor's skills in assigning the accurate diagnosis and its impact towards the quality of clinical coding were not addressed by this study. This study only focused on the availability of the information written by the doctors in the discharge summaries by using information written in medical records as the gold standard.

VI CONCLUSIONS AND RECOMMENDATIONS

6.1 Introduction

This chapter reiterates the important findings of the study. Recommendations for a better quality of clinical coding in UKMMC are also identified. This study has proven that the clinical coding errors which majorly caused by the incomplete documentation of primary reference of clinical coding would potentially impact the hospital revenue in UKMMC.

6.2 Conclusions of Study's Findings

This study demonstrated an extensive incidence of clinical coding errors due to incomplete discharge summary is occurring in UKMMC. The clinical coding errors rate reported by this study was as high as 89.4% covering 415 of the selected cases. The findings of this study highlighted the usage of discharge summaries as the primary reference of clinical coding process as the most important factor relating to the high coding errors rate in

UKMMC. Subsequently, in line with the existing literature, this study found that the clinical coding errors have caused a substantial amount of potential loss of revenue towards UKMMC. This study highlighted that the potential hospital revenue escalated by 39.1% from RM 1, 672, 922 before the re-coding process to RM 2, 327, 226 after the audit.

It could be concluded from the disccusion of this study's findings that, to increase the quality of clinical coding in UKMMC, the high level of awareness on the importance of clinical coding among every level of hospital's staff is imperative. This includes the hospital managers, the coders and the doctors. However, whilst a supportive hospital managers, high knowledgeable coders and highly cooperative doctors are critical, the overriding need for improvement of clinical coding lies in the quality of the primary reference of the clinical coding process. During the literature reviews in Chapter II, this study has raised the question on the reliability of the discharge summaries as the primary reference during the clinical coding process. Accordingly, this study found that the quality of discharge summaries in UKMMC is significantly low relating to the extensive number of under-coded cases.

The information written in the discharge summaries was proven to be less specific in comparisons to the information written in the patient's medical records. This is especially involving the information of secondary diagnosis. The output of this study has suggested that the root caused of the extensive number of under-coded cases is due to the lack of specificity of the information written in the discharge summaries. As the consequences of the lack of reporting of secondary diagnosis, more than 40.0% of the selected cases were assigned to the wrong severity level before the commencement of this study. It is also important to reiterates that the majority of the cases were re-assigned to a higher level of severity after the evaluation of by the Independent Senior Coder.

The multivariate analysis using the multiple logistic regression shows that the most influential factor relating to the wrong assignment of hospital tariff in UKMMC is the wrong assignment of severity level due to the clinical coding errors. Accordingly, the output of this study has highlighted that potential loss of revenue among cases with errors in the assignment of severity level has reached more than RM600,000.00. This has raised the attention on the improvement's programme of quality of clinical coding in UKMMC especially the quality of secondary diagnosis code. This study's recommendations on the improvement of the quality of the quality of clinical coding are discussed in the next sub-topic.

6.3 Recommendations

The reformation of healthcare financing through casemix system as the provider payment tool requires a high quality of clinically coded data to ensure the accuracy of the hospital tariff assigned to the patient. In preparing UKMMC towards this reformation, a significant restructuring of the clinical coding process is highly required. Subsequently, from the findings and reflection of this study's findings, the efforts of improving the quality of clinical coding in UKMMC lies on the cooperation of three essential personnel namely hospital managers, doctors and coders. Apart from that, the improvement of the quality of the primary reference of clinical coding process is also imperative. Accordingly, from the findings of this study, the recommendations of the improvement of the quality of clinical coding would be according to this four important element namely, hospital managers, doctors, coders and primary reference of the clinical coding process. Next sub-topic would elaborate in details on the recommendations of this study for the quality improvement of clinical coding in UKMMC.

6.3.1 Hospital Managers

In improving the quality of clinical coding, it is important for the hospital managers to be aware of the importance of clinical coding and its consequences towards the hospital governance. Thus, this study would suggest for the hospital managers to implement casemix system in the governance of UKMMC officially. From the official implementation of casemix system, the clinical coding process would become one of the crucial elements in executing this system. Subsequently, it would increase the importance of clinical coding in the hospital governance. From here, specific rules and guidelines in conducting clinical coding process could be constituted, a regular monitoring programme could be performed and also would enable an adequate budget allocation for the clinical coding programme.

With the vital role to play by clinical coding data in casemix system, it would increase the urgency to constitute specific rules and guidelines of the clinical coding process in UKMMC. For example, the hospital managers could officially announce mandate on the selection of the best documentation as the primary reference of clinical coding. This would help the hospital's staff to maintain a good quality of the selected primary reference. Another recommendation on the constitution of the clinical coding's rules and guidelines is, the hospital managers could provide a list of the secondary diagnosis that is unnecessary to be reported due to its regular role as comorbidity and not as complication. This is believed could reduce the time consumed by the doctors during the documentation process mainly on the reporting of the secondary diagnosis code.

In improving the quality of clinical coding in UKMMC, a continuous monitoring of the clinical coding process by the hospital managers is also recommended. The monitoring programme may include the monitoring of the primary reference of clinical coding and monitoring of the clinical coding process conducted by the clinical coders. The continuous monitoring of the elements of clinical coding could help the hospital managers in identifying problems that may occur during the clinical coding process.

Lastly, an adequate allocation of clinical coding programmes by the hospital managers could be beneficial in improving the quality of clinical coding in UKMMC. For instance, the adequate allocation given by the hospital managers could help the clinical coding unit to purchase the latest nosology of the clinical coding process. This would subsequently improve coder's knowledge of the updated clinical coding codes. Apart from this, an adequate fundings given by the hospital managers could help to facilitate clinical coding's training in order to increase coder's knowledge of the clinical coding.

6.3.2 Coders

From the output of this study, there are three major recommendations to improve the quality of clinical coding in UKMMC through coders. This may include the effort to increase coder's knowledge regularly, trained coders according to speciality and reduce unnecessary job task that is unrelated to clinical coding.

The quality of clinical coding lies on the coder's ability in conducting the clinical coding process. Therefore, it is essential for the coders to receive a regular clinical coding's training. For instance, a three monthly clinical coding workshop could be conducted by the hospital to increase coder's knowledge of clinical coding rules and guidelines. The regular clinical coding workshop also could continuously refresh coder's awareness on the clinical coding regulations and guidelines.

The improvement of the quality of clinical coding through coder also could be made by trained the coders according to speciality. Focusing on acquiring clinical codings' rules and guidelines in many specialities could also link to the low quality of clinical coding. Therefore it is recommended to train coders according to speciality. This may help to prepare the coders in becoming the subject matter of expert on the clinical coding rules and guidelines on the particular speciality. This subsequently may result in a high quality of clinical coding.

Another recommendation to increase the quality of clinical coding is by reducing clinical coder's clerical and administrative task. It would be beneficial if the clinical coders could focus on the clinical coding task only without being actively involved in other tasks that is unrelated to the clinical coding. Apart from the full focus given during the clinical coding process, the reduction of unrelated coding work also could help the clinical coders in mastering the clinical coding's skills in a faster timeline.

6.3.3 Doctors

To improve the quality of clinical coding in UKMMC, doctors active involvement in the clinical coding process is critical. The doctor's active participation in the clinical coding process is facilitated by the high level of awareness on the importance of clinical coding. Subsequently, among the recommendations that could be provided by this study is to embed the concept of clinical coding in the early year of doctor's service. Also, conducting a regular clinical coding roadshow to the department could also increase the level of awareness of the clinical coding. Lastly, the effort in improving the quality of clinical coding could also be conducted by including the documentation task as one of the variables in calculating doctor's key performance indicator (KPI).

Firstly, it is recommended to expose doctors towards the importance of clinical coding at the early year of their service. For instance, during the first orientation of the houseman before commencing their clinical job, the critical role of clinical coding need to be exposed. The junior doctors need aware that the culture of reporting the accurate and specific condition of the patient regardless of any medical documents is important in maintaining a good quality of service. Therefore this study also would suggest for the hospital managers to conduct a one day workshop specifically on the importance of clinical coding and documentation among the junior doctors before they officially commence their clinical job in the hospital.

Secondly, to increase the quality of clinical coding in UKMMC, a regular roadshow on the importance of complete documentation and accurate clinical coding could be conducted. For instance, from the regular monitoring by the hospital managers, it would be easier to identify the departments with most problems in executing proper clinical coding. From here a regular roadshow could be conducted in the particular department to help them in resolving the clinical coding issue.

Lastly, the high awareness on the clinical coding could be achieved by putting an adequate weigh on the documentation task among the doctors. For instance, the complete documentation could be among the variable of doctor's KPI. This would encourage the doctors to report accurate and specific patient's condition that would subsequently increase the quality of clinical coding in UKMMC.

6.3.4 Primary Reference of Clinical Coding

Apart from this 3 personnel, good quality of clinical coding also lies in the excellent quality of primary reference of clinical coding. From the output of the data analysis, this study also recommends the improvement of the quality of clinical coding to be conducted parallel with the improvement of the quality of the primary reference of clinical coding. This includes the selection of primary reference of clinical coding, usage of abbreviation, consistency in reporting patient's condition and also timely documentation.

Firstly, this study would recommend for the clinical coding process to be conducted by using the patient's medical records as the primary reference. Current practice in UKMMC using the discharge summary has resulted in excessive under-coding issue. To eliminate this issue, it is imperative for the primary reference of clinical coding process shifted from the discharge summary to the patient's medical records as evidently information written in the medical record is more specific and accurate than in the discharge summary.

Secondly, clear rules and guidelines need to be constituted during the documentation process by the doctors. For example, the hospital managers could provide a list of frequently used abbreviations and medical terminology to the doctors and coders. During the documentation process, it is recommended for the doctors to comply with the list given by the hospital managers. This would help to increase the consistency among doctors in documenting patient's clinical condition. Subsequently, the consistency inputs given by the doctors could help coders in accurately conducting the clinical coding process without having any erroneous assumptions towards doctors input.

Lastly, to improve the quality of clinical coding, it is critical for the primary reference of the clinical coding process to be produced timely. When the documentation is ready timely, it will become easier for the coders to rectify with the doctors if there are any ambiguities in the documentation provided to the coders. This would subsequently increase the quality of clinical coding in UKMMC.

References

Adams, D.L., Norman, H. & Burroughs, V.J. 2002. Addressing medical coding and billing part II: a strategy for achieving compliance. A risk management approach for reducing coding and billing errors. *Journal of the National Medical Association* *94*(6): 430–47. http://www.pubmedcentral.nih.gov/articlerender.fcgi?artid=2594405&tool=pmcentrez&rendertype=abstract. [30 March 2013].

Adeleke, I.T., Ajayi, O.O., Jimoh, A.B., Adebisi, A.A., Omokanye, S.A. & Jegede, M.K. 2014. Current clinical coding practices and implementation of ICD-10 in Africa: A survey of Nigerian hospitals. *American Journal of Health Research* *3*(3): 38–46. http://www.researchgate.net/publication/270275007_Current_clinical_coding_practices_and_implementation_of_ICD-10_in_Africa_A_survey_of_Nigerian_hospitals. [15 September 2014].

Averill, R.F., Muldoon, J.H., Vertrees, J.C., Ph, D. & Goldfield, N.I. 1998. The Evolution of Casemix Measurement Using Diagnosis Related Groups (DRGs). Report No. .

Bajaj, Y., Crabtree, J. & Tucker, a. G. 2007. Clinical coding: how accurately is it done? *Clinical Governance: An International Journal* *12*(3): 159–169.

Beckley, I.C.A., Nouraei, R. & Carter, S.S.C. 2009. Payment by results: Financial implications of clinical coding errors in urology. *BJU International 104*(8): 1043–1046.

Bernama. Voluntary health insurance scheme will be introduced next year. *Malay Mail Online*, 2017 http://www.themalaymailonline.com/malaysia/article/voluntary-health-insurance-scheme-will-be-introduced-next-year. [30 June 2017]

Bhangu, A., Nepogodiev, D., Taylor, C., Durkin, N. & Patel, R. 2012. Accuracy of clinical coding from 1210 appendicectomies in a British district general hospital. *International Journal of Surgery 10*(3): 144–147. http://dx.doi.org/10.1016/j.ijsu.2012.01.007.

Bhasker, D. & Coatesworth, A. 2016. How much are coding errors costing us? *The Bulletin of the Royal College of Surgeons of England 98*(5): 209–210. http://publishing.rcseng.ac.uk/doi/10.1308/rcsbull.2016.210.

Bramley, M. & Reid, B. 2007. Evaluation standards for clinical coder training. *The HIM Journal 36*(3): 20–30.

Bramley, M. & Reid, B.A. 2005. Clinical coder training initiatives in Ireland. *The HIM Journal 34*(2): 40–46.

Burns, E.M., Rigby, E., Mamidanna, R., Bottle, a., Aylin, P., Ziprin, P. & Faiz, O.D. 2012. Systematic review of discharge coding accuracy. *Journal of Public Health 34*(1): 138–148.

Busse, R., Geissler, A., Aaviksoo, A., Cots, F., Hakkinen, U., Kobel, C., Mateus, C., Or, Z., O'Reilly, J., Serden, L., Street, A., Tan, S.S. & Quentin, W. 2011. Diagnosis related groups in Europe: moving towards transparency, efficiency, and quality in hospitals. Report No. . *BMC*

Health Services Research. http://books.google.com/books?id=k6InVQ6aKwoC&pgis=1. [6 June 2013]

Byrne, E., Fernando, B., Kalra, D. & Sheikh, A. 2011. The benefits and risks of structuring and coding of patient histories in the electronic clinical record: Protocol for a systematic review. *Informatics in Primary Care* 18(3): 197–203.

Callen, J., McIntosh, J. & Li, J. 2010. Accuracy of medication documentation in hospital discharge summaries: A retrospective analysis of medication transcription errors in manual and electronic discharge summaries. *International Journal of Medical Informatics* 79(1): 58–64.

Campbell, S.E., Campbell, M.K., Grimshaw, J.M. & Walker, a E. 2001a. A systematic review of discharge coding accuracy. *Journal of Public Health Medicine* 23(3): 205–11. http://www.ncbi.nlm.nih.gov/pubmed/11585193.

Campbell, S.E., Campbell, M.K., Grimshaw, J.M. & Walker, A.E. 2001b. A systematic review of discharge coding accuracy. *Journal of Public Health Medicine* 23(3): 205–11. http://www.ncbi.nlm.nih.gov/pubmed/11585193.

Chen, G., Faris, P., Hemmelgarn, B., Walker, R.L. & Quan, H. 2009. Measuring agreement of administrative data with chart data using prevalence unadjusted and adjusted kappa. *BMC Medical Research Methodology* 9(1): 1–8.

Chin, N., Perera, P., Roberts, A. & Nagappan, R. 2013. Review of medical discharge summaries and medical documentation in a metropolitan hospital: Impact on diagnostic-related groups and Weighted Inlier Equivalent Separation. *Internal Medicine Journal* 43(7): 767–771.

Chiu GA & Woodwards, R. 2011. Surginote: Improving the Accuracy and Quality of Operation Note-Keeping. *Bulletin of The Royal College of Surgeons of England* 93(5): 1–6.

Chok, L., Bachli, E.B., Steiger, P., Bettex, D., Cottini, S.R., Keller, E., Maggiorini, M. & Schuepbach, R.A. 2018. Effect of diagnosis related groups implementation on the intensive care unit of a Swiss tertiary hospital: a cohort study. *BMC Health Services Research* 18(1): 84.

Cresswell, K., Morrison, Z., Sheikh, A. & Kalra, D. 2012. "there are too many, but never enough": Qualitative case study investigating routine coding of clinical information in depression. *PLoS ONE* 7(8): 1–10.

Curtis, K., Bollard, L. & Dickson, C. 2002. Coding errors and the trauma patient--is nursing case management the solution? *Australian Health Review : A Publication of the Australian Hospital Association* 25(4): 73–80.

Dinescu, A., Fernandez, H., Ross, J.S. & Karani, R. 2012. Audit and feedback: an intervention to improve discharge summary completion. *Hospital Medicine* 6(1): 28–32.

Donoghue, M. 1992. The Prevalence and Cost of Documentation and Coding Errors. *Australian Medical Record Journal* 22(3): 91–97.

Dowling, J., Coordinator, C. & John, S. 1995. The strategy of casemix. *Australian Health Review* 18(4): 105–115.

Elizabeth Goldman, L., Chu, P.W., Osmond, D. & Bindman, A. 2011. The accuracy of present-on-admission reporting in administrative data. *Health Services Research* 46(6 PART 1): 1946–1962.

Ellen, S., Lacey, C., Kouzma, N., Sauvey, N. & Carroll, R. 2006. Data Collection in Consultation– Liaison Psychiatry:

An Evaluation of Casemix. *Australasian Psychiatry* 14(1): 43-45.

Farhan, J., Al-Jummaa, S., Alrajhi, A. a, Al-Rajhi, A., Al-Rayes, H. & Al-Nasser, A. 2005. Documentation and coding of medical records in a tertiary care center: a pilot study. *Annals of Saudi Medicine* 25(1): 46-9.

Fisher, E.S., Whaley, F.S., Kmushat, W.M., Malenka, D.J., Fleming, C., Baron, J.A. & Hsia, D.C. 1991. The Accuracy of Medicare's Hospital Claims Data : Progress Has Been Made, but Problems Remain. *American Journal of Public Health* 82(2): 243-248.

Ghaffari, S., Doran, C., Wilson, A. & Aibett, C. 2010. Trailing Diagnostic Related Group Classification in Iranian Health System : a case study examining the feasibility of introducing casemix. *Eastern Mediterranean Health Journal* 16(5): 460-466.

Gibson, N. & Bridgman, S.A. 1998. A novel method for the assessment of the accuracy of diagnostic codes in general surgery. *Annals of the Royal College of Surgeons of England* 80(4): 293-296.

Goldfield, N. 2010. The Evolution of Diagnosis Related Groupe (DRGs): From Its Beginnings in Case-Mix and Resource Use Theory, to Its Implementation for Payment and Now for Its Current Utilization for Quality Within and Ourside the Hospital. *Quality Manage Health Care* 19(1): 3-16.

Gong, Z., Duckett, S.J., Legge, D.G. & Pei, L. 2004. Describing Chinese hospital activity with diagnosis related groups (DRGs). *Health Policy* 69(1): 93-100. http://linkinghub.elsevier.com/retrieve/pii/S0168851003002264 [21 January 2014].

Haliasos, N., Rezajooi, K., O'neill, K.S., Van Dellen, J., Hudovsky, A. & Nouraei, S. 2010. Financial and clinical governance implications of clinical coding accuracy in neurosurgery: a multidisciplinary audit. *British Journal of Neurosurgery* 24(2): 191–5. http://www.ncbi.nlm.nih.gov/pubmed/20210533 [25 March 2014].

Hassan.A, K., H, S. & D.W, C. 2002. Coding errors: a comparative analysis of hospital and prospectively collected departmental data. *British Journal of Urology International* 89: 178–80.

Hennessy, D.A., Quan, H., Faris, P.D. & Beck, C.A. 2010. Do coder characteristics influence validity of ICD-10 hospital discharge data? *BMC Health Services Research* 10(99).

Hensen, P., Fürstenberg, T., Luger, T. a, Steinhoff, M. & Roeder, N. 2005. Case mix measures and diagnosis-related groups: opportunities and threats for inpatient dermatology. *Journal of the European Academy of Dermatology and Venereology : JEADV* 19(5): 582–8. http://www.ncbi.nlm.nih.gov/pubmed/16164713 [12 July 2013].

Heywood, N.A., Gill, M.D., Charlwood, N., Brindle, R., Kirwan, C.C., Allen, N., Charleston, P., Coe, P., Cunningham, J., Duff, S., Forrest, L., Hall, C., Hassan, S., Hornung, B., al Jarabah, M., Jones, A., Mbuvi, J., Mclaughlin, T., Nicholson, J., Overton, J., Rees, A., Sekhar, H., Smith, J., Smith, S., Sung, N., Tarr, N., Teasdale, R. & Wilkinson, J. 2016. Improving accuracy of clinical coding in surgery: collaboration is key. *Journal of Surgical Research* 204(2): 490–495.

Hopfe, M., Stucki, G., Marshall, R., Twomey, C.D., Üstün, T.B. & Prodinger, B. 2016. Capturing patients' needs in casemix: a systematic literature review on the value of adding functioning information in reimbursement systems. *BMC Health Services Research* 16(1): 40.

Horwitz, L.I., Jenq, G.Y., Brewster, U.C., Chen, C., Kanade, S., Van Ness, P.H., Araujo, K.L.B., Ziaeian, B., Moriarty, J.P., Fogerty, R.L. & Krumholz, H.M. 2013. Comprehensive quality of discharge summaries at an academic medical center. *Journal of Hospital Medicine* 8(8): 436-443.

Hywel Dda University, H.B. 2014. Clinical Coding Audit Assignment Report 2013 / 14. Report No. http://www.wales.nhs.uk/sitesplus/documents/862/Attach7ciiiMiAAClinicalCoding AuditAssignmentReportHDUHB2013-2014.pdf. [1 January 2015]

Jaafar, S., Mohd Noh, K., Muttalib, K.A., Othman, N.H., Healy, J., Maskon, K., Abdullah, A.R., Zainuddin, J., Bakar, A.A., Rahman, S.S.A., Ismail, F., Chew, Y.Y., Baba, N. & Said, Z.M. 2013. Malaysia Health System Review. Report No. . *Health Systems in Transition.* http://www.wpro.who.int/asia_pacific_observatory/hits/series/Malaysia_Health_Systems_Review2013.pdf. [1 January 2015]

Jameson, S. & Reed, M.R. 2007. Payment by results and coding practice in the National Health Service. The importance for orthopaedic surgeons. *The Journal of Bone and Joint Surgery. British Volume* 89(11): 1427-1430.

Jegers, M., Kesteloot, K., De Graeve, D. & Gilles, W. 2002. A typology for provider payment systems in health care. *Health Policy* 60(3): 255-273.

Jewish Healthcare, F. & Pittsburgh Regional, H.I. 2007. Incentives For Excellence: Rebuilding the healthcare payment system from the ground up. Report No. http://jhf.org/admin/uploads/jhf-roots-20070901.pdf. [12 June 2013]

Johnson, T., Kane, J.M., Odwazny, R. & McNutt, R. 2014. Association of the position of a hospital-acquired condition diagnosis code with changes in medicare severity diagnosis-related group assignment. *Journal of Hospital Medicine* 9(11): 707–713.

Julie Levin Alexander. 2004. *Guide to Medical Billing and Coding*. (G. Joan & G. Bornwen, Eds.) 2nd Editio. New Jersey: Publishing ICDC.

K.H., T., K., K. & G.S.H., Y. 2006. Epidemiology of pre-eclampsia and eclampsia at the KK Women's and Children's Hospital, Singapore. *Singapore Medical Journal* 47(1): 48–53.

Kind, A.J.H., Thorpe, C.T., Sattin, J.A., Walz, S.E. & Smith, M.A. 2012. Provider characteristics, clinical-work processes and their relationship to discharge summary quality for sub-acute care patients. *Journal of General Internal Medicine* 27(1): 78–84.

Kirkman, M.A., Mahattanakul, W., Gregson, B.A. & Mendelow, A.D. 2009. The accuracy of hospital discharge coding for hemorrhagic stroke. *Acta Neurologica Belgica* 109(2): 114–119.

Kripalani, S., Lefevre, F., Phillips, C.O., Williams, M. V, Basaviah, P. & Baker, D.W. 2007. Deficits in Communication and Information Transfer Between Hospital-Based and Primary Care Physicians. *American Medical Association* 297(8): 831–841.

Lehtonen, T. 2007. DRG-based prospective pricing and case-mix accounting-Exploring the mechanisms of successful implementation. *Management Accounting Research 18*(3): 367–395.

Lorence, D.P. & Ibrahim, I.A. 2003. Disparity in Coding Concordance - Do Pyhsicians and Coders Agree?.pdf. *Jourma; of Health Care FInance 29*(4): 43–53.

Lorence, D.P. & Richards, M. 2002. Variation in coding influence across the USA: Risk and reward in reimbursement optimization. *Journal of Management in Medicine 16*(6): 422–435. http://www.emeraldinsight.com/10.1108/02689230210450981 [12 September 2013].

Lowe, A. 2001. Casemix accounting systems and medical coding. *Journal of Organizational Change Management 14*(1): 79–100.

Lydon-Rochelle, M.T., Holt, V.L., Nelson, J.C., Cárdenas, V., Gardella, C., Easterling, T.R. & Callaghan, W.M. 2005. Accuracy of reporting maternal in-hospital diagnoses and intrapartum procedures in Washington State linked birth records. *Paediatric and Perinatal Epidemiology 19*(6): 460–471.

Ma, C. to A. 1994. Health Care Payment Systems: Cost and Quality Incentives. *Journal of Economics & Management Strategy 3*(1): 93–112.

Mahfouz, C., Bonney, A., Mullan, J. & Rich, W. 2017. An Australian discharge summary quality assessment tool: A pilot study. *Australian Family Physician 46*(1): 57–63.

Maria, A., Rhonda, A., Danita, A., Sheila, B., Elizabeth, B., Gloryanne, B., Christine Catalan, B., Kathy, D., Michelle, D., Rose, D., Cheryl, E., Paula, F., Gail, G., Susan, G., Chad, G., Bill, H., Robin, H., Marilyn, J., Jenna, J., Christine Karaman, M., Collette, L., Eve-Ellen, M.,

Gail, M., Carol, Os., Sheila, P., Richard, P., Chuck, T., Kathleen, W., Susan, W. & MeChelle, W. 2010. Clinical Documentation Improvement Toolkit American Health Information Management Association. Report No. . *American Health Information Management Association.*

Marini, G. & Street, A. 2007. A transaction costs analysis of changing contractual relations in the English NHS. *Health Policy 83*(1): 17–26.

Mathauer, I. & Wittenbecher, F. 2013. Hospital payment systems based on diagnosis-related groups: experiences in low- and middle-income countries. *Bulletin of the World Health Organization 91*(10): 746–756A.

Mayo, A.M. & Duncan, D. 2004. Nurse perceptions of medication errors: what we need to know for patient safety. *Journal of Nursing Care Quality 19*(3): 209–17. http://www.ncbi.nlm.nih.gov/pubmed/15326990.

McClellan, M. & Rivlin, A.M. 2014. Improving Health While Reducing Cost Growth : What is Possible ? Report No. . *The Future of U.S. Health Care Spending Conference.* https://www.ncbi.nlm.nih.gov/nlmcatalog/101664544. [15 September 2014]

Mckenzie, K., Walker, S., Besenyei, A., Aitken, L.M. & Allison, B. 2005. Reviewed articles Assessing the concordance of trauma registry data and hospital records. *Health Care Management Science 34*(1): 3–7.

Mehrdad, F., Sheikhtaheri Abbas. & Sadoughi, F. 2010. Effective factors on accuracy of principal diagnosis coding based on International Classification of Diseases, the 10th revision (ICD-10). *International Journal of Information Management 30*(1): 78–84. http://linkinghub.elsevier.com/retrieve/pii/S0268401209000887 [23 May 2013].

Min, C.C. 2013. Health Spending : The Malaysian Experience Malaysia Socio-Economic Indicators. Report No. http://www.mof.go.jp/pri/research/seminar/fy2015/tff2015_s2_04.pdf.

Moshiri, H., Aljunid, S.M., Mohd Amin, R. & Ahmed, Z. 2010. Impact of Implementation of Case-mix System on Efficiency of a Teaching Hospital in Malaysia. *Global Journal of Health Science* 2(2): 91.

Murphy, P. 2012. Interventional procedures : physician involvement enhances. *Royal College of Physicians* 2012.

Neuhaus, V., Bot, A.G.J., Swellengrebel, C.H.J., Jain, N.B., Warner, J.J.P. & Ring, D.C. 2014. Treatment choice affects inpatient adverse events and mortality in older aged inpatients with an isolated fracture of the proximal humerus. *Journal of Shoulder and Elbow Surgery* 23(6): 800–806.

Nouraei, S. a. R., Hudovsky, A., Frampton, a. E., Mufti, U., White, N.B., Wathen, C.G., Sandhu, G.S. & Darzi, A. 2015. A Study of Clinical Coding Accuracy in Surgery. *Annals of Surgery* 261(6): 1.

Nouraei, S. a. R., Virk, J.S., Hudovsky, A., Wathen, C., Darzi, A. & Parsons, D. 2016. Accuracy of clinician-clinical coder information handover following acute medical admissions: implication for using administrative datasets in clinical outcomes management. *Journal of Public Health* 38(2): 352–362.

Nouraei, S. a R., O'Hanlon, S., Butler, C.R., Hadovsky, A., Donald, E., Benjamin, E. & Sandhu, G.S. 2009. A multidisciplinary audit of clinical coding accuracy in otolaryngology: Financial, managerial and clinical governance considerations under payment-by-results. *Clinical Otolaryngology 34*(1): 43–51.

O'Malley, K.J., Cook, K.F., Price, M.D., Wildes, K.R., Hurdle, J.F. & Ashton, C.M. 2005. Measuring diagnoses: ICD code accuracy. *Health Services Research 40*(5 Pt 2): 1620–39. http://www.pubmedcentral.nih.gov/articlerender.fcgi?artid=1361216&tool=pmcentrez&rendertype=abstract [4 September 2013].

Or., Z. 2014. Implementation of DRG Payment in France: Issues and recent developments. *Health Policy 117*(2): 146–150.

Palmer, G. & Reid, B. 2001. Evaluation of the performance of diagnosis-related groups and similar casemix systems: methodological issues. *Health Services Management Research : An Official Journal of the Association of University Programs in Health Administration / HSMC, AUPHA 14*(2): 71–81.

Paranjothy, S., Frost, C. & Thomas, J. 2005. How much variation in CS rates can be explained by case mix differences? *BJOG: An International Journal of Obstetrics and Gynaecology 112*(5): 658–666.

Paul, A., Michel, J. & Marius, F. 2008. Improving the quality of the coding of primary diagnosis in standardized discharge summaries. *Health Care Manage Science 11*: 147–151.

Peng, M., Southern, D.A., Williamson, T. & Quan, H. 2016. Under-coding of secondary conditions in coded hospital health data: Impact of co-existing conditions, death status and number of codes in a record. *Health Informatics Journal* 1–8. http://jhi.sagepub.com/content/early/2016/05/08/1460458216647089?papetoc. [15 January 2017]

Pine, M., Jordan, H.S., Elixhauser, A., Fry, D.E., Hoaglin, D.C., Jones, B., Meimban, R., Warner, D. & Gonzales, J. 2009. Modifying ICD-9-CM coding of secondary diagnoses to improve risk-adjustment of inpatient mortality rates. *Medical Decision Making : An International Journal of the Society for Medical Decision Making* 29(1): 69–81. http://www.ncbi.nlm.nih.gov/pubmed/18812585. [12 April 2013]

Ping, C., Annette, G., Kerin, M.R. & Lindsay, P. 2009. The risk and consequences of clinical miscoding due to inadequate medical documentation : a case study of the impact on health services funding. *Health Information Management Journal* 38(1).

Pocklington, C. & Al-Dhahir, L. 2011. A comparison of methods of producing a discharge summary: Handwritten vs. electronic documentation. *British Journal of Medical Practitioners* 4(3).

Pongpirul, K. & Robinson, C. 2013. Hospital manipulations in the DRG system : a systematic scoping review. *Asian Biomedicine* 7(3): 301–310.

Pongpirul, K., Walker, D.G., Rahman, H. & Robinson, C. 2011. DRG coding practice: a nationwide hospital survey in Thailand. *BMC Health Services Research* 11(1): 290. http://www.pubmedcentral.nih.gov/articlerender.fcgi?artid=3213673&tool=pmcentrez&rendertype=abstract [18 July 2013].

Pongpirul, K., Walker, D.G., Winch, P.J. & Robinson, C. 2011. A qualitative study of DRG coding practice in hospitals under the Thai Universal Coverage Scheme. *BMC Health Services Research* 11(1): 71. http://www.biomedcentral.com/1472-6963/11/71 [12 June 2013].

Preda, A.L., Chiriac, N.D. & Musat, S.N. 2012. Aspects of clinical coding. *Management in Health 16*(3): 19–21.

Preston, A.M., Chua, W.-F. & Neu, D. 1997. The Diagnosis-Related Group-Prospective Payment System and the problem of the government of rationing health care to the elderly. *Accounting, Organizations and Society 22*(2): 147–164. http://linkinghub.elsevier.com/retrieve/pii/S0361368296000116. [12 June 2013]

Preyra, C. 2004. Coding response to a case-mix measurement system based on multiple diagnoses. *Health Services Research 39*(4 Pt 1): 1027–45.

Radu, C.-P., Chiriac, D.N. & Vladescu, C. 2010. Changing Patient Classification System for Hospital Reimbursement in Romania. *Croatian Medical Journal 51*(3): 250–258. http://www.ncbi.nlm.nih.gov/pmc/articles/PMC2897082/ [21 January 2014].

Razik, A., Venkat-Raman, V. & Haddad, F. 2013. Assessing the Accuracy of Clinical Coding in Orthopaedic Day Surgery Patients. *The Bulletin of the Royal College of Surgeons of England 95*(1): 14–16. http://publishing.rcseng.ac.uk/. [15 March 2014]

Reid, B. & Sutch, S. 2008. Comparing diagnosis-related group systems to identify design improvements. *Health Policy 87*(1): 82–91.

Reid, B.A., Ridoutt, L., O'Connor, P. & Murphy, D. 2017a. Best practice in the management of clinical coding services: Insights from a project in the Republic of Ireland, Part 1. *Health Information Management Journal 46*(2): 69–77. http://journals.sagepub.com/. [11 December 2017]

Reid, B.A., Ridoutt, L., O'Connor, P. & Murphy, D. 2017b. Best practice in the management of clinical coding services: Insights from a project in the Republic of Ireland, Part 1. *Health Information Management Journal* 46(2): 69–77. http://journals.sagepub.com/. [16 September 2017]

Robinson, J.C. 2001. Theory and practice in the design of physician payment incentives. *The Milbank Quarterly* 79(2): 149–177, III.

Robyn, P.J., Sauerborn, R. & Bärnighausen, T. 2013. Provider payment in community-based health insurance schemes in developing countries: A systematic review. *Health Policy and Planning* 28(2): 111–122.

Roger France, F.H. 2003. Case mix use in 25 countries: A migration success but international comparisons failure. *International Journal of Medical Informatics* 70(2–3): 215–219.

Romano, P.S., Yasmeen, S., Schembri, M.E., Keyzer, J.M. & Gilbert, W.M. 2005. Coding of perineal lacerations and other complications of obstetric care in hospital discharge data. *Obstetrics and Gynecology* 106(4): 717–725.

Rosenberg, M.A. & Browne, M.J. 2001. The Impact of the Inpatient Prospective Payment System and Diagnosis-Related Groups. *North American Actuarial Journal* 5(4): 84–94.

Rosenstein, A.H., O'Daniel, M., White, S. & Taylor, K. 2009. Medicare's value-based payment initiatives: impact on and implications for improving physician documentation and coding. *American Journal of Medical Quality : The Official Journal of the American College of Medical Quality* 24(3): 250–258.

Roszita, I., Nur, A.M., Zafirah, A.R.S.A. & Aljunid, S.M. 2017. Estimation of cost of diagnostic laboratory services using Activity Based Costing (ABC) for implementation of Malaysia Diagnosis Related Group (MY-DRG®) in a teaching hospital. *Malaysian Journal of Public Health Medicine 17*(2): 1–8.

Rudman, W.J. 2000. Coding and Documentation of Domestic Violence http://vawnet.org/publisher/family-violence-prevention-fund.

Santos, S., Murphy, G., Baxter, K. & Robinson, K.M. 2008. Organisational factors affecting the quality of hospital clinical coding. *Health Information Management 37*(1): 25–37.

Saperi, S., Amrizal, M.N., Rohaizat, Y., Zafar, A. & Syed, A. 2005. Implementation Of Casemix In Hospital UKM : The Progress. *Malaysia Journal of Public Health Medicine 5*(Supplement 2).

Schreyögg, J., Stargardt, T., Tiemann, O. & Busse, R. 2006. Methods to determine reimbursement rates for diagnosis related groups (DRG): A comparison of nine European countries. *Health Care Management Science 9*: 215–223.

Shepheard, J. 2010. Health information management and clinical coding workforce issues. *Health Information Management Journal 39*(3): 37–41.

Sherri, A., Therese, C. & Tesesa, S. 2003. Overview of inpatient coding.pdf. *American Journal Health System Pharmacy* http://ovidsp.tx.ovid.com/sp-3.23.0a/ovidweb.cgi?WebLinkFrameset=1&S=KHMAFPDJFCDDILKFNCHKDCMCDKOMAA00&returnUrl=ovidweb.cgi?&Full+Text=L%7CS.sh.22.23%7C0%7C00043627-200311016 00004&S=KHMAFPDJFCDDIL

KFNCHKDCMCDKOMAA00&directlink=http://ovidsp.tx.ovid.com\/ov. [16 Septembr 2016]

Shin, E., Dow, W.H., Kaluzny, A.D., Park, Y. & Park, K. 2003. Disease coding errors by health care organizations : effects of a government quality intervention. *International Journal of Health Planning and Management 18*: 151–159.

Silverman, E. & Skinner, J. 2004. Medicare upcoding and hospital ownership. *Journal of Health Economics 23*(2): 369–89. http://www.ncbi.nlm.nih.gov/pubmed/15019762 [6 September 2013].

Singh, G., Harvey, R., Dyne, A., Said, A. & Scott, I. 2015. Hospital discharge summary scorecard: A quality improvement tool used in a tertiary hospital general medicine service. *Internal Medicine Journal 45*(12): 1302–1305.

Sivaselvam, B.S. UKM Granted Autonomy UKM Granted Autonomy. *UKM News Portal*, 26 January: 1–2. Kuala Lumpur http://www.ukm.my/news/index.php/en/extras/959-ukm-granted-autonomy-.html. [16 May 2013]

Soonman, K. 2003. Payment system reform for health care providers in Korea. *Health Policy and Planning 18*(1): 84–92.

Stanfill, M.H., Williams, M., Fenton, S.H., Jenders, R.A. & Hersh, W.R. 2010. A systematic literature review of automated clinical coding and classification systems. *Journal of the American Medical Informatics Association 17*(6): 646–651.

Tai, T.W., Anandarajah, S., Dhoul, N. & de Lusignan, S. 2007. Variation in clinical coding lists in UK general practice: A barrier to consistent data entry? *Informatics in Primary Care 15*(3): 143–150.

Tang, K.L., Lucyk, K. & Quan, H. 2017. Coder perspectives on physician-related barriers to producing high-quality administrative data: a qualitative study. *CMAJ Open* 5(3): E617–E622.

Thabrany, H. 2008. Politics of National Health Insurance of Indonesia : A New Era of Universal Coverage. In *7th European Conference on Health Economics*. p. 20. [15 August 2016]

Tucker, D., Parry, M. & Packham, I. 2016. Financial ramifications of inaccurate clinical coding in two common orthopaedic procedures. *The Bulletin of the Royal College of Surgeons of England* 98(1): 34–37.

Turner-Stokes, L., Sutch, S. & Dredge, R. 2012. Healthcare tariffs for specialist inpatient neurorehabilitation services: rationale and development of a UK casemix and costing methodology. *Clinical Rehabilitation* 26(3): 264–279.

UNU IIGH. 2008. No Title http://unuiigh-casemixonline.org/. [15 April 2013]

Van Walraven, C. & Demers, S. V. 2001. Coding diagnoses and procedures using a high-quality clinical database instead of a medical record review. *Journal of Evaluation in Clinical Practice* 7(3): 289–297.

Wallis, K.L., Malic, C.C., Littlewood, S.L., Judkins, K. & Phipps, A.R. 2009. Surviving "Payment by Results": A simple method of improving clinical coding in burn specialised services in the United Kingdom. *Burns* 35(2): 232–236.

Weingart, S.N., Davis, R.B. & Iezzoni, L.I. 2002. Discrepancies Between Explicit and Implicit Review : Physician and Nurse Assessments of Complications and Quality Objective Methods Description of the CSP Chart

Abstraction Instruments : Explicit Review. *Health Services Research 37*(2): 483–498.

Wockenfuss, R., Frese, T., Herrmann, K., Claussnitzer, M. & Sandholzer, H. 2009. Three- and four-digit ICD-10 is not a reliable classification system in primary care. *Scandinavian Journal of Primary Health Care 27*(3): 131–6. http://www.pubmedcentral.nih.gov/articlerender.fcgi?artid=3413183&tool=pmcentrez&rendertype=abstract [5 March 2014].

Yao, P., Wiggs, B.R., Gregor, C., Sigurnjak, R. & Dodek, P. 1999. Discordance between physicians and coders in assignment of diagnoses. *International Journal for Quality in Health Care 11*(2): 147–153.

Zafirah, S.A., Nur, A.M., Puteh, S.E.W. & Aljunid, S.M. 2018. Potential loss of revenue due to errors in clinical coding during the implementation of the Malaysia diagnosis related group (MY-DRG®) Casemix system in a teaching hospital in Malaysia. *BMC Health Services Research 18*(1): 38.

Zafirah, S.A., Nur, A.M., Wp, S.E. & Aljunid, S.M. 2017. Incidence of Clinical Coding Errors and Implications on Casemix Reimbursement in a Teaching Hospital in Malaysia. *Malaysia Journal of Public Health Medicine 17*(2): 19–28.

Appendix A
STUDY TOOLS

Data Abstraction Checklist by Independent Coder

Date Abstracted :
Patient Name :
Patient Medical Record Number:

1. DIAGNOSIS

No	Validated **Primary Diagnosis** by Independent Coder	Validated **Primary Diagnosis CODE** by Independent Coder	Remarks
1.			

No	Validated **Secondary Diagnosis** by Independent Coder	Validated **Secondary Diagnosis CODE** by Independent Coder	Remarks
1.			
2.			
3.			
4.			
5.			
6.			
7.			
8.			
9.			
10.			
11.			
12.			
13.			
14.			
15.			

2. Procedure

No	Validated **Primary Procedure** by Independent Coder	Validated **Primary Procedure CODE** by Independent Coder	Remarks
1.			

No	Validated **Secondary Procedure** by Independent Coder	Validated **Secondary Procedure CODE** by Independent Coder	Remarks
1.			
2.			
3.			
4.			
5.			
6.			
7.			
8.			
9.			
10.			
11.			
12.			
13.			
14.			
15.			
16.			
17.			
18.			

Checklist for 14 Casemix Variables (per patient per episode)

No	Item	Complete	Incomplete	None
1.	**Patient's Identifier** • Patient Name			
	• Medical Record Number			
2.	**Age** *Age in years* *Age in days (less for one year old babies*			
3.	**Gender** *Male* *Female* *Unknown*			
4.	**Birth date** *DD/MM/YY*			
5.	**Birth Weight** *For neonatal only (28 days and below)* *Stated in gram*			
6.	**Admission Date** *DD/MM/YY*			
7.	**Discharge Date** *DD/MM/YY*			
8.	**Length of stay (LOS)** *Written in days*			
9.	**Discharge Category** *Home/transfer acute facility/against medical advice/died/other or unknown*			
10.	**Patient type (3 category)** *Inpatient/ outpatient or ambulatory/undesignated*			
11.	**Principal Diagnosis** *The main reason patient is*			

Appendix B

LIST OF TOP 50 ASSIGNED PRIMARY DIAGNOSIS CODE

No.	Code	Description	Non Error Case	Error Case	Total
1.	O32.1	Maternal care for breech presentation	0	6	6
2.	O68.0	Labour and delivery complicated by fetal heart rate anomaly	0	6	6
3.	K35.9	Acute appendicitis, unspecified	3	2	5
4.	O03.4	Spontaneous abortion : incomplete, without complication	2	3	5
5.	O24.4	Diabetes mellitus arising in pregnancy	0	5	5
6.	O42.0	Premature rupture of membranes, onset of labour within 24 hours	0	5	5
7.	O42.1	Premature rupture of membranes, onset of labour after 24 hours	1	4	5
8.	O44.1	Placenta praevia with haemorrhage	1	4	5
9.	I12.0	Hypertensive renal disease with renal failure	0	4	4
10.	K35.0	Acute appendicitis with generalized peritonitis	0	4	4
11.	N40	Hyperplasia of prostate	1	3	4

12.	O32.2	Maternal care for transverse and oblique lie	0	4	4
13.	O82.1	Delivery by emergency caesarean section	1	3	4
14.	P07.3	Other preterm infants	0	4	4
15.	P55.1	ABO isoimmunization of fetus and newborn	0	4	4
16.	A41.9	Sepsis, unspecified	0	3	3
17.	A90	Dengue fever [classical dengue]	0	3	3
18.	D64.9	Anaemia, unspecified	0	3	3
19.	H27.0	Aphakia	1	2	3
20.	J38.0	Paralysis of vocal cords and larynx	1	2	3
21.	K40.2	Bilateral inguinal hernia, without obstruction or gangrene	1	2	3
22.	K80.5	Calculus of bile duct without cholangitis or cholecystitis	0	3	3
23.	N20.0	Calculus of kidney	2	1	3
24.	N35.9	Urethral stricture, unspecified	0	3	3
25.	O41.0	Oligohydramnios	0	3	3
26.	O63.1	Prolonged second stage (of labour)	0	3	3
27.	O68.1	Labour and delivery complicated by meconium in amniotic fluid	0	3	3
28.	P22.0	Respiratory distress syndrome of newborn	1	2	3
29.	P24.0	Neonatal aspiration of meconium	0	3	3
30.	Q37.9	Unspecified cleft palate with unilateral cleft lip	1	2	3
31.	A08.0	Rotaviral enteritis	1	1	2
32.	C20	Malignant neoplasm of rectum	0	2	2
33.	D25.9	Leiomyoma of uterus, unspecified	0	2	2
34.	E87.1	Hypo-osmolality and hyponatraemia	0	2	2
35.	G40.9	Epilepsy, unspecified	0	2	2
36.	I20.0	Unstable angina	0	2	2
37.	I25.1	Atherosclerotic heart disease	0	2	2
38.	I25.9	Chronic ischaemic heart disease, unspecified	0	2	2

39.	J44.1	Chronic obstructive pulmonary disease with acute exacerbation, unspecified	0	2	2
40.	J46	Status asthmaticus	0	2	2
41.	K40.3	Unilateral or unspecified inguinal hernia, with obstruction, without gangrene	0	2	2
42.	K56.1	Intussusception	1	1	2
43.	K61.0	Anal abscess	0	2	2
44.	K92.2	Gastrointestinal haemorrhage, unspecified	0	2	2
45.	L02.2	Cutaneous abscess, furuncle and carbuncle of trunk	0	2	2
46.	N61	Inflammatory disorders of breast	0	2	2
47.	O02.1	Missed abortion	0	2	2
48.	O61.0	Failed medical induction of labour	0	2	2
49.	O69.0	Labour and delivery complicated by prolapse of cord	1	1	2
50.	O70.1	Second degree perineal laceration during delivery	0	2	2

Appendix C

LIST OF TOP 50 ASSIGNED SECONDARY DIAGNOSIS CODE

No.	Code	Description	Non Error Case	Error Case	Total
1.	O34.2	Maternal care due to uterine scar from previous surgery	1	12	13
2.	O82.0	Delivery by elective caesarean section	1	12	13
3.	D64.9	Anaemia, unspecified	1	11	12
4.	O81.4	Vacuum extractor delivery	0	11	11
5.	O42.0	Premature rupture of membranes, onset of labour within 24 hours	0	9	9
6.	O99.0	Anaemia complicating pregnancy, childbirth and the puerperium	0	9	9
7.	Z38.0	Singleton, born in hospital	1	8	9
8.	I25.9	Chronic ischaemic heart disease, unspecified	0	8	8
9.	E86	Volume depletion	1	6	7
10.	N18.1	Chronic kidney disease, stage 1	0	7	7
11.	O99.2	Endocrine, nutritional and metabolic diseases complicating pregnancy, childbirth and the puerperium	0	7	7

12.	P70.4	Other neonatal hypoglycaemia	0	7	7
13.	A41.9	Sepsis, unspecified	0	6	6
14.	E66.9	Obesity, unspecified	0	6	6
15.	I25.1	Atherosclerotic heart disease	0	6	6
16.	I48	Atrial fibrillation and flutter	1	5	6
17.	J45.9	Asthma, unspecified	0	6	6
18.	N17.9	Acute renal failure, unspecified	0	6	6
19.	O75.7	Vaginal delivery following previous caesarean section	0	6	6
20.	P36.9	Bacterial sepsis of newborn, unspecified	1	5	6
21.	P70.1	Syndrome of infant of a diabetic mother	2	4	6
22.	Z51.1	Chemotherapy session for neoplasm	2	4	6
23.	O23.4	Unspecified infection of urinary tract in pregnancy	0	5	5
24.	O98.8	Other maternal infectious and parasitic diseases complicating pregnancy, childbirth and the puerperium	0	5	5
25.	P22.1	Transient tachypnoea of newborn	0	5	5
26.	Z53.8	Procedure not carried out for other reasons	0	5	5
27.	G81.9	Hemiplegia, unspecified	1	3	4
28.	I95.9	Hypotension, unspecified	0	4	4
29.	M51.3	Other specified intervertebral disc degeneration	1	3	4
30.	O41.0	Oligohydramnios	0	4	4
31.	O47.1	False labour at or after 37 completed weeks of gestation	0	4	4
32.	O61.0	Failed medical induction of labour	0	4	4
33.	O99.5	Diseases of the respiratory system complicating pregnancy, childbirth and the puerperium	0	4	4
34.	P05.1	Small for gestational age	0	4	4
35.	P07.3	Other preterm infants	0	4	4
36.	P12.0	Cephalhaematoma due to birth injury	0	4	4
37.	P22.0	Respiratory distress syndrome of newborn	0	4	4

38.	P92.8	Other feeding problems of newborn	1	3	4
39.	Z30.2	Sterilization	0	4	4
40.	D25.9	Leiomyoma of uterus, unspecified	0	3	3
41.	D55.0	Anaemia due to glucose-6-phosphate dehydrogenase [G6PD] deficiency	0	3	3
42.	E78.0	Pure hypercholesterolaemia	0	3	3
43.	G40.9	Epilepsy, unspecified	0	3	3
44.	G47.3	Sleep apnoea	0	3	3
45.	I12.0	Hypertensive renal disease with renal failure	0	3	3
46.	J06.9	Acute upper respiratory infection, unspecified	1	2	3
47.	J18.9	Pneumonia, unspecified	0	3	3
48.	N40	Hyperplasia of prostate	0	3	3
49.	O14.9	Pre-eclampsia, unspecified	0	3	3
50.	O30.0	Twin pregnancy	1	2	3

Appendix D

LIST OF TOP 50 ASSIGNED PRIMARY PROCEDURE CODE

No.	Code	Description	Non Error Case	Error Case	Total
1.	72.71	Vacuum extraction with episiotomy	0	6	6
2.	13.41	Phacoemulsification and aspiration of cataract	2	3	5
3.	51.1	Diagnostic procedures on biliary tract	0	5	5
4.	72.79	Other vacuum extraction	0	5	5
5.	86.22	Excisional debridement of wound, infection, or burn	1	4	5
6.	99.04	Transfusion of packed cells	0	5	5
7.	47.01	Laparoscopic appendectomy	1	3	4
8.	47.09	Other appendectomy	2	2	4
9.	60.18	Other diagnostic procedures on prostate and periprostatic tissue	0	4	4
10.	73.4	Medical induction of labour	0	4	4
11.	75.34	Other fetal monitoring	0	4	4
12.	88.72	Diagnostic ultrasound of heart	1	3	4
13.	74.1	Low cervical caesarean section	0	4	4

14.	34.04	Insertion of intercostal catheter for drainage	0	3	3
15.	45.13	Other endoscopy of small intestine	0	3	3
16.	73.3	Failed forceps	0	3	3
17.	88.19	Other x-ray of abdomen	0	3	3
18.	88.79	Other diagnostic ultrasound	0	3	3
19.	8.2	Excision or destruction of lesion or tissue of eyelid	0	2	2
20.	13.71	Insertion of intraocular lens prosthesis at time of cataract extraction, one-stage	0	2	2
21.	18.11	Otoscopy	0	2	2
22.	39.27	Arteriovenous for renal dialysis	0	2	2
23.	49.01	Incision of perianal abscess	0	2	2
24.	53	Repair of hernia	0	2	2
25.	53.1	Other bilateral repair of inguinal hernia	1	1	2
26.	55.03	Percutaneous nephrostomy without fragmentation	0	2	2
27.	74.2	Extraperitoneal caesarean section	0	2	2
28.	86.07	Insertion of totally implantable vascular access device [VAD]	0	2	2
29.	87.17	Other x-ray of skull	0	2	2
30.	88.01	Computerized axial tomography of abdomen	0	2	2
31.	88.21	Skeletal x-ray of shoulder and upper arm	0	2	2
32.	88.71	Diagnostic ultrasound of head and neck	0	2	2
33.	92.29	Other radiotherapeutic procedure	0	2	2
34.	6.4	Complete thyroidectomy	1	0	1
35.	6.81	Complete parathyroidectomy	0	1	1
36.	11.64	Other penetrating keratoplasty	1	0	1
37.	12.12	Other iridotomy	0	1	1
38.	12.4	Excision or destruction of lesion of iris and ciliary body	0	1	1

39.	12.5	Facilitation of intraocular circulation	0	1	1
40.	13.59	Other extracapsular extraction of lens	0	1	1
48.	38.59	Ligation and stripping of varicose veins; lower limb veins	0	1	1
49.	39.5	Other repair of vessels	0	1	1
50.	39.53	Repair of arteriovenous fistula	0	1	1

Appendix E

LIST OF TOP 50 ASSIGNED SECONDARY PROCEDURE CODE

No.	Code	Description	Non Error Case	Error Case	Total
1.	66.39	Other bilateral destruction or occlusion of fallopian tubes	0	5	5
2.	87.03	Computerized axial tomography of head	0	5	5
3.	88.19	Other x-ray of abdomen	0	6	5
4.	99.83	Other phototherapy	0	5	5
5.	86.22	Excisional debridement of wound, infection, or burn	1	3	4
6.	87.79	Other x-ray of male genital organs	1	3	4
7.	90.99	Microscopic examination of specimen from lower gastrointestinal tract and of stool, other microscopic examination	0	4	4
8.	93.39	Other physical therapy therapeutic procedures	0	4	4
9.	69.09	Other dilation and curettage of uterus	1	2	3
10.	74.1	Low cervical caesarean section	0	3	3

11.	75.69	Repair of other current obstetric laceration	0	3	3
12.	88.01	Computerized axial tomography of abdomen	0	3	3
13.	88.76	Diagnostic ultrasound of abdomen and retroperitoneum	0	3	3
14.	88.78	Diagnostic ultrasound of gravid uterus	0	3	3
15.	89.26	Gynecological examination	0	3	3
16.	96.6	Enteral infusion of concentrated nutritional substances	0	3	3
17.	22.19	Other diagnostic procedures on nasal sinuses	0	2	2
18.	36.06	Insertion of non-drug-eluting coronary artety stent(s)	0	2	2
19.	40	Operations on lymphatic system	0	2	2
20.	54.11	Exploratory laparotomy	0	2	2
21.	54.21	Laparoscopy	0	2	2
22.	88.27	Skeletal x-ray of thigh, knee, and lower leg	0	2	2
23.	88.74	Diagnostic ultrasound of digestive system	0	2	2
24.	93.57	Application of other wound dressing	0	2	2
25.	8.61	Reconstruction of eyelid with skin flap or graft	0	1	1
26.	8.89	Other eyelid repair	0	1	1
27.	13.19	Other intracapsular extraction of lens	1	0	1
28.	14.73	Mechanical vitrectomy by anterior approach	0	1	1
29.	16.09	Other orbitotomy	0	1	1
30.	18.11	Otoscopy	0	1	1
31.	38.93	Venous catheterization, not elsewhere classified	0	1	1
32.	41.31	Biopsy of bone marrow	0	1	1
33.	45.23	Colonoscopy	0	1	1
34.	46.01	Exteriorization of small intestine	0	1	1

35.	51.43	Insertion of choledochohepatic tube for decompression	0	1	1
36.	51.82	Pancreatic sphincterotomy	0	1	1
37.	54	Other operations on abdominal region	0	1	1
38.	55.02	Nephrostomy	0	1	1
39.	55.87	Correction of ureteropelvic junction	0	1	1
40.	57.32	Other cystoscopy	0	1	1
48.	67.12	Other cervical biopsy	0	1	1
49.	68.16	Closed biopsy of uterus	0	1	1
50.	75.4	Manual removal of retained placenta	0	1	1

Appendix F

LIST OF TOP 50 CASES WITH HIGHEST POTENTIAL LOSS OF REVENUE

No.	Hospital Tariff Before Audit	Hospital Tariff After Audit	Potential Loss Due to Coding Errors	Original MY-DRG Group	Description	New MY-DRG Group	Description
1.	RM6,099.09	RM24,547.17	RM18,448.08	J-4-21-II	Respiratory System Signs, Symptoms & Other Disorders- Moderate	M-4-21-III	Other Musculoskeletal System & Connective Tissue Disorders - Severe
2.	RM2,822.00	RM20,747.07	RM17,925.07	P-8-17-II	Neonate, Birthweight >2499 Grams Without Complex Operation- Moderate	P-8-12-II	Neonate, Birthweight 1500 1999 Grams Without Complex Operation - Moderate
3.	RM2,822.00	RM20,747.07	RM17,925.07	P-8-17-II	Neonate, Birthweight >2499 Grams Without Complex Operation - Moderate	P-8-12-II	Neonate, Birthweight 1500 1999 Grams Without Complex Operation - Moderate
4.	RM4,565.00	RM21,772.03	RM17,207.03	P-8-16-III	Neonate, Birthweight >2499 Grams With Congenital/Perinatal Sepsis - Severe	P-8-13-III	Neonate, Birthweight 2000 2499 Grams Without Complex Operation - Severe
5.	RM14,193.00	RM30,723.31	RM16,530.31	M-1-03-II	Spinal Fusion Procedures - Moderate	M-1-03-III	Spinal Fusion Procedures - Severe
6.	RM2,238.07	RM18,029.87	RM15,791.80	I-4-15-I	Peripheral & Other Vascular Diseases - Mild	M-1-02-II	Amputation - Moderate

7.	RM2,925.37	RM18,441.07	RM15,515.70	I-4-10-III	Acute Myocardial Infarction	J-1-20-III	Simple Respiratory System Operations - Severe
8.	RM1,829.80	RM15,649.54	RM13,819.74	D-4-13-II	Anaemia Excluding Sickle Cell Anaemia With Crisis - Moderate	D-1-20-II	Other Procedures Of Blood And Blood Forming Organs - Moderate
9.	RM4,979.09	RM16,624.04	RM11,644.95	N-1-40-II	Urethral & Transurethral Operations - Moderate	N-1-20-III	Upper Urinary Tract Operation - Severe
10.	RM2,375.00	RM13,802.96	RM11,427.96	I-4-15-II	Peripheral & Other Vascular Diseases - Moderate	M-1-30-III	Operation Of Foot - Severe
11.	RM3,917.03	RM14,767.32	RM10,850.29	O-6-10-I	Caesarean Section -Mild	O-6-10-III	Caesarean Section - Severe
12.	RM4,857.50	RM13,194.82	RM8,337.32	U-4-13-I	Epiglottitis, Upper Respiratory Tract Infection, Laryngotracheitis & Otitis Media - Mild	U-1-20-II	Other Ear, Nose, Mouth & Throat Operations - Moderate
13.	RM5,518.00	RM13,802.96	RM8,284.96	H-1-30-I	Intraocular & Lens Operations - Mild	M-1-30-III	Operation Of Foot - Severe
14.	RM3,170.00	RM11,372.56	RM8,202.56	K-1-13-I	Appendix Operation - Mild	K-1-10-II	Simple Small & Large Bowel Operation - Moderate
15.	RM6,130.26	RM13,459.23	RM7,328.97	F-4-11-II	Major Depression - Moderate	F-4-13-II	Bipolar Disorders Including Mania - Moderate
16.	RM4,530.00	RM11,278.66	RM6,748.66	L-1-50-I	Breast Operations - Mild	L-1-50-II	Breast Operations - Moderate
17.	RM5,778.00	RM11,984.16	RM6,206.16	N-1-20-II	Upper Urinary Tract Operation - Moderate	B-1-11-II	Complex Operations Of Biliary Tract - Moderate
18.	RM1,412.00	RM7,531.60	RM6,119.60	P-8-17-I	Neonate, Birthweight >2499 Grams Without Complex Operation- Mild	P-8-13-II	Neonate, Birthweight 2000 2499 Grams Without Complex Operation - Moderate

No.				
19.	RM1,412.00	RM7,531.60	RM6,119.60	P-8-17-I	Neonate, Birthweight>2499 Grams Without Complex Operation - Mild
20.	RM1,412.00	RM7,531.60	RM6,119.60	P-8-17-I	Neonate, Birthweight >2499 Grams Without Complex Operation - Mild
21.	RM1,726.00	RM7,536.31	RM5,810.31	K-1-40-I	Other Operation Of Digestive System - Mild
22.	RM2,094.00	RM7,531.60	RM5,437.60	P-8-08-I	Neonate, Birthweight >2499 Grams With Respiratory Distress Syndrome & Congenital Pneumonia – Mild
23.	RM2,094.00	RM7,531.60	RM5,437.60	P-8-08-I	Neonate, Birthweight >2499 Grams With Respiratory Distress Syndrome & Congenital Pneumonia - Mild
24.	RM2,822.00	RM7,531.60	RM4,709.60	P-8-17-II	Neonate, Birthweight >2499 Grams Without Complex Operation - Moderate
25.	RM2,933.00	RM7,531.60	RM4,598.60	P-8-08-II	Neonate, Birthweight >2499 Grams With Respiratory Distress Syndrome & Congenital Pneumonia - Moderate
26.	RM4,431.63	RM8,958.30	RM4,526.67	W-1-01-II	Pelvic Evisceration, Hysterectomy & Vulvectomy - Moderate
27.	RM7,408.10	RM11,842.89	RM4,434.79	S-4-13-III	Complications Of Treatment & Procedures - Severe
				P-8-13-II	Neonate, Birthweight 2000 2499 Grams Without Complex Operation - Moderate
				P-8-13-II	Neonate, Birthweight 2000 2499 Grams Without Complex Operation - Moderate
				K-1-20-II	Complex Intestinal Operation – Moderate
				P-8-13-II	Neonate, Birthweight 2000 2499 Grams Without Complex Operation - Moderate
				P-8-13-II	Neonate, Birthweight 2000 2499 Grams Without Complex Operation - Moderate
				P-8-13-II	Neonate, Birthweight 2000 2499 Grams Without Complex Operation - Moderate
				P-8-13-II	Neonate, Birthweight 2000 2499 Grams Without Complex Operation - Moderate
				K-1-20-III	Complex Intestinal Operation - Severe
				N-1-12-III	Dialysis Device Procedure - Severe

28.	RM1,359.41	RM5,777.64	RM4,418.23	N-4-16-I	Other Renal & Urinary Tract Diseases - Mild	N-1-20-II	Upper Urinary Tract Operation - Mild
29.	RM3,888.43	RM8,219.10	RM4,330.67	D-4-10-III	Agranulocytosis - Severe	U-4-13-III	Epiglottitis, Upper Respiratory Tract Infection, Laryngotracheitis & Otitis Media - Severe
30.	RM3,292.00	RM7,531.60	RM4,239.60	P-8-17-III	Neonate, Birthweight >2499 Grams Without Complex Operation - Severe	P-8-13-II	Neonate, Birthweight 2000 2499 Grams Without Complex Operation - Moderate
31.	RM2,149.17	RM6,098.51	RM3,949.34	P-8-14-I	Neonate, Birthwt >2499 Grams With Complex Congenital Abnormalities - Mild	J-4-12-III	Pulmonary Embolism - Severe
32.	RM1,757.78	RM5,557.71	RM3,799.93	E-4-13-I	Other Diseases Of Endocrine System - Mild	U-4-13-II	Epiglottitis, Upper Respiratory Tract Infection, Laryngotracheitis & Otitis Media - Moderate
33.	RM1,275.02	RM4,857.50	RM3,582.48	G-4-22-I	Multiple Sclerosis & Cerebellar Ataxia - Mild	U-4-13-I	Epiglottitis, Upper Respiratory Tract Infection, Laryngotracheitis & Otitis Media - Mild
34.	RM2,834.00	RM6,310.69	RM3,476.69	H-1-30-I	Intraocular & Lens Operations - Mild	H-1-30-II	Intraocular & Lens Operations - Moderate
35.	RM1,412.00	RM4,752.83	RM3,340.83	P-8-17-I	Neonate, Birthweight >2499 Grams Without Complex Operation	M-4-18-II	Other Disorder Of Bones & Joints - Moderate
36.	RM2,833.60	RM5,844.16	RM3,010.56	S-4-16-I	Burns - Mild	S-4-16-II	Burns - Moderate

37.	RM1,823.00	RM4,564.62	RM2,741.62	P-8-15-I	Neonate, Birthweight >2499 Grams With Aspiration Syndrome - Mild
				G-4-22-III	Seizure - Severe
38.	RM2,933.00	RM5,633.97	RM2,700.97	P-8-08-II	Neonate, Birthweight >2499 Grams With Respiratory Distress Syndrome & Congenital Pneumonia - Moderate
				P-8-12-I	Neonate, Birthweight 1500 1999 Grams Without Complex Operation - Mild
39.	RM2,614.74	RM5,260.86	RM2,646.12	O-6-13-I	Vaginal Delivery - Mild
				O-6-10-II	Caesarean Section - Moderate
40.	RM2,614.74	RM5,260.86	RM2,646.12	O-6-13-I	Vaginal Delivery - Mild
				O-6-10-II	Caesarean Section - Moderate
41.	RM2,614.74	RM5,260.86	RM2,646.12	O-6-13-I	Vaginal Delivery - Mild
				O-6-10-II	Caesarean Section - Moderate
42.	RM2,614.74	RM5,260.86	RM2,646.12	O-6-13-I	Vaginal Delivery - Mild
				O-6-10-II	Caesarean Section - Moderate
43.	RM2,614.74	RM5,260.86	RM2,646.12	O-6-13-I	Vaginal Delivery - Mild
				O-6-10-II	Caesarean Section - Moderate
44.	RM2,292.81	RM4,877.96	RM2,585.15	C-4-14-I	Other Neoplasm Including Secondary Neoplasm - Mild
				M-1-60-I	Other Operations Of Musculoskeletal System & Connective Tissue - Mild
45.	RM2,614.74	RM5,077.90	RM2,463.16	O-6-13-I	Vaginal Delivery - Mild
				W-4-12-II	Other Diseases Of Female Reproductive System - Moderate
46.	RM2,820.56	RM5,260.86	RM2,440.30	O-6-12-I	Vaginal Delivery With Other Procedure Excluding Sterilization &/ Or Dilation & Curettage - Mild
				O-6-10-II	Caesarean Section - Moderate
47.	RM2,786.68	RM5,207.49	RM2,420.81	K-4-18-III	Other Digestive System Disorders – Severe
				I-1-20-II	Other Operations Of Circulatory System - Moderate
48.	RM2,079.00	RM4,432.63	RM2,353.63	N-1-12-I	Dialysis Device Procedure - Mild
				N-1-12-II	Dialysis Device Procedure – Moderate
49.	RM1,435.50	RM3,703.99	RM2,268.49	N-4-10-I	Renal & Urinary Tract Neoplasm & Kidney Failure – Mild
				Z-4-12-II	Other Factors Influencing Health Status - Mdoerate
50.	RM3,004.23	RM5,260.86	RM2,256.63	O-6-13-II	Vaginal Delivery - Moderate
				O-6-10-II	Caesarean Section - Moderate

www.ingramcontent.com/pod-product-compliance
Lightning Source LLC
Chambersburg PA
CBHW020722180526
45163CB00001B/71